Comprehensive Gynecology and Obstetrics

Series Editor

Ikuo Konishi
National Kyoto Medical Center
Kyoto
Japan

Hidetaka Katabuchi
Department of Obstetrics and Gynecology
Kumamoto University
Kumamoto
Japan

This series presents the current and future perspectives of medical science in gynecology and obstetrics. The authors fully describe the current understanding of a disease including clinical features, imaging, pathology, and molecular biology, and also include the historical aspects and theories for exploring the etiology of the disease. Also, recent developments in diagnostic strategy, medical treatment, surgery, radiotherapy, prevention, and better health-care methods are clearly shown. Thus, each volume in the series focuses on the scientific basis for the pathogenesis of a disease and provides clinical applications that make it possible to offer personalized treatment for each patient.Over the past 20 years, physicians have been working to develop a standard treatment and publish clinical guidelines for a disease based on epidemiological evidence, mainly through the use of randomized clinical trials and meta-analyses. Recently, however, comprehensive genomic and genetic analyses have revealed the differences and variations in biological characteristics even among patients with the same diagnosis and have been focusing on personalized therapy. Now all physicians and patients are entering a new world of "precision medicine" through the use of genomic evidence. We are confident that readers will greatly benefit from the contents of the series with its purview of the exciting and promising future of gynecology and obstetrics.

More information about this series at http://www.springer.com/series/13621

Hidetaka Katabuchi
Editor

Frontiers in Ovarian Cancer Science

Springer

Editor
Hidetaka Katabuchi
Department of Obstetrics and Gynecology
Kumamoto University
Kumamoto
Japan

ISSN 2364-1932 ISSN 2364-219X (electronic)
Comprehensive Gynecology and Obstetrics
ISBN 978-981-10-4159-4 ISBN 978-981-10-4160-0 (eBook)
DOI 10.1007/978-981-10-4160-0

Library of Congress Control Number: 2017950491

Printed on acid-free paper

This Springer imprint is published by Springer Nature
The registered company is Springer Nature Singapore Pte Ltd.
The registered company address is: 152 Beach Road, #21-01/04 Gateway East, Singapore 189721, Singapore

Preface

The ovaries are not only reproductive organs that hold the ova, which are a source of life, but also endocrine organs that produce female sex steroid hormones. Diverse germ cell tumors and sex-cord tumors develop from respective precursor cells. Although epithelial tumors, which constitute the most common type of ovarian tumors, have long been thought to arise from the ovarian surface epithelium, a new theory has emerged indicating that they can arise within the tubal fimbriae in serous tubal intraepithelial cancer (STIC) as precursor cells. In 2014, the World Health Organization revised its histological classifications of gynecological tumors for the first time in 13 years based on these findings, issuing the *WHO Classification of Tumours of Female Reproductive Organs*. Rapid advances in molecular biology have resulted in a new classification of epithelial ovarian cancer into two types through the addition of precursors and known molecular genetic alterations to the conventional histological type. A new point of view for the diagnosis and prevention of epithelial ovarian cancer was introduced when two genes responsible for hereditary breast–ovarian cancer, which accounts for approximately 5–10% of cases of epithelial ovarian cancer, were identified.

Clinically, over the past 30 years, a markedly increasing trend in cases of epithelial ovarian cancer has been seen in developed Western countries. Epithelial ovarian cancer is now the eighth most common disease among women worldwide and the seventh leading cause of death. For cases of epithelial ovarian cancer, half of which are progressive cancer cases, it is important to implement multimodal therapy with surgery and chemotherapy. As various international clinical trials on chemotherapy with platinum agents and taxane are under way, new and innovative treatments such as neoadjuvant chemotherapy (NAC) are beginning to be clinically applied. In addition to the introduction of molecular-targeted therapy, the current feasibility of immunotherapy has made it possible to anticipate improvement in the long-term prognosis. However, as no marked improvement in prognosis for cases of progressive ovarian cancer is expected, the most important clinical issue is the treatment of recurrent ovarian cancer, with the basis of treatment being the early introduction of palliative medicine. Moreover, the introduction of the concept of oncofertility is an important issue for young patients, while treatment strategies for elderly patients, whose number is increasing with the aging population, must not be neglected.

On this topic, we scientifically studied ovarian cancer and summarized the basic principles and frontline clinical management in Chap. 17. I take pride in the fact that all authors are highly renowned in their field worldwide. I sincerely hope that this book becomes a must-have resource not only for basic scientists and gynecologic oncologists but also for many doctors, ranging from those in the younger generation who have just started engaging in research or clinical care to experienced gynecologists.

Kumamoto, Japan Hidetaka Katabuchi

Contents

Epidemiology and Etiology of Ovarian Cancer

1

Hiroyuki Nomura, Naomi Iwasa, Tomoko Yoshihama, Yoshiko Nanki, and Daisuke Aoki

Abstract

The median age of patients diagnosed with ovarian cancer is 63 years in the United States, and the risk for developing this cancer increases with age. The age-adjusted incidence rate of ovarian cancer is 11.9 per 100,000 females, which is relatively low, and it ranks 17th among all cancers. On the other hand, the mortality from this cancer is relatively high, and the age-adjusted mortality is 7.5 per 100,000 females. Both the annual incidence rate and the mortality have been declining in recent years, reflecting advances in treatment. From a global viewpoint, the incidence rate is higher in developed countries (especially in Northern Europe) compared to developing countries.

Although the cause of ovarian cancer is still unknown, several risk factors related to its development have been identified. The most important factors are the family history and genetic background, which account for approximately 10% of ovarian cancer. Hereditary breast and ovarian cancer and Lynch syndrome are associated with mutations of certain genes. Other causes of ovarian cancer that have been suggested include continuous ovulation, excessive gonadotropin stimulation, excessive hormone stimulation, and pelvic inflammation. Ovarian cancer occurs more frequently among nulliparous women and infertile women, while it is less frequent among women with a history of oral contraceptive use, pregnancy, or breastfeeding.

Keywords

Ovarian cancer • Incidence rate • Mortality • Risk factor

H. Nomura, M.D., Ph.D. • N. Iwasa, M.D. • T. Yoshihama, M.D. • Y. Nanki, M.D.
D. Aoki, M.D., Ph.D. (✉)
Department of Obstetrics and Gynecology, Keio University School of Medicine,
35 Shinanomachi, Shinjuku-ku, Tokyo, Japan
e-mail: aoki@z7.keio.jp

H. Katabuchi (ed.), *Frontiers in Ovarian Cancer Science*, Comprehensive Gynecology and Obstetrics, DOI 10.1007/978-981-10-4160-0_1

1.1 Introduction

Ovarian cancer is uncommon and often advanced at the time of diagnosis and has a poor prognosis. The prevalence of ovarian cancer is influenced by the social background, demographic factors, racial and ethnic factors, and lifestyle factors. The survival rate of ovarian cancer patients has improved with the development and standardization of new treatments. It is important to be aware of epidemiological trends in the diagnosis and treatment of ovarian cancer. This section provides an outline of the age distribution of ovarian cancer, annual changes of the incidence rate and mortality, and international comparisons, as well as information about epidemiology and etiology with a focus on risk factors.

1.2 General Epidemiology of Ovarian Cancer

Ovarian cancer includes various tumors that arise from the ovaries, and its histological classification is based on the classification of the World Health Organization (WHO) [1]. Superficial epithelial/stromal tumors account for approximately 80% of all ovarian tumors. These tumors contain epithelial and interstitial tissues in various proportions, and the tumor components are normally derived from the epidermis. Sex cord-stromal tumors are derived from granulosa cells and Sertoli cells, theca cells differentiating from the interstitium, or Leydig cells and account for approximately 5% of all ovarian tumors. Germ cell tumors are derived from germ cells or extraembryonic tissues and comprise approximately 15–20% of all ovarian tumors. Although ovarian cancer occurs in all age groups, the histological types vary with age (Table 1.1) [2]. While malignant germ cell tumors are most frequent in young women aged 20 years or younger, malignant epithelial tumors are frequent in older women aged 50 years or older.

Some patients with ovarian cancer have a positive family history or genetic background, and the disease is called familial ovarian cancer in a broad sense if a patient has a relative with ovarian cancer. If a patient has a family history of ovarian cancer in close relatives or a number of relatives with this cancer, it is called familial or hereditary ovarian cancer, including hereditary breast and ovarian cancer (HBOC) and Lynch syndrome. Hereditary ovarian cancer is estimated to account for approximately 10% of all ovarian cancer [3, 4].

Globally, it has been reported that approximately 200,000 women are diagnosed with ovarian cancer and 125,000 women die of this cancer every year [5, 6].

Table 1.1 Primary ovarian neoplasms related to age (From ref. 2)

Type	<20 years	20–50 years	>50 years
Coelomic epithelium	29%	71%	81%
Germ cell	59%	14%	6%
Specialized gonadal stroma	8%	5%	4%
Non-specific mesenchyme	4%	10%	9%

1.3 Current Status and Changes of Ovarian Cancer Incidence Rate

The "number of cases (or number of deaths)" is the "number of cases (or deaths) newly diagnosed during a certain period (usually 1 year) in a target population," and it is often expressed as the "incidence rate (mortality)." However, in diseases such as cancer for which age is considered to be a contributing factor, the age-stratified incidence rate (or mortality) is important, and therefore the "age-specific incidence rate (or mortality)" is calculated. When comparing incidence rate (or mortality) between different regions or periods, it is difficult to perform accurate comparison due to differences in the age distribution of the target populations. To overcome this problem, the "age-adjusted incidence rate (or mortality)" is often calculated, which is the incidence rate (or mortality) adjusted for the age-specific population of the standard population, in order for the age composition to be the same as that of the standard population.

The detailed trends of cancer prevalence and mortality are reported by the Surveillance, Epidemiology, and End Results (SEER) program compiled by the National Cancer Institute (NCI) in the United States [7]. Although SEER is based on data from the United States, it can be used as a relatively general reference since the racial composition of the population is diverse in the United States.

According to the 2009–2013 data, the age-adjusted incidence rate of ovarian cancer is 11.9 per 100,000 females. According to the 2010–2012 data, the lifetime risk of ovarian cancer for women is 1.3% (approximately 1 out of every 78 females). The population of women in the United States is approximately 160 million (2015 data) [8], and the estimated annual number of patients developing ovarian cancer in the United States is 22,280 (as of 2016), while it is estimated that there were a total of 195,767 patients with ovarian cancer in 2013. The cancer causing the highest age-adjusted incidence rate for women is breast cancer, and the incidence rate is 125.0 per 100,000 females. The incidence rate due to ovarian cancer is less than one tenth of that caused by breast cancer, and it is ranked 17th among all cancers affecting women in terms of the estimated annual number of patients, accounting for only 1.3% of new cancers annually (Table 1.2).

Table 1.2 Estimated new cases and deaths compared to other cancers: ovarian cancer (From ref. 7)

Common types of cancer		Estimated new cases 2016	Estimated deaths 2016
1	Breast cancer (female)	246,660	40,450
2	Lung and bronchus cancer	224,390	158,080
3	Prostate cancer	180,890	26,120
4	Colon and rectum cancer	134,490	49,190
5	Bladder cancer	76,960	16,390
6	Melanoma of the skin	76,380	10,130
7	Non-Hodgkin lymphoma	72,580	20,150
8	Thyroid cancer	64,300	1,980
9	Kidney and renal pelvis cancer	62,700	14,240
10	Leukemia	60,140	24,400
—		—	—
17	Ovarian cancer	22,280	14,240

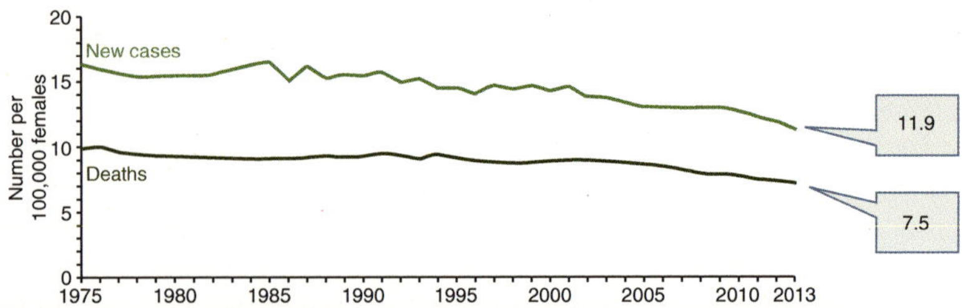

Year	1975	1980	1985	1990	1995	2000	2004	2008
5-Year relative survival	33.7%	38.2%	38.7%	40.4%	42.2%	43.0%	44.3%	46.2%

1975–2013, All races, females. Rates are age-adjusted.

Fig. 1.1 Trends of age-adjusted incidence rate, mortality, and 5-year relative survival rate: ovarian cancer (From ref. 7)

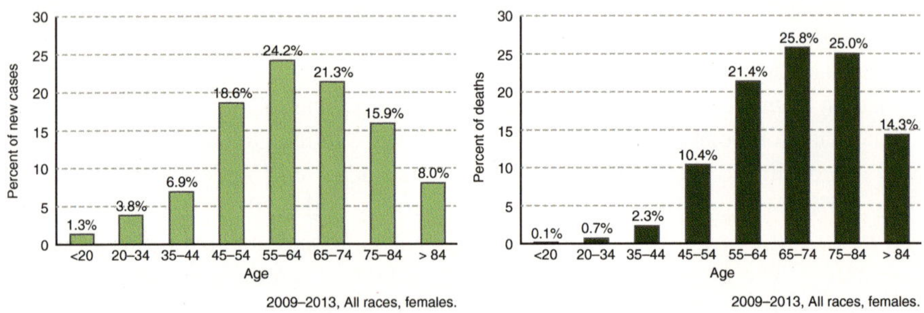

Fig. 1.2 Percentage of new cases and deaths by age group: ovarian cancer (From ref. 7)

Thus, ovarian cancer is relatively infrequently in proportion to all cancers. The annual age-adjusted incidence rate of ovarian cancer has been decreasing, as it was 16.3 per 100,000 females in 1975, 15.4 in 1990, 13.0 in 2005, and 11.9 in 2013 (Fig. 1.1).

The median age of women diagnosed with ovarian cancer is 63 years. As for the age-specific incidence, 1.3% of women with ovarian cancer are diagnosed at 19 years or younger, 3.8% at 20–34 years, 6.9% at 35–44 years, 18.6% at 45–54 years, 24.2% at 55–64 years, 21.3% at 65–74 years, 15.9% at 75–84 years, and 8.0% at 85 years or older (Fig. 1.2). Thus, the prevalence of ovarian cancer increases with age, and it increases rapidly from the age of 45 years. Patients who are 45 or older comprise 88% of the total number of patients, with a peak at 55–64 years. These points suggest that aging is an important factor in the development of ovarian cancer.

As for racial/ethnic background, the age-adjusted incidence rate per 100,000 females is 12.5 for whites, 9.6 for blacks, 9.3 for Asian/Pacific islanders, 10.4 for American Indians/Alaskan natives, 10.6 for Hispanics, and 12.0 for non-Hispanics. Thus, ovarian cancer incidence rate tends to be lower among blacks and Asians, while it is higher among whites and non-Hispanics (Fig. 1.3).

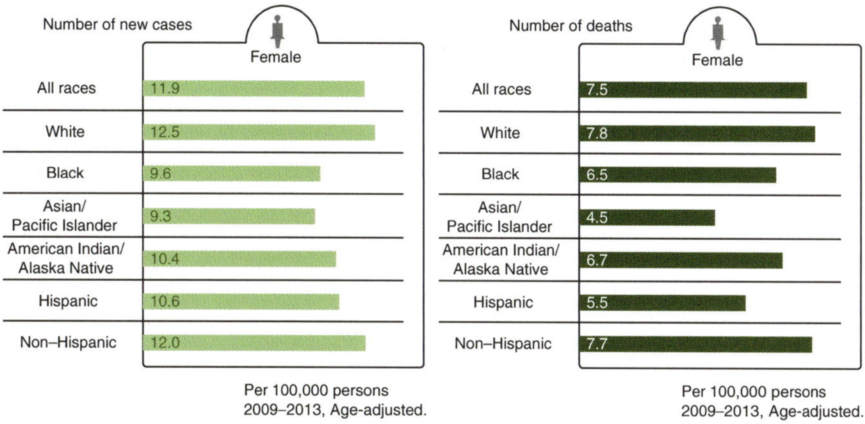

Fig. 1.3 Age-adjusted incidence rate and mortality by race/ethnicity: ovarian cancer (From ref. 7)

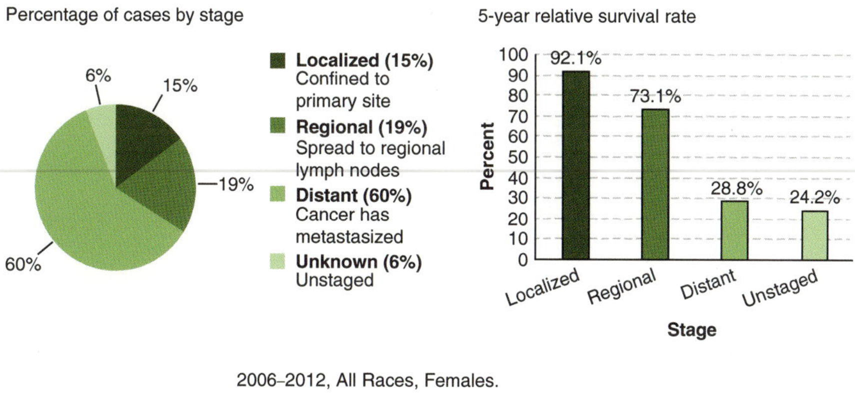

Fig. 1.4 Percentage of cases and 5-year relative survival rate by stage at diagnosis: ovarian cancer (From ref. 7)

Ovarian cancer is confined to the ovary at diagnosis in 15% of patients, while it has spread to regional lymph nodes in 19% and has spread or metastasized beyond the primary site in 60% (the details are unknown in 6%), indicating that more than half of all patients have advanced disease at diagnosis (Fig. 1.4). In older women, ovarian cancer is diagnosed at a relatively more advanced stage than in young women.

On the other hand, the trends of cancer prevalence and mortality in Japan are reported by the Cancer Registry and Statistics in Cancer Information Service, National Cancer Center, Japan [9], and the annual report of the Committee on Gynecologic Oncology, Japan Society of Obstetrics and Gynecology (JSOG) [10]. As of 2012, the age-adjusted incidence rate of ovarian cancer was 8.3 per 100,000 females. That of all sites of female cancer was 265.8 per 100,000 females, and that of breast cancer was 64.3 per 100,000 females, which was the highest in female cancers. Ovarian cancer is ranked seventh among all sites of female cancers and accounting for 3.1% of new cancers. In Japan, the annual age-adjusted incidence rate of ovarian cancer has doubled in these 30 years. Patients aged 60–69, 50–59, and 40–49 years accounted for 26.9%, 24.6%, and 21.5%, respectively, of all patients whose treatment was initiated in 2013. Women in their 50s and 60s were predominantly affected by ovarian cancer, same as the report on SEER. The distribution of surgical stages is as follows: stage I (confined to primary site) accounted for 42.2%, stage II (spread to pelvic cavity) accounted for 9.8%, stage III (spread to regional lymph nodes and/or peritoneal cavity) accounted for 28.2%, and stage IV (metastasize to distant organs) accounted for 8.3% of all patients. Neoadjuvant chemotherapy was administered to 10.9% of patients.

1.4 Current Status and Changes of Ovarian Cancer Mortality

According to SEER [7], the age-adjusted mortality rate of ovarian cancer was 7.5 per 100,000 females in 2009–2013. Based on the 2006–2012 data, the 5-year survival rate of ovarian cancer patients was 46.2%, indicating that more than half of these patients die within 5 years. In the United States, 14,240 patients are predicted to die of ovarian cancer in 2016 (Table 1.2). Ovarian cancer accounts for 2.4% of all cancer deaths, which is high in proportion to the number of patients with this tumor. When compared to the 5-year survival rate of 89.7% for breast cancer and the 40,450 estimated annual deaths (21.5 per 100,000 females) from this cancer, which has the highest estimated annual incidence, the higher risk of death from ovarian cancer becomes obvious. However, the annual age-adjusted mortality due to ovarian cancer is decreasing, as it was 9.8 per 100,000 females in 1975, 9.3 in 1990, 8.7 in 2004, and 7.5 in 2013. In addition, the 5-year survival rate is increasing, since it was 33.7% in 1975, 40.4% in 1990, and 46.2% in 2008 (Fig. 1.1). This improvement is thought to be due to advances in operative treatment and to the development and standardization of novel chemotherapy regimens.

The median age at which patients die of ovarian cancer is 70 years. As for the age-specific mortality, 0.1% of patients die at 19 years or younger, 0.7% at 20–34 years, 2.3% at 35–44 years, 10.4% at 45–54 years, 21.4% at 55–64 years, 25.8% at 65–74 years, 25.0% at 75–84 years, and 14.3% at 85 years or older (Fig. 1.2). The ovarian cancer mortality is in proportion to the incidence of this cancer and thus increases with age to a peak at 55–64 years.

With respect to the influence of racial/ethnic background, the age-adjusted mortality per 100,000 females is 7.8 for whites, 6.5 for blacks, 4.5 for Asian/Pacific islanders, 6.7 for American Indians/Alaskan natives, 5.5 for Hispanics, and 7.7 for non-Hispanics. Thus, mortality tends to be lower in Asian/Pacific islanders and Hispanics compared with the incidence of this cancer (Fig. 1.3).

The 5-year survival rate at the time of diagnosis of ovarian cancer is 92.1% if the tumor is confined to the ovary, 73.1% if it has spread to regional lymph nodes, 28.8% if it has spread or metastasized beyond the region, and 24.2% when the details are unknown. Therefore, the prognosis is poorer as the disease becomes more advanced, and the overall prognosis is poor because many patients have advanced disease at the time of diagnosis (Fig. 1.4).

According to the Cancer Registry and Statistics in Japan [9], the age-adjusted mortality rate of ovarian cancer was 3.1 per 100,000 females in 2014. That of all sites of female cancer is 63.0 per 100,000 females, and that of breast cancer is 8.9 per 100,000 females. Ovarian cancer is ranked eighth among all sites of female cancers and accounting for 4.9% of all female cancer deaths. Based on the 2006–2008 data, the 5-year survival rate of ovarian cancer patients was 58.0%. Those in 1993–1996, in 1997–1999, in 2000–2002, and in 2003–2005 are 49.4%, 52.0%, 53.3%, and 55.0%, respectively. The 5-year survival rate also has been gradually improving in Japan. According to the annual report of JSOG for patients whose treatment was initiated in 2008 [10], the 5-year survival rates were 90.5% in stage I patients, 73.3% in stage II patients, 47.8% in stage III patients, and 30.2% in stage IV patients. Patients with serous carcinoma had a significantly poorer prognosis compared with those with mucinous carcinoma, endometrioid carcinoma, and clear cell carcinoma.

1.5 International Comparison of Ovarian Cancer Incidence Rate and Mortality

The International Agency for Research on Cancer (IARC), which is an agency of the World Health Organization (WHO), has reported the trends for the incidence and death from ovarian cancer based on data from 184 countries [11]. As of 2012, the age-adjusted regional ovarian cancer incidence rate is 8.0–9.9 per 100,000 females in Europe, North America, and Oceania versus 4.8–5.6 in Africa, South America, and Asia, being somewhat higher in Western countries (Fig. 1.5). Also as of 2012, the age-adjusted regional ovarian cancer mortality is 4.9–5.4 per 100,000 females in Europe, North America, and Oceania versus 3.0–3.8 in Africa, South America, and Asia, showing a relatively higher number of deaths in South America and Africa compared to the incidence in these regions (Fig. 1.5). The age-adjusted incidence rate in developed countries is 9.1 per 100,000 females, and it is 5.0 per 100,000 females in developing countries, while the age-adjusted mortality is 5.0 and 3.1 per 100,000 females, respectively, suggesting higher incidence rate and mortality from ovarian cancer in developed countries.

When comparing representative countries from each region, including annual changes (Fig. 1.6), ovarian cancer incidence rate is highest in countries from Northern and Eastern Europe (such as Denmark, Norway, and the Czech Republic), followed by Western Europe and North America, but the overall incidence rate tends to be low. While ovarian cancer incidence rate is generally low in Asia and Central or South America, it is increasing in Brazil and Japan. As for ovarian cancer mortality, it is decreasing markedly in Western countries but remains unchanged in other regions where the mortality has previously been lower (Fig. 1.6).

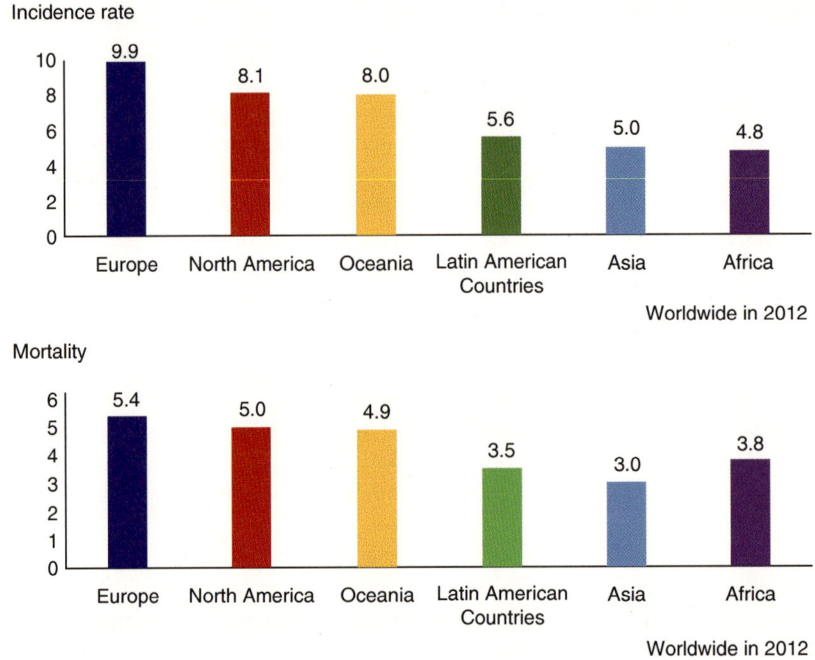

Fig. 1.5 Estimated age-adjusted incidence rate and mortality by regions: ovarian cancer (From ref. 9)

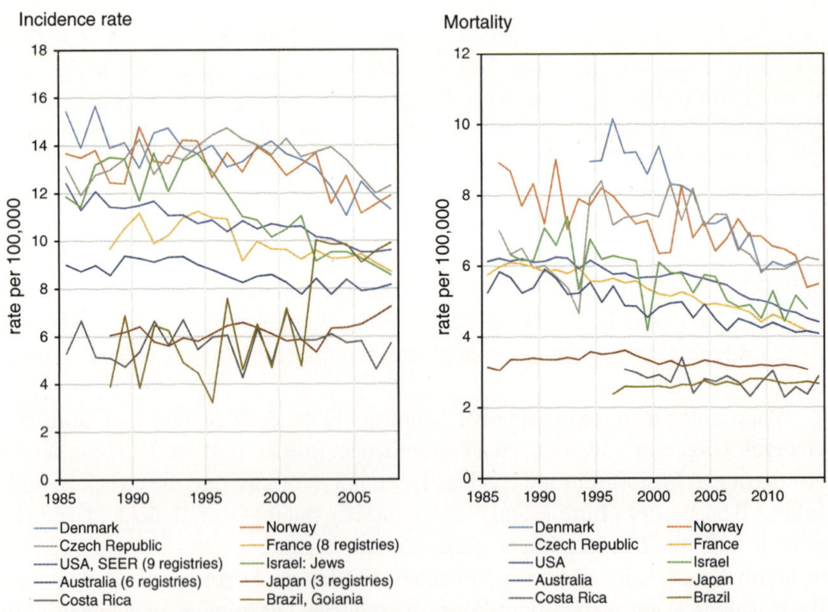

Fig. 1.6 Time trends of age-adjusted incidence rate and mortality: ovarian cancer (From ref. 9)

Although the risk of ovarian cancer is influenced by geographical and racial factors, global differences may become smaller in the future due to environmental factors and population mobility.

1.6 Risk Factors for Ovarian Cancer

The details of the etiology of ovarian cancer are unknown at present, although several environmental, biological, and genetic risk factors have been identified (Table 1.3) [12].

There have been many reports of familial ovarian cancer, and a family history of breast cancer or ovarian cancer is the most important known risk factor for this tumor [13, 14]. In particular, the relative risk is increased by threefold or more for a female who has a first-degree relative with ovarian cancer (e.g., mother, daughter, or sister) [15]. In the case of hereditary ovarian cancer, the influence of cancer-related gene mutations is considered to be significantly stronger than other factors. The characteristic feature of hereditary breast and ovarian cancer (HBOC) is the presence of multiple family members with early-onset breast cancer or ovarian cancer. HBOC is caused by mutation of *BRCA1* or *BRCA2*, which functions as tumor suppressor genes. The lifetime risk of developing ovarian cancer is 30% for women with *BRCA1* mutation and 27% for those with *BRCA2* mutation [16, 17]. Lynch syndrome is characterized by the presence of a family member with early-onset

Table 1.3 Risk factors for epithelial ovarian cancer (From ref. 10)

Increased	Decreased	Indeterminate
Hereditary	Reproductive	Fertility drugs
– Family history of ovarian cancer	– Multiparity	Exercise
– Personal history of breast cancer	– Breastfeeding	Cigarette smoking
– Alteration in *BRCA1* or *BRCA2*	Hormonal	
– Lynch syndrome	– Oral contraceptives	
Reproductive	– Progestins	
– Advanced age	Surgery	
– Nulligravida	– Hysterectomy	
– Infertility	– Tubal ligation	
Hormonal		
– Early age at menarche		
– Late age at natural menopause		
– Hormone replacement therapy		
– Estrogen		
– Androgens		
Inflammatory		
– Perineal talc exposure		
– Endometriosis		
– Pelvic inflammatory disease		
Lifestyle		
– Obesity		
Geography		
– Extremes in latitude		

Table 1.4 Factors suggestive of an inherited predisposition to breast and/or ovarian cancer (From ref. 18)

HBOC	– Personal history of both breast and ovarian cancer – Personal history of ovarian cancer and a close relative with breast cancer at ≤50 years or ovarian cancer at any age – History of ovarian cancer at any age combined with Ashkenazi Jewish ancestry
	– History of breast cancer at ≤50 years and a close relative with ovarian or male breast cancer at any age – Women of Ashkenazi Jewish ancestry and breast cancer at ≤40 years – Women with a first-degree or second-degree relative with a known *BRCA1* or *BRCA2* mutation – Women with bilateral breast cancer (particularly if the first cancer was at ≤50 years) – Women with breast cancer at ≤50 years and a close relative with breast cancer at ≤50 years – Women of Ashkenazi Jewish ancestry with breast cancer at ≤50 years – Women with breast or ovarian cancer at any age and two or more close relatives with breast cancer at any age (particularly if at least one breast cancer was at ≤50 years)
Lynch	– Women with endometrial or colorectal cancer who have At least three relatives with a Lynch/HNPCC-associated cancer (colorectal cancer, cancer of the endometrium, small bowel, ureter, or renal pelvis) in one lineage One affected individual should be a first-degree relative of the other two At least two successive generations should be affected At least one HNPCC-associated cancer should be diagnosed before age 50 – Women with synchronous or metachronous endometrial and colorectal cancer with the first cancer diagnosed before age 50

colon cancer, endometrial cancer, or other gastrointestinal or urinary tract cancers, and these patients sometimes develop ovarian cancer as well. This syndrome is caused by mutation of DNA mismatch repair genes (*MLH1*, *MSH2*, *MSH6*, or *PMS2*), and the lifetime risk of ovarian cancer is 9–12% [18, 19]. In patients with a family history of certain cancers, a genetic background should be suspected, and genetic counseling and testing should be performed (Table 1.4) [20]. Note that the details of hereditary ovarian cancer are described in the following section.

Regarding the etiology of sporadic ovarian cancer, which accounts for the majority of this disease, continuous ovulation, excessive gonadotropin stimulation, excessive hormone stimulation, and pelvic inflammation have all been proposed as causes [21].

There is a theory that trauma to the ovarian epithelium through repeated ovulation is a factor contributing to the development of ovarian tumors, and it is thought that DNA damage occurs in epithelial cells during the course of repeated ovulation and epithelial repair, possibly leading to carcinogenesis. Ovarian cancer is more frequent among unmarried, nulliparous, or infertile women, as well as women who have used ovulation inducers [22–24]. On the other hand, ovarian cancer is less frequent among women with a history of oral contraceptive use, pregnancy, or breastfeeding. In other words, ovarian cancer occurs less frequently among women in whom ovulation has been inhibited either artificially or naturally [25, 26]. Although a long lifetime ovulatory period may also be a risk factor, there is no stable relationship between the age of first menstruation, first birth, or menopause and the risk of ovarian cancer.

In addition, high levels of gonadotropins and steroid hormones are considered to have a role in ovarian carcinogenesis. It is thought that inclusion cysts formed within the ovaries due to ovulation may undergo genetic transformation due to stimulation by steroid hormones such as estrogen. Considering that ovarian tumors are less frequent around puberty and more frequent around menopause [27], involvement of endocrinological factors is further suggested. It is also suspected that high steroid hormone levels in the tumor microenvironment may possibly facilitate malignant transformation. A diet high in animal fat, increased cholesterol intake, and resulting obesity (high body mass index) are also considered to increase the risk of ovarian cancer [28]. This may possibly be related to increased levels of endogenous steroid hormones (androgens and estrogens) associated with high fat intake. The reduced risk of ovarian cancer due to the use of oral contraceptives may be related to inhibition of ovulation and a decrease of gonadotropins [25]. In contrast, hormone replacement therapy (HRT) after menopause may be a risk factor for ovarian cancer along with breast cancer, endometrial cancer, and liver cancer [29–32].

With respect to pelvic inflammation, it is thought that as with ovulation, DNA damage triggered during repair of the ovarian epithelium due to inflammation may lead to tumorigenesis. Exogenous substances such as talc and asbestos may also possibly increase the risk of ovarian cancer [33], while tubal ligation and hysterectomy are thought to be related to a lower risk of ovarian cancer because these procedures prevent carcinogenic substances from reaching the ovaries [34]. However, the incidence of ovarian cancer in patients undergoing these operations could be reduced by intraoperative examination of the ovaries and removal of asymptomatic early ovarian cancer, so the direct effect is unclear. Among internal factors, pelvic inflammatory disease (PID) is considered to increase the risk of ovarian cancer [35], and there is also a risk of precancerous change associated with endometriosis [36].

Conclusion

Both the incidence rate and mortality of ovarian cancer were increasing in the past but have stabilized or been decreasing in recent years. Regional differences seem to be decreasing in developed countries along with advances in and standardization of surgical treatment and chemotherapy, better understanding of risk factors, and widespread use of oral contraceptives. On the other hand, there are still regional differences based on racial/ethnic differences, and genetic background of this cancer has been attracting attention in recent years. As differences in the response to treatment may also be related to such differences, close attention must be paid to future epidemiological trends.

References

1. Kurman RJ, Carcangiu ML, Herrington CS, Young RH, editors. WHO classification of tumours of female reproductive organs. 4th ed. Geneva: World Health Organization; 2014.
2. DiSaia PJ, Creasman WT, editors. Clinical gynecologic oncology. 8th ed. Amsterdam: Elsevier; 2012. p. 314–9.

3. Smith SA, Richards WE, Caito K, Hanjani P, Markman M, DeGeest K, et al. BRCA1 germline mutations and polymorphisms in a clinic-based series of ovarian cancer cases: a gynecologic oncology group study. Gynecol Oncol. 2001;83:586–92.
4. Daly MB, Axilbund JE, Bryant E, Buys S, Eng C, Friedman S, et al. Genetic/familial high-risk assessment: breast and ovarian. J Natl Compr Cancer Netw. 2006;4:156–76.
5. Sankaranarayanan R, Ferlay J. Worldwide burden of gynaecological cancer: the size of the problem. Best Pract Res Clin Obstet Gynaecol. 2006;20:207–25.
6. Parkin DM, Bray F, Ferlay J, Pisani P. Global cancer statistics, 2002. CA Cancer J Clin. 2005;55:74–08.
7. Cancer Statistics. National Cancer Institute, Surveillance, Epidemiology, and End Results Program. http://seer.cancer.gov/. Accessed 20 Aug 2016.
8. World Population Prospects. UNITED NATIONS. 2016. https://esa.un.org/unpd/wpp/. Accessed 4 Sep 2016.
9. Hori M, Matsuda T, Shibata A, Katanoda K, Sobue T, Nishimoto H, et al. Cancer incidence and incidence rates in Japan in 2009: a study of 32 population-based cancer registries for the monitoring of cancer incidence in Japan (MCIJ) project. Jpn J Clin Oncol. 2015;45:884–91.
10. Saito T, Katabuchi H. Annual report of the committee on gynecologic oncology, Japan Society of Obstetrics and Gynecology: patient annual report for 2013 and treatment annual report for 2008. J Obstet Gynaecol Res. 2016;42:1069–79.
11. Cancer Statistics Resources. International Agency for Research on Cancer. 2016. https://www.iarc.fr/. Accessed 22 Aug 2016.
12. Hunn J, Rodriguez GC. Ovarian cancer: etiology, risk factors, and epidemiology. Clin Obstet Gynecol. 2012;55:3–23.
13. Schildkraut JM, Thompson WD. Familial ovarian cancer: a population-based case-control study. Am J Epidemiol. 1988;128:456–66.
14. Koch M, Gaedke H, Jenkins H. Family history of ovarian cancer patients: a case-control study. Int J Epidemiol. 1989;18:782–5.
15. Schildkraut JM, Risch N, Thompson WD. Evaluating genetic association among ovarian, breast, and endometrial cancer: evidence for a breast/ovarian cancer relationship. Am J Hum Genet. 1989;4:521–9.
16. Whittemore AS, Gong G, Itnyre J. Prevalence and contribution of BRCA1 mutations in breast cancer and ovarian cancer: result from three U.S. population-based case-control studies of ovarian cancer. Am J Hum Genet. 1997;60:496–504.
17. Ford D, Easton DP, Stratton M, Narod S, Goldgar D, Devilee P, et al. Genetic heterogeneity and penetrance analysis of the BRCA1 and BRCA2 genes in breast cancer families. Am J Hum Genet. 1998;62:676–89.
18. Aarnio M, Sankila R, Pukkala E, Salovaara R, Aaltonen LA, de la Chapelle A, et al. Cancer risk in mutation carriers of DNA-mismatch-repair genes. Int J Cancer. 1999;81:214–8.
19. Dunlop MG, Farrington SM, Carothers AD, Wyllie AH, Sharp L, Burn J, et al. Cancer risk associated with germline DNA mismatch repair gene mutations. Hum Mol Genet. 1997;6:105–10.
20. Schorge JO, Modesitt SC, Coleman RL, Cohn DE, Kauff ND, Duska LR, et al. SGO white paper on ovarian cancer: etiology, screening and surveillance. Gynecol Oncol. 2010;119:7–17.
21. Landen CN Jr, Birrer MJ, Sood AK. Early events in the pathogenesis of epithelial ovarian cancer. J Clin Oncol. 2008;26:995–1005.
22. Titus-Ernstoff L, Perez K, Cramer DW, Harlow BL, Baron JA, Greenberg ER. Menstrual and reproductive factors in relation to ovarian cancer risk. Br J Cancer. 2001;84:714–21.
23. Rossing MA, Tang MT, Flagg EW, Weiss LK, Wicklund KG. A case-control study of ovarian cancer in relation to infertility and the use of ovulation-inducing drugs. Am J Epidemiol. 2004;160:1070–8.
24. Jensen A, Sharif H, Frederiksen K, Kjaer SK. Use of fertility drugs and risk of ovarian cancer: Danish population based cohort study. BMJ. 2009;338:b249.
25. Tworoger SS, Fairfield KM, Colditz GA, Rosner BA, Hankinson SE. Association of oral contraceptive use, other contraceptive methods, and infertility with ovarian cancer risk. Am J Epidemiol. 2007;166:894–901.

26. Hinkula M, Pukkala E, Kyyronen P, Kauppila A. Incidence of ovarian cancer of grand multiparous women – a population-based study in Finland. Gynecol Oncol. 2006;103:207–11.
27. Goodman MT, Howe HL, Tung KH, Hotes J, Miller BA, Coughlin SS, et al. Incidence of ovarian cancer by race and ethnicity in the United States, 1992-1997. Cancer. 2003;97:2676–85.
28. Olsen CM, Green AC, Whiteman DC, Sadeghi S, Kolahdooz F, Webb PM. Obesity and the risk of epithelial ovarian cancer: a systematic review and meta-analysis. Eur J Cancer. 2007;43:690–709.
29. Lacey JV Jr, Brinton LA, Leitzmann MF, Mouw T, Hollenbeck A, Schatzkin A, et al. 1 menopausal hormone therapy and ovarian cancer risk in the national institutes of health-AARP diet and health study cohort. J Natl Cancer Inst. 2006;98:1397–405.
30. Rossing MA, Cushing-Haugen KL, Wicklund KG, Doherty JA, Weiss NS. Menopausal hormone therapy and risk of epithelial ovarian cancer. Cancer Epidemiol Biomark Prev. 2007;16:2548–56.
31. Neves-E-Castro M. An analysis of ovarian cancer in the million women study. Gynecol Endocrinol. 2007;23:410–3.
32. Wernli KJ, Newcomb PA, Hampton JM, Trentham-Dietz A, Egan KM. Hormone therapy and ovarian cancer: incidence and survival. Cancer Causes Control. 2008;19:605–13.
33. Huncharek M, Geschwind JF, Kupelnick B. Perineal application of cosmetic talc and risk of invasive epithelial ovarian cancer: a meta-analysis of 11,933 subjects from sixteen observational studies. Anticancer Res. 2003;23:1955–60.
34. Hankinson SE, Hunter DJ, Colditz GA, Willett WC, Stampfer MJ, Rosner B, et al. Tubal ligation, hysterectomy, and risk of ovarian cancer. A prospective study. JAMA. 1993;270:2813–8.
35. Lin HW, Tu YY, Lin SY, Su WJ, Lin WL, Lin WZ, et al. Risk of ovarian cancer in women with pelvic inflammatory disease: a population-based study. Lancet Oncol. 2011;12:900–4.
36. Sayasneh A, Tsivos D, Crawford R. Endometriosis and ovarian cancer: a systematic review. ISRN Obstet Gynecol. 2011;2011:1403–10.

Hereditary Ovarian Cancer

2

Masayuki Sekine and Takayuki Enomoto

Abstract

Hereditary ovarian cancer, approximately 20% of epithelial ovarian cancers, occurs as part of several genetically distinct syndromes, hereditary breast and ovarian cancer (HBOC), Lynch syndrome (hereditary nonpolyposis colorectal cancer, HNPCC), and so on. HBOC are caused by mutations in the *BRCA1/2* genes, and the penetrance of the genes for ovarian cancer was estimated to be 8–62% in different populations. A high-grade serous carcinoma is a major histological subtype, although endometrioid and clear cell carcinomas also have been reported in the *BRCA*-related ovarian cancers. Germline mutations in *BRCA1/2* are responsible for approximately 15% of epithelial ovarian cancers. *BRCA1/2* mutation-positive women with ovarian cancer showed more favorable survival outcomes compared with mutation-negative women due to higher response rates to platinum regimens.

Ovarian cancer screening with transvaginal ultrasound and CA-125 has not been shown to be sufficiently sensitive or specific, so risk-reducing salpingo-oophorectomy (RRSO) after completion of childbearing has been recommended for *BRCA1/2* mutation carriers. RRSO for ovarian and breast cancer was associated with 80% and 50% risk reduction in *BRCA1/2* mutation carriers, respectively. An oral contraceptive significantly reduced the risk for ovarian cancer by approximately 50% for the mutation carriers. So far, more than 20 genes are known to be involved in pathogenesis of hereditary ovarian cancer. The NCCN Guidelines recommend RRSO in *BRCA1/2*, MMR genes, *BRIP1, and RAD51C/D* mutation carriers.

M. Sekine, M.D., Ph.D. (✉) • T. Enomoto, M.D., Ph.D.
Department of Obstetrics and Gynecology, Niigata University Graduate School of Medical and Dental Sciences, Niigata, Japan
e-mail: masa@med.niigata-u.ac.jp

H. Katabuchi (ed.), *Frontiers in Ovarian Cancer Science*, Comprehensive Gynecology and Obstetrics, DOI 10.1007/978-981-10-4160-0_2

Poly (ADP-ribose) polymerase (PARP) inhibitors cause cancer cell death in *BRCA*-mutated cancers by synthetic lethality. Olaparib was the first PARP inhibitor approved in the EU and USA for the treatment of advanced ovarian cancer patients with a germline *BRCA* mutation. Several trials are ongoing for the inhibitors in other populations such as patients with homologous recombination deficiency.

Keywords
BRCA1 • *BRCA2* • Hereditary breast and ovarian cancer (HBOC) • Risk-reducing salpingo-oophorectomy (RRSO) • Homologous recombination deficiency (HRD) • Poly (ADP-ribose) polymerase (PARP) inhibitors

2.1 Introduction

Ovarian cancer is the most lethal disease in gynecological malignancy. A positive family history of ovarian cancer is one of the strongest and most consistent of the risk factors for the development of the disease. It has been reported that first-degree relatives of ovarian cancer patients were found to be at a two- to fourfold increased risk for developing the disease [1, 2].

Now, approximately 20% of ovarian cancers have been related to hereditary conditions [3]. Hereditary ovarian cancer occurs as part of several genetically distinct syndromes, hereditary breast and ovarian cancer (HBOC), hereditary nonpolyposis colorectal cancer (HNPCC), and so on. HBOC caused by inherited mutations of *BRCA1/2* and HNPCC caused by the mismatch repair genes are predicted to be responsible for about 65–75% and 10–15% of hereditary ovarian cancer, respectively. Furthermore, other suppressor genes and oncogenes have been related with hereditary ovarian cancer [4–7]. So far, more than 20 genes are known to be involved in pathogenesis of hereditary ovarian cancer; however, unknown susceptibility genes and their mutations appear to exist [8].

We reviewed the available published data regarding clinical and molecular features and management (i.e., surveillance, chemoprevention, risk-reducing surgery, and molecular targeting agents) of hereditary ovarian cancer, especially *BRCA*-related hereditary breast and ovarian cancer.

2.2 Hereditary Breast and Ovarian Cancer (HBOC): *BRCA*-Related Breast and Ovarian Cancer

2.2.1 Clinical and Molecular Features of HBOC

Hereditary breast and ovarian cancer (HBOC) is caused by mutations in the *BRCA1/2* genes [9, 10]. *BRCA1/2* genes are tumor suppresser genes and involved in DNA repair of double-strand DNA breaks and the regulation of cell-cycle checkpoints in response to DNA damage [11, 12]. The *BRCA1* gene is located on short arm of chromosome 17, and the *BRCA2* gene on long arm of chromosome 13. The frequency of pathogenic mutations in *BRCA1/2* genes has been estimated to be 1/300 and 1/800, respectively [13–15].

It has been estimated that more than 90% of hereditary breast and ovarian cancer families are related to germline mutation of *BRCA1/2* genes in Western countries [16]; on the other hand, approximately 80% of breast and ovarian cancer families in Japan are based on the mutation [17]. In analysis of hereditary ovarian cancer families, *BRCA1/2* mutations were detected in 41.9% of families in which there were at least two ovarian cancer cases [18]. In Japanese population, among the 55 ovarian cancer families without breast cancer patients, 24 families were carrying germline mutations in *BRCA1/2* (24/55, 43.6%); however, in 27 breast-ovarian cancer families, 21 families were positive with the mutation (21/27, 77.8%) [17]. About half of families showing a genetic predisposition to ovarian cancer did not have identifiable BRCA1/2 mutations, so other gene mutations predisposing a patient to ovarian cancer are likely to exist [19, 20].

Germline mutations in *BRCA1/2* are responsible for more than 10% of epithelial ovarian cancers [21, 22]. Among 1915 patients with ovarian cancer, 280 (15%) had mutations in *BRCA1* ($n = 182$) or *BRCA2* ($n = 98$) [22]. Histological characteristics by BRCA1/2 mutation status in this large mutational analysis were summarized in Table 2.1 [22]. The *BRCA1/2* mutation prevalence was 11–16% in high-grade serous carcinoma [22, 23]. In analysis of invasive ovarian cancer, 13–20% of the patients have a germline mutation of *BRCA1/2* [24–27]. In Japan, Sakamoto et al. reported that 12 of the 95 unselected women with ovarian cancer (12.6%), including 5 in the *BRCA1* (5.3%) and 7 in the *BRCA2* (7.4%), had deleterious mutations and all cases with *BRCA* mutation were diagnosed at advanced stage and had high-grade serous carcinoma [28]. Table 2.2 demonstrates histological and molecular subtypes of epithelial ovarian cancer [29].

Table 2.1 Histological characteristics by BRCA1/2 mutation status

	High-grade serous	Low-grade serous	High-grade endometrioid	Low-grade endometrioid	Clear cell	Mucinous	Unspecified carcinoma
No.	1501	70	64	14	58	16	166
BRCA1 (%)	10.3	4.3	6.3	0	6.9	0	8.4
BRCA2 (%)	5.7	1.4	4.7	0	0	0	5.4
BRCA1/2 (%)	16.0	5.7	10.9	0	6.9	0	13.9

Table 2.2 Histological and molecular subtypes of epithelial ovarian cancer

	High-grade serous	Low-grade serous	High-grade endometrioid	Low-grade endometrioid	Clear cell	Mucinous
Genomic alterations	*TP53* *BRCA1/2* Other HRR genes	*BRAF* *KRAS* *PTEN* *PIK3CA*	*BRCA1/2*	*PTEN* *PIK3CA* *CTNNB1* *ARID1A* *BRAF*	*ARID1A* *PIK3CA*	*KRAS* *CDKN2A* *PIK3CA* *BRAF* *TP53*
Copy number alterations	–	–	–	–	*ERBB2*	*ERBB2*

HRR homologous recombination repair

Several founder mutations have been observed in the specific population, for example, the 187delAG and 5385insC mutations in *BRCA1* and the 6174delT mutation in *BRCA2* have been identified in the Ashkenazi Jewish population [30, 31]. In Japanese population, it was reported that the L63X and Q934X mutations in *BRCA1* were the founder mutations with high frequency in hereditary ovarian cancer families [17], and it has been reported that the L63X is a founder mutation with the highest frequency in Japanese breast cancer families [32, 33].

The penetrance of *BRCA1/2* gene mutation in ovarian cancer is lower than that in breast cancer. A lifetime risk for ovarian cancer in *BRCA* mutation carriers was estimated to be 8–62% in different populations; however, that for breast cancer was 41–90%. A meta-analysis of these published data showed the average cumulative risks for breast and ovarian cancer by age 70 years for *BRCA1* mutation carriers were 57% and 40%, respectively. For *BRCA2* mutation carriers, they were 49% and 18%, respectively, in the meta-analysis [5, 24, 34–42]. In a recent prospective study, the estimated average cumulative risks for breast and ovarian cancer by age 70 years for *BRCA1* mutation carriers were 60% and 59%, respectively. In addition, for BRCA2 mutation carriers, they were 55% and 16.5%, respectively [39]. A subsequent alteration or silencing in the second copy of the gene without the hereditary mutation is believed to be necessary for the initiation of cancer development, so the risk of breast and ovarian cancer with *BRCA1/2* mutations is various, even within families with the same mutation. In an international observational study of 19,581 carriers of *BRCA1* mutations and 11,900 carriers of *BRCA2* mutations in 33 countries on 6 continents, 12% of the *BRCA1* mutation carriers and 6% of the *BRCA2* mutation carriers were diagnosed with ovarian cancer, and 46% of the *BRCA1* mutation carriers and 52% of the *BRCA2* mutation carriers were diagnosed with breast cancer [43]. As described above, *BRCA1/2* mutation carriers have a high risk for both breast cancer and an ovarian cancer, so there was a need to consider more intensive screening and prevention strategies such as chemoprevention and prophylactic surgery.

It has been reported that some pathological features are observed more frequently in breast and ovarian cancer patients with *BRCA1/2* mutation. For example, breast cancers with *BRCA1/2* mutation are characterized as ER/PR and HER2 negative: triple negative [44–49]. In ovarian cancers with *BRCA1/2* mutation, high-grade serous carcinoma is a major histological subtype, although endometrioid and clear cell carcinomas also have been reported in the *BRCA*-related ovarian cancers [21, 25–27, 50–53]. Mucinous type is very rare in the population [25, 27]. In Japanese hereditary breast and ovarian cancer families, the major histological type of *BRCA*-associated ovarian cancers was serous carcinoma in 81% of tumors, and only one case was clearcell carcinoma. No tumor with mucinous carcinoma occurred in these families [17]. Mucinous carcinomas appear to be related to other gene mutations; *KRAS* and *TP53* [54]. Borderline epithelial ovarian tumors are not associated with a *BRCA1/2* mutation [21]. Although non-epithelial ovarian carcinomas are not significantly associated with a *BRCA1/2* mutation, sex cord tumors may be associated with Peutz-Jeghers syndrome, and Sertoli-Leydig cell tumors are caused by germline mutations in the *DICER1* gene [55–61].

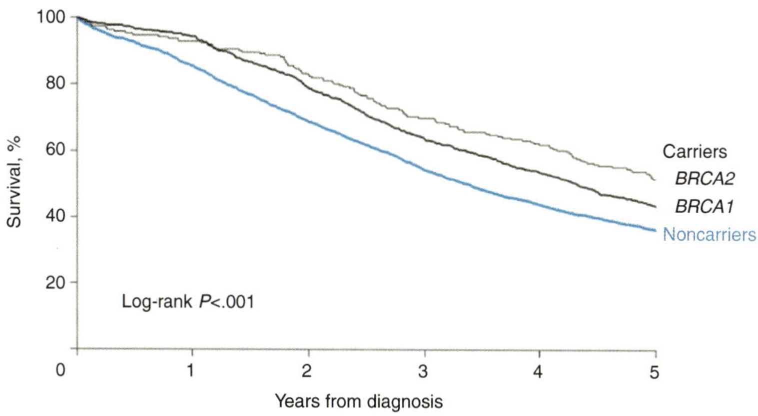

No. at risk						
Noncarriers	1047	1687	1540	1395	1225	1044
Carriers						
BRCA1	327	593	569	490	408	342
BRCA2	117	199	192	179	164	125

Fig. 2.1 Association between *BRCA1/2* mutations and survival in women with invasive epithelial ovarian cancer. *BRCA1* and *BRCA2* mutation carriers showed a more favorable survival than non-carriers (for *BRCA1*, HR = 0.78 [95% CI, 0.68–0.89], $P < 0.001$, and for *BRCA2*, HR = 0.61 [95% CI, 0.50–0.76], $P < 0.001$) in a pooled analysis from 26 observational studies that included invasive epithelial ovarian cancer cases from *BRCA1/2* mutation carriers (n = 1213) and noncarriers (n = 2666). Kaplan-Meier analysis was adjusted for year of diagnosis and study [63]

Several studies have reported that *BRCA* mutation-positive women with ovarian cancer showed more favorable survival outcomes compared with mutation-negative women [62–67]. Figure 2.1 indicates that *BRCA1/2* mutation carriers showed a more favorable survival than noncarriers (for BRCA1, HR = 0.78 [95% CI, 0.68–0.89], $P < 0.001$, and for BRCA2, HR = 0.61 [95% CI, 0.50–0.76], $P < 0.001$) in a pooled analysis from 26 observational studies that included invasive epithelial ovarian cancer cases from *BRCA1/2* mutation carriers (n = 1213) and noncarriers (n = 2666) [63]. The 5-year overall survival was 36% for noncarriers, 44% for *BRCA1* carriers, and 52% for *BRCA2* carriers. In a population-based case-control study of women with invasive epithelial (non-mucinous) ovarian cancer (n = 1001), patients carrying germline mutations of *BRCA1/2* had improved rates of progression-free survival (median, 20 months vs 16 months; not statistically significant) and overall survival (median, 62 months vs 55.5 months; $P = 0.031$) [62]. Survival outcomes appear to be most favorable for *BRCA2* mutation carriers [63]. An observational study of 1915 women with ovarian cancer from the University of Washington (UW) gynecologic tissue bank and from the Gynecologic Oncology Group (GOG) phase III clinical trials (n = 1345) showed that patients with a *BRCA2* mutation from the GOG trials had significantly longer progression-free survival (HR, 0.60; 95% CI, 0.45–0.79; $P < 0.001$) and OS (HR, 0.39; 95% CI, 0.25–0.60; $P < 0.001$), compared with those without mutations [22].

BRCA mutation carriers appeared to be more responsive to cytotoxic chemotherapy compared with noncarrier patients [68]. Several studies have shown a higher response rate to platinum regimens and longer treatment-free intervals between relapses in *BRCA* mutation carriers compared with noncarriers [62, 63, 66, 69–71]. These clinical features of BRCA-associated ovarian cancer are attributed to homologous recombination repair deficiency in the absence of *BRCA1/2* function, which results in an impaired ability of tumor cells to repair platinum-induced double-strand breaks [66, 70, 72]. Thereby conferring increased chemosensitivity and increased sensitivity to poly (ADP-ribose) polymerase (PARP) enzyme inhibition and other DNA-damaging chemotherapeutic agents such as pegylated liposomal doxorubicin (PLD) [68].

2.2.2 Ovarian Cancer Screening for Surveillance

Ovarian cancer screening with transvaginal ultrasound and CA-125 has not been shown to be sufficiently sensitive or specific. So far, there is no evidence that these screening are appropriate methods of substituting for ovarian cancer risk-reducing surgery [73, 74]. In recent large randomized controlled trial, the UK Collaborative Trial of Ovarian Cancer Screening (UKCTOCS), which assessed multimodality screening with ultrasound and CA-125 versus either ultrasound alone or no screening, showed that a significant mortality reduction was not observed after a median of 11 years of follow-up; however, a prespecified analysis of death from ovarian cancer of multimodality screening versus no screening with exclusion of prevalent cases showed significantly different death rates ($P = 0.021$) [75, 76]. In this trial, the cases with increased risk of familial ovarian cancer were included in exclusion criteria. The NCCN Guidelines recommend that ovarian cancer screening with transvaginal ultrasound and CA-125 may be considered starting at age 30–35 years by the doctor's discretion for women who have not selected the risk-reducing surgery [13]. GOG-0199 is a two-arm, prospective, nonrandomized study for managing the risk of ovarian cancer in high-risk women. One arm is women who elected RRSO, and the other is those who chose the ROCA (risk of ovarian cancer algorithm) surveillance using transvaginal ultrasound and CA-125. This 5-year follow-up period ended in November 2011 and the data has been analyzed [77].

2.2.3 Risk-Reducing Salpingo-Oophorectomy (RRSO)

The risk for ovarian cancer in *BRCA1/2* mutation carriers is generally considered to be lower than the risk for breast cancer. However, due to the absence of reliable methods of early detection and the poor prognosis associated with advanced ovarian cancer, RRSO after completion of childbearing has been recommended for *BRCA1/2* mutation carriers. The NCCN Guidelines recommend RRSO for women with

BRCA1/2 mutation, typically between ages 35 and 40 years for women with a *BRCA1* mutation [13]. For women with a *BRCA2* mutation who have undergone efforts to maximize their breast cancer prevention (i.e., bilateral mastectomy), it is reasonable to delay RRSO until between ages 40 and 45 years since ovarian cancer onset tends to be later in women with a *BRCA2* mutation [78]. RRSO should only be considered upon completion of childbearing.

The effectiveness of RRSO in reducing the risk for ovarian cancer in *BRCA1/2* mutation carriers has been reported in various studies. In a meta-analysis including ten studies, RRSO was associated with a statistically significant reduction in the risk of *BRCA*-associated ovarian or fallopian tube cancer (HR = 0.21; 95% CI = 0.12–0.39) [78]. In an international observational study of 5783 women with a *BRCA1/2* mutation, risk-reducing oophorectomy was associated with an 80% reduction (HR, 0.20; 95% CI, 0.13–0.30) in the risk of ovarian, fallopian tube, or peritoneal cancer in *BRCA1/2* carriers and a 77% reduction in all-cause mortality (HR, 0.23; 95% CI, 0.13–0.39) [78]. RRSO reduces mortality at all ages in *BRCA1* mutation carriers; however, RRSO is not associated with reduced mortality in those at the ages of more than 61 in *BRCA2* mutations carriers [78]. Furthermore, in prospective, multicenter cohort study of 2482 women with *BRCA1/2* mutations, RRSO was associated with lower all-cause mortality (10% vs 3%; HR, 0.40 [95% CI, 0.26–0.61]), breast cancer-specific mortality (6% vs 2%; HR, 0.44 [95% CI, 0.26–0.76]), and ovarian cancer-specific mortality (3% vs 0.4%; HR, 0.21 [95% CI, 0.06–0.80]) [79]. We have to take care that 1–4.3% risk of a primary peritoneal cancer has remained after RRSO [80–84]. The ovarian cancer risk and management were shown in Table 2.3 [13].

Many studies have reported that RRSO reduced the risk for breast cancer in *BRCA1/2* mutation carriers [80, 81, 83, 85, 86]. In a meta-analysis of all reports of RRSO published between 1999 and 2007, RRSO was associated with a statistically significant reduction in risk of breast cancer in *BRCA1/2* mutation carriers (HR = 0.49; 95% confidence interval [CI] = 0.37–0.65), *BRCA1* mutation carriers (HR = 0.47; 95% CI = 0.35–0.64), and *BRCA2* mutation carriers (HR = 0.47; 95%

Table 2.3 Ovarian cancer risk and management

	Ovarian cancer risk	Management
BRCA1	Increased risk of OC	Consider RRSO at 35–40 year
BRCA2	Increased risk of OC	Consider RRSO at 45–50 year
MMR genes	Increased risk of OC	Consider RRSO and hysterectomy at completion of childbearing
BRIP1	Increased risk of OC	Consider RRSO at 45–50 year
RAD51C	Increased risk of OC	**Consider RRSO at 45–50 year**
RAD51D	Increased risk of OC	**Consider RRSO at 45–50 year**
PALB2	**Insufficient evidence for OC risk**	—
TP53	**No increased risk of OC**	—

MMR mismatch repair, *OC* ovarian cancer, *RRSO* risk-reducing salpingo-oophorectomy

CI = 0.26–0.84) [80]. Results of a prospective cohort study suggest that RRSO may be associated with a greater reduction in breast cancer risk for *BRCA2* mutation carriers compared with *BRCA1* mutation carriers [87]. Reductions in breast cancer risk for *BRCA1/2* mutation carriers following RRSO may be associated with decreased hormonal exposure due to resection of the ovaries. In an international case-control study of 1439 patients with breast cancer and 1866 matched controls derived from a registry of *BRCA1/2* mutation carriers, the risk reduction was greater if the oophorectomy was performed before age 40 (OR = 0.36; 95% CI, 0.20–0.64 for *BRCA1* carriers) than after age 40 (OR = 0.53; 95% CI, 0.30–0.91), and no significant reduction was found for women aged 51 years or older in breast cancer risk [86]. However, the hazard ratio for breast cancer-specific mortality in *BRCA1/2* mutation carriers was 0.76 (95% CI, 0.32–1.78; $P = 0.53$) for women with estrogen receptor-positive breast cancer and 0.07 (95% CI, 0.01–0.51; $P = 0.009$) for women with estrogen receptor-negative breast cancer [88].

RRSO is an opportunity for occult gynecologic cancer detection in *BRCA1/2* mutation carriers. In studies of women with a *BRCA1/2* mutation who underwent RRSO, occult gynecologic carcinomas and ovarian, tubal, or peritoneal cancer were identified in 4.5–9% of cases, and tubal intraepithelial carcinoma (TIC) was detected in 5–8% of cases [84, 89–92]. The fimbriae or distal tube was reported to be the predominant site of origin for these early malignancies found in patients with *BRCA1/2* mutations [89, 92, 93].

In a prospective cohort of 462 women with *BRCA1/2* mutation carriers, short-term hormone replacement therapy (HRT) in women undergoing RRSO does not negate the protective effect of bilateral prophylactic oophorectomy on subsequent breast cancer risk in BRCA1/2 mutation carriers [94]. Moreover, results of a case-control study of BRCA1 mutation carriers showed no association between use of HRT and increased breast cancer risk in postmenopausal *BRCA1* mutation carriers [95]. However, there is no randomized study of the issue, so the use of HRT in *BRCA1/2* mutation carriers undergoing RRSO should be carried out carefully [96, 97].

Salpingectomy has been performed in premenopausal women, and there have been some evidence regarding the safety and feasibility of this procedure [98, 99]. However, there is limited data regarding its efficacy in reducing the risk for ovarian cancer [100, 101]. In addition, *BRCA1/2* mutation carriers undergoing salpingectomy alone may not get the 50% reduction in breast cancer risk of *BRCA1/2* carriers following oophorectomy. Hence, the salpingectomy alone has not been recommended as the standard risk-reducing surgery in *BRCA1/2* mutation carriers at this time.

The NCCN Guidelines recommend RRSO protocol [102]: (1) Perform operative laparoscopy. (2) Survey upper abdomen, bowel surfaces, omentum, appendix (if present), and pelvic organs. (3) Biopsy any abnormal peritoneal findings. (4) Obtain pelvic washing for cytology. (5) Perform total BSO, removing 2 cm of proximal ovarian vasculature/IP ligament, all tube up to the cornua, and all peritoneum surrounding the ovaries and tubes, especially peritoneum underlying areas of adhesion between tube and/or ovary and the pelvic sidewall. (6) Engage in minimal instrument handling of the tubes and ovaries to avoid traumatic exfoliation of cells. (7) Both ovaries and tubes should be placed in an endobag for retrieval from the pelvis. (8) Both ovaries and tubes should be processed according to SEE-FIM protocol [103]. (9) If occult malignancy or STIC is identified, provide referral to gynecologic oncologist. (10) The prevention benefits of salpingectomy alone are not yet proven. If considered, the fallopian tube from the fimbria to its insertion into the uterus should be removed.

Japan Society of Gynecologic Oncology guidelines 2015 for the treatment of ovarian cancer described procedures for the examination and management of HBOC. In the guidelines, it was recommended that RRSO only be performed by a gynecologic oncologist who is a member of the Japan Society of Gynecologic Oncology in cooperation with a clinical geneticist at a medical facility with an established genetic counseling system and cooperative pathologists, after review and approval by the institutional ethics committee [104]. In addition, the Gynecologic Oncology Committee of Japan Society of Obstetrics and Gynecology have proposed the requirement of RRSO for *BRCA1/2* mutation carriers in more detail [105].

2.2.4 Chemoprevention

As regards the effect of oral contraceptives (OC) in *BRCA1/2* mutation carriers, two meta-analyses showed significant reduction of the risk for ovarian cancer. In analysis of *BRCA1/2* mutation carriers with (n = 1503) and without (n = 6315) ovarian cancer, OC use significantly reduced the risk for ovarian cancer by approximately 50% for both the *BRCA1* mutation carriers (RR, 0.51; 95% CI, 0.40–0.65) and *BRCA2* mutation carriers (RR, 0.52; 95% CI, 0.31–0.87) [106]. The other including one cohort study (N = 3181) and three case-control studies (1096 cases and 2878 controls) also showed an inverse association between OC use and ovarian cancer (OR, 0.58; 95% CI, 0.46–0.73), and the risks appeared to decrease with longer duration of oral contraceptive use [107]. Two meta-analyses showed that OC use is not significantly associated with breast cancer risk in *BRCA1/2* mutation carriers [106, 108]. However, case-control studies in the analyses on the effect of OC use on breast cancer risk in *BRCA1/2* mutation carriers have showed conflicting results.

2.3 Genes Other than *BRCA1/2* Involved in Hereditary Ovarian Cancer

2.3.1 Mismatch Repair Genes (Lynch Syndrome)

Ovarian cancer is a component tumor of Lynch syndrome that is associated with germline mutations in mismatch repair genes (*MLH1*, *MSH2*, *MSH6*, *MLH3*, and *PMS2*) [109]. Lynch syndrome, also known as hereditary nonpolyposis colon cancer (HNPCC), accounts for 10–15% of all hereditary ovarian cancers [109] and is at increased risk for endometrial and ovarian cancers: up to 60% and 24%, respectively

[110–113]. The loss of function of one of the mismatch repair proteins results in the accumulation of repeated nucleotide sequences phenotypically expressed as microsatellite instability (MSI). Several oncogenes and tumor suppressor genes contain microsatellites; impairment of MMR could cause mutations in many genes implicated in ovarian tumorigenesis [114–118]. *BRCA*-related ovarian cancers are associated with non-mucinous tumors; on the other hand, Lynch syndrome-associated ovarian cancers appear to be associated with both non-mucinous and mucinous tumors. Ovarian cancers in Lynch syndrome are mostly endometrioid or clear cell [119–123]. The cumulative lifetime risk of ovarian cancer is estimated to be 6–10% in *MSH2* and *MLH1* mutation carriers. An average age of diagnosis was 51 years in families associated with *MLH1* mutations and 45 years in families associated with *MSH2* mutations [113, 124, 125]. Lynch syndrome-associated ovarian cancers were more likely at diagnosis to be of low grade and early stage and generally showed a better prognosis [124, 126, 127]. Total abdominal hysterectomy and/or bilateral salpingo-oophorectomy are options that may be considered for risk reduction in women with mutation of mismatch repair genes who have completed childbearing [128–132]. No evidence has been showed to support routine transvaginal ultrasound and CA-125 testing in these mutation carriers because they have not been shown to be sufficiently sensitive or specific [128, 133–137].

2.3.2 Homologous Recombination Deficiency (HRD)-Related Genes

Homologous recombination (HR) plays in a repair of double-strand breaks (DSBs) [29]. A lot of proteins involved in homologous recombination are recognized to also contribute to hereditary cancer risk, e.g., BRCA1/2, ATM, PALB2, RAD51C, RAD51D, CHEK2, BARD1, Mre11, RAD50, NBS1, BRIP1, and Fanconi anemia proteins [3]. These proteins interact with BRCA1/2 proteins in the DNA repair and the maintenance of genomic stability. It has been hypothesized that genes coding for these proteins would be alternative candidates for ovarian cancer susceptibility. The Cancer Genome Atlas (TCGA) has showed that around half of high-grade serous ovarian cancers have aberrations in homologous recombination repair (See Fig. 7.1) [138, 139]. These patients with mutation of HRD-related gene are at increased risk for both ovarian and breast cancers, similar to *BRCA1/2* mutation carriers. In addition, these tumors present a specific phenotype similar to *BRCA*-related ovarian cancers [7], including sensitivity to platinum agents and improved survival rates [71, 72]. The survival was similar for women with mutations in *BRCA1* and other HRD-related genes (Fig. 2.2) [22].

RAD51 genes are involved in homologous recombination, and this biallelic mutation can cause a Fanconi anemia-like phenotype [140]. *RAD51C* and *RAD51D* have been shown to be associated with increased risk for ovarian cancer [140]. In 1915 unselected ovarian cancer cases, 1.1% of patients had either a *RAD51C* or *RAD51D* mutation [22]. In cases from 1100 German families with gynecological malignancies, Meindl et al. identified six monoallelic pathogenic mutations in

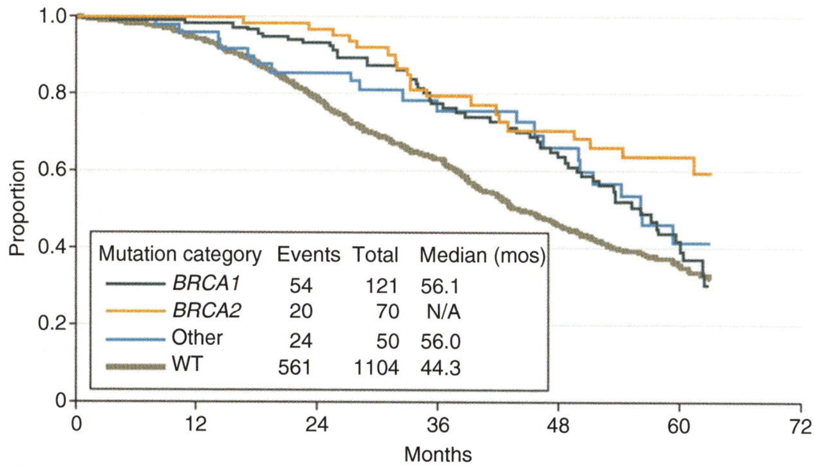

No. at risk

BRCA1	121	118	104	63	50	19
BRCA2	70	69	63	41	32	18
Other	50	47	41	28	21	9
WT	1104	1039	832	435	293	153

Fig. 2.2 Overall survival by mutation category in advanced ovarian cancers. The survival was similar for women with mutations in *BRCA1* and other HRD-related genes in GOG 218 and GOG 262. GOG indicates Gynecologic Oncology Group; NA indicates not applicable; other indicates the genes *BRIP1*, *PALB2*, *RAD51C*, *RAD51D*, and *BARD1*; WT indicates wild type [22]

RAD51C that confer an increased risk for breast and ovarian cancer [141]. Loveday et al. reported that 8 inactivating *RAD51D* mutations were identified in unrelated individuals from 911 breast-ovarian cancer families, and the mutations confer a 6.3-fold increased risk of ovarian cancer but cause only a small increase in breast cancer risk (RR = 1.32) [142]. The analyses from the same trial including 1132 probands with a family history of ovarian cancer and 1156 controls also showed that *RAD51C* was associated with an increased risk for ovarian cancer (RR, 5.88; 95% CI, 2.91–11.88; $P < 0.001$) [143]. In a case-control analysis of 3429 ovarian cancer cases and 2772 controls, both *RAD51C* (OR, 5.2; 95% CI, 1.1–24; $P = 0.035$) and *RAD51D* (OR, 12.0; 95% CI, 1.5–90; $P = 0.019$) were associated with an increased risk for ovarian cancer [144]. The NCCN Guidelines recommend that RRSO in *RAD51C* and *RAD51D* mutation carriers is considered beginning at ages 45–50; however, further analyses are needed to confirm recommendation age of RRSO in these mutation carriers [13].

BRIP1, *BRCA1*-interacting protein C-terminal helicase 1, is a DNA helicase and defective in Fanconi anemia complementation group J. In 1915 unselected ovarian cancer cases, 1.4% of patients had a mutation in *BRIP1* [22]. In analysis of Icelandic 656 ovarian cancer cases and 3913 controls, *BRIP1* frameshift mutation confers an increase in ovarian cancer risk (OR, 8.13; 95% CI, 4.74–13.95; $P < 0.001$) [145]. In addition, an analysis of 3236 invasive ovarian cancer patients, 3431 controls, and 2000 unaffected high-risk women from a clinical screening trial of ovarian cancer (UKFOCSS) showed that *BRIP1* is associated with a significant increased risk for ovarian cancer and relative risks associated with *BRIP1* mutations were 11.22 for invasive ovarian cancer (95% CI, 3.22–34.10; $P < 0.001$) and 14.09 for high-grade serous disease (95% CI, 4.04–45.02; $P < 0.001$) [146]. The cumulative lifetime risk of developing ovarian cancer by age 80 in *BRIP1* mutation carriers is estimated to be 5.8% (95% CI, 3.6–9.1) [146]. The NCCN Guidelines recommend that RRSO in *BRIP1* mutation carriers be considered beginning at ages 45–50; however, their cumulative risk exceeds that of a woman with a first-degree relative with a non-*BRCA*-related ovarian cancer in around age 50–55 years. Further prospective trials are needed to confirm recommendation age of RRSO in these mutation carriers [13].

PALB2, partner and localizer of *BRCA2*, is a Fanconi anemia gene and an integral component of the *BRCA* complex required for homologous recombination repair [147]. *PALB2* mutations have been detected in 1–4% of families negative for *BRCA* mutations [148]. Norquist et al. reported that 12 patients had germline mutations of *PALB2* in analysis of 1915 ovarian cancer patients [22]. In sequence analysis of genomic DNA of 1144 familial breast cancer patients with wild-type sequences at *BRCA1* and *BRCA2*, *PALB2* heterozygotes were 1.3-fold more likely to have a relative with ovarian cancer ($P = 0.18$) [6]. Overall, significantly less ovarian cancer is seen in *PALB2* families when compared with *BRCA1* and *BRCA2* families; therefore, it remains to be seen whether ovarian cancer risk is truly increased in individuals who are *PALB2* mutation carriers or not [148].

2.4 PARP Inhibitors

Poly (ADP-ribose) polymerase (PARP) inhibitors cause cancer cell death in BRCA-mutated cancers by synthetic lethality. Olaparib was the first PARP inhibitor approved in the European Union and the USA for the treatment of advanced ovarian cancer patients with a germline *BRCA* mutation. The FDA approved olaparib for the patients who have received treatment with three or more lines of chemotherapy [149, 150]. Recent data suggest that olaparib is especially active in patients with platinum-sensitive recurrent ovarian cancer; on the other hand, a lower response rate is observed in patients showing resistance or refractory to platinum agent [151–156].

Maintenance monotherapy with olaparib significantly prolonged progression-free survival versus placebo in patients with platinum-sensitive recurrent serous ovarian cancer. In a randomized, double-blind, phase 2 study, median PFS was significantly longer in the olaparib group than in the placebo group of patients with a *BRCA* mutation (11.2 months [95% CI, 8.3 to not calculable] vs 4.3 months [3.0–5.4]; HR 0.18 [0.10–0.31]; $P < 0.0001$); however, overall survival did not significantly differ between two groups (HR 0.88 [95% CI, 0.64–1.21]; $P = 0.44$). Interestingly, in the patients with wild-type *BRCA*, median PFS was also significantly longer in the olaparib group than in the placebo group (7.4 months [5.5–10.3] vs 5.5 months [3.7–5.6]; HR 0.54 [0.34–0.85]; $P = 0.0075$) [157]. A recent trial of monotherapy with olaparib showed that the overall response rate was 34% in women with recurrent advanced ovarian cancer [149, 158].

A combination of olaparib plus paclitaxel and carboplatin followed by maintenance monotherapy significantly improved progression-free survival versus paclitaxel plus carboplatin alone in patients with platinum-sensitive, recurrent, high-grade serous ovarian cancer in a randomized phase 2 study. Progression-free survival was significantly longer in the olaparib plus chemotherapy group (median 12.2 months [95% CI, 9.7–15.0]) than in the chemotherapy-alone group (median 9.6 months [95% CI, 9.1–9.7]) (HR 0.51 [95% CI, 0.34–0.77]; $P = 0.0012$), especially in patients with *BRCA* mutations (HR 0.21 [0.08–0.55]; $P = 0.0015$) [159].

Multiple PARP inhibitors, olaparib, veliparib, talazoparib, rucaparib, and niraparib, have been evaluated in clinical trials. Current study is extending the use of PARP inhibitors beyond *BRCA* mutations, and several trials are ongoing for the inhibitors in other populations such as patients with HR deficiency [160, 161].

Conclusions

We reviewed the recent data regarding clinical and molecular features and management of hereditary ovarian cancer. RRSO after completion of childbearing has been recommended for *BRCA1/2* mutation carriers due to the absence of reliable methods of early detection and the poor prognosis associated with advanced ovarian cancer. The effectiveness of RRSO in reducing the risk for breast and ovarian cancer in *BRCA1/2* mutation carriers has been reported in various studies, and RRSO was associated with lower all-cause mortality. Genetic counseling in RRSO for *BRCA1/2* mutation carriers should include discussion of extent of cancer risk reduction, risks associated with surgeries, reconstructive options, and risks associated with premature menopause (e.g., osteoporosis, cardiovascular disease, vasomotor symptoms, and sexual concerns), management of menopausal symptoms, and discussion of reproductive desires.

In Japan, *BRCA1/2* genetic testing has been available as a routine clinical examination for patients with epithelial ovarian cancer; however, there are too few genetic counselors to do the counseling sufficiently. Therefore, genetic testing has not been widely performed in Japan. It is important to organize a system which can usually perform a genetic counseling in every cancer treatment centers.

Olaparib was the first PARP inhibitor approved in the EU and USA for the treatment of advanced ovarian cancer patients with a germline *BRCA* mutation. Multiple PARP inhibitors, olaparib, veliparib, talazoparib, rucaparib, and niraparib, have been evaluated in clinical trials. It has been shown that around half of high-grade serous ovarian cancers have aberrations in homologous recombination repair. Current study is extending the use of PARP inhibitors beyond BRCA mutations, and several trials are ongoing for the inhibitors in other populations such as patients with HR deficiency. Further clinical studies are needed to extend the use of PARP inhibitors to non-*BRCA*-mutated ovarian cancers.

References

1. Goldgar DE, Easton DF, Cannon-Albright LA, Skolnick MH. Systematic population-based assessment of cancer risk in firstdegree relatives of cancer probands. J Natl Cancer Inst. 1994;86:1600–8.
2. Schildkraut JM, Risch N, Thompson WD. Evaluating genetic association among ovarian, breast, and endometrial cancer: evidence for a breast/ovarian cancer relationship. Am J Hum Genet. 1989;45:521–9.
3. Toss A, Tomasello C, Razzaboni E, Contu G, Grandi G, Cagnacci A, Schilder RJ, Cortesi L. Hereditary ovarian cancer: not only BRCA 1 and 2 genes. Biomed Res Int. 2015;2015:341723.
4. Walsh T, Casadei S, Lee MK, et al. Mutations in 12 genes for inherited ovarian, fallopian tube, and peritoneal carcinoma identified by massively parallel sequencing. Proc Natl Acad Sci U S A. 2011;108:18032–7.
5. Walsh T, Casadei S, Coats KH, et al. Spectrum of mutations in BRCA1, BRCA2, CHEK2, and TP53 in families at high risk of breast cancer. JAMA. 2006;295:1379–88.
6. Casadei S, Norquist BM, Walsh T, et al. Contribution of inherited mutations in the BRCA2-interacting protein PALB2 to familial breast cancer. Cancer Res. 2011;71:2222–9.
7. Engel NJ, Gordon P, Thull DL, et al. A multidisciplinary clinic for individualizing management of patients at increased risk for breast and gynecologic cancer. Familial Cancer. 2012;11:419–27.
8. Liliac L, Amalinei C, Balan R, Grigoras A, Caruntu I-D. Ovarian cancer: insights into genetics and pathogeny. Histol Histopathol. 2012;27:707–19.
9. Miki Y, Swensen J, Shattuck-Eidens D, et al. A strong candidate for the breast and ovarian-cancer susceptibility gene BRCA1. Science. 1994;266:66–71.
10. Wooster R, Bignell G, Lancaster J, Swift S, Seal S, Mangion J, Collins N, Gregory S, Gumbs C, Micklem G. Identification of the breast cancer susceptibility gene BRCA2. Nature. 1995;378:789–92.
11. Yun MH, Hiom K. Understanding the functions of BRCA1 in the DNA-damage response. Biochem Soc Trans. 2009;37:597–604.
12. Cipak L, Watanabe N, Bessho T. The role of BRCA2 in replicationcoupled DNA interstrand cross-link repair in vitro. Nat Struct Mol Biol. 2006;13:729–33.
13. NCCN Clinical Practice Guidelines in Oncology (NCCN Guidelines) Genetic/Familial High-Risk Assessment: Breast and Ovarian Version 2.2017.
14. American College of Obstetricians and Gynecologists; ACOG Committee on Practice Bulletins—Gynecology; ACOG Committee on Genetics; Society of Gynecologic Oncologists. ACOG Practice Bulletin No. 103: hereditary breast and ovarian cancer syndrome. Obstet Gynecol. 2009;113:957–66.
15. Whittemore AS. Risk of breast cancer in carriers of BRCA gene mutations. N Engl J Med. 1997;337:788–9.
16. Ford D, Easton DF, Stratton M, et al. Genetic heterogeneity and penetrance analysis of the BRCA1 and BRCA2 genes in breast cancer families. The Breast Cancer Linkage Consortium. Am J Hum Genet. 1998;62:676–89.
17. Sekine M, Nagata H, Tsuji S, et al. Mutational analysis of BRCA1 and BRCA2 and clinicopathologic analysis of ovarian cancer in 82 ovarian cancer families: two common founder mutations of BRCA1 in Japanese population. Clin Cancer Res. 2001;7:3144–50.
18. Kast K, Rhiem K, Wappenschmidt B, et al. Prevalence of BRCA1/2 germline mutations in 21 401 families with breast and ovarian cancer. J Med Genet. 2016;53:465–71.
19. Gayther SA, Russell P, Harrington P, et al. The contribution of germline BRCA1 and BRCA2 mutations to familial ovarian cancer: no evidence for other ovarian cancer-susceptibility genes. Am J Hum Genet. 1999;65:1021–9.
20. Sekine M, Nagata H, Tsuji S, et al. Localization of a novel susceptibility gene for familial ovarian cancer to chromosome 3p22-p25. Hum Mol Genet. 2001;10:1421–9.

21. Jazaeri AA, Lu K, Schmandt R, et al. Molecular determinants of tumor differentiation in papillary serous ovarian carcinoma. Mol Carcinog. 2003;36:53–9.
22. Norquist BM, Harrell MI, Brady MF, et al. Inherited mutations in women with ovarian carcinoma. JAMA Oncol. 2016;2:482–90.
23. Song H, Cicek MS, Dicks E, et al. The contribution of deleterious germline mutations in BRCA1, BRCA2 and the mismatch repair genes to ovarian cancer in the population. Hum Mol Genet. 2014;23:4703–9.
24. Risch HA, McLaughlin JR, Cole DE, et al. Population BRCA1 and BRCA2 mutation frequencies and cancer penetrances: a kin-cohort study in Ontario, Canada. J Natl Cancer Inst. 2006;98:1694–706.
25. Pal T, Permuth-Wey J, Betts JA, et al. BRCA1 and BRCA2 mutations account for a large proportion of ovarian carcinoma cases. Cancer. 2005;104:2807–16.
26. Schrader KA, Hurlburt J, Kalloger SE, et al. Germline BRCA1 and BRCA2 mutations in ovarian cancer: utility of a histology-based referral strategy. Obstet Gynecol. 2012;120:235–40.
27. Zhang S, Royer R, Li S, et al. Frequencies of BRCA1 and BRCA2 mutations among 1,342 unselected patients with invasive ovarian cancer. Gynecol Oncol. 2011;121:353–7.
28. Sakamoto I, Hirotsu Y, Nakagomi H, Ouchi H, Ikegami A, Teramoto K, Amemiya K, Mochizuki H, Omata M. BRCA1 and BRCA2 mutations in Japanese patients with ovarian, fallopian tube, and primary peritoneal cancer. Cancer. 2016;122:84–90.
29. Ledermann JA, Drew Y, Kristeleit RS. Homologous recombination deficiency and ovarian cancer. Eur J Cancer. 2016;60:49–58.
30. Foulkes WD. Inherited susceptibility to common cancers. N Engl J Med. 2008;359:2143–53.
31. Metcalfe KA, Poll A, Royer R, et al. Screening for founder mutations in BRCA1 and BRCA2 in unselected Jewish women. J Clin Oncol. 2010;28:387–91.
32. Sugano K, Nakamura S, Ando J, et al. Cross-sectional analysis of germline BRCA1 and BRCA2 mutations in Japanese patients suspected to have hereditary breast/ovarian cancer. Cancer Sci. 2008;99:1967–76.
33. Nakamura S, Takahashi M, Tozaki M, Nakayama T, Nomizu T, Miki Y, Murakami Y, Aoki D, Iwase T, Nishimura S, Yamauchi H, Ohsumi S, Baba S, Shimizu T. Prevalence and differentiation of hereditary breast and ovarian cancers in Japan. Breast Cancer. 2015;22:462–8.
34. Anglian Breast Cancer Study Group. Prevalence and penetrance of BRCA1 and BRCA2 mutations in a population-based series of breast cancer cases. Br J Cancer. 2000;83:1301–8.
35. Antoniou A, Pharoah PD, Narod S, et al. Average risks of breast and ovarian cancer associated with BRCA1 or BRCA2 mutations detected in case series unselected for family history: a combined analysis of 22 studies. Am J Hum Genet. 2003;72:1117–30.
36. Chen S, Parmigiani G. Meta-analysis of BRCA1 and BRCA2 penetrance. J Clin Oncol. 2007;25:1329–33.
37. Ford D, Easton DF, Bishop DT, et al. Risks of cancer in BRCA1- mutation carriers. Breast Cancer Linkage Consortium. Lancet. 1994;343:692–5.
38. King MC, Marks JH, Mandell JB. Breast and ovarian cancer risks due to inherited mutations in BRCA1 and BRCA2. Science. 2003;302:643–6.
39. Mavaddat N, Peock S, Frost D, et al. Cancer risks for BRCA1 and BRCA2 mutation carriers: results from prospective analysis of EMBRACE. J Natl Cancer Inst. 2013;105:812–22.
40. van den Broek AJ, van't Veer LJ, Hooning MJ, et al. Impact of age at primary breast cancer on contralateral breast cancer risk in BRCA1/2 mutation carriers. J Clin Oncol. 2016;34:409–18.
41. Finch A, Beiner M, Lubinski J, et al. Salpingo-oophorectomy and the risk of ovarian, fallopian tube, and peritoneal cancers in women with a BRCA1 or BRCA2 mutation. JAMA. 2006;296:185–92.
42. Risch HA, McLaughlin JR, Cole DE, et al. Prevalence and penetrance of germline BRCA1 and BRCA2 mutations in a population series of 649 women with ovarian cancer. Am J Hum Genet. 2001;68:700–10.
43. Rebbeck TR, Mitra N, Wan F, et al. Association of type and location of BRCA1 and BRCA2 mutations with risk of breast and ovarian cancer. JAMA. 2015;313:1347–61.

44. Atchley DP, Albarracin CT, Lopez A, et al. Clinical and pathologic characteristics of patients with BRCA-positive and BRCA-negative breast cancer. J Clin Oncol. 2008;26:4282–8.
45. Eerola H, Heikkila P, Tamminen A, et al. Relationship of patients' age to histopathological features of breast tumours in BRCA1 and BRCA2 and mutation-negative breast cancer families. Breast Cancer Res. 2005;7:R465–9.
46. Lakhani SR, Reis-Filho JS, Fulford L, et al. Prediction of BRCA1 status in patients with breast cancer using estrogen receptor and basal phenotype. Clin Cancer Res. 2005;11:5175–80.
47. Lakhani SR, Van De Vijver MJ, Jacquemier J, et al. The pathology of familial breast cancer: predictive value of immunohistochemical markers estrogen receptor, progesterone receptor, HER-2, and p53 in patients with mutations in BRCA1 and BRCA2. J Clin Oncol. 2002;20:2310–8.
48. Lee E, McKean-Cowdin R, Ma H, et al. Characteristics of triplenegative breast cancer in patients with a BRCA1 mutation: results from a population-based study of young women. J Clin Oncol. 2011;29:4373–80.
49. Young SR, Pilarski RT, Donenberg T, et al. The prevalence of BRCA1 mutations among young women with triple-negative breast cancer. BMC Cancer. 2009;9:86.
50. Berchuck A, Heron KA, Carney ME, et al. Frequency of germline and somatic BRCA1 mutations in ovarian cancer. Clin Cancer Res. 1998;4:2433–7.
51. Bjorge T, Lie AK, Hovig E, et al. BRCA1 mutations in ovarian cancer and borderline tumours in Norway: a nested case-control study. Br J Cancer. 2004;91:1829–34.
52. Lakhani SR, Manek S, Penault-Llorca F, et al. Pathology of ovarian cancers in BRCA1 and BRCA2 carriers. Clin Cancer Res. 2004;10:2473–81.
53. Press JZ, De Luca A, Boyd N, et al. Ovarian carcinomas with genetic and epigenetic BRCA1 loss have distinct molecular abnormalities. BMC Cancer. 2008;8:17.
54. Rechsteiner M, Zimmermann AK, Wild PJ, et al. TP53 mutations are common in all subtypes of epithelial ovarian cancer and occur concomitantly with KRAS mutations in the mucinous type. Exp Mol Pathol. 2013;95:235–41.
55. Werness BA, Ramus SJ, DiCioccio RA, et al. Histopathology, FIGO stage, and BRCA mutation status of ovarian cancers from the Gilda Radner Familial Ovarian Cancer Registry. Int J Gynecol Pathol. 2004;23:29–34.
56. Ayadi-Kaddour A, Bouraoui S, Bellil K, et al. Colonic adenocarcinoma and bilateral malignant ovarian sex cord tumor with annular tubules in Peutz-Jeghers syndrome. Pathologica. 2004;96:117–20.
57. Clements A, Robison K, Granai C, et al. A case of Peutz-Jeghers syndrome with breast cancer, bilateral sex cord tumor with annular tubules, and adenoma malignum caused by STK11 gene mutation. Int J Gynecol Cancer. 2009;19:1591–4.
58. Kondi-Pafiti A, Bakalianou K, Iavazzo C, et al. Endometrial carcinoma and ovarian sex cord tumor with annular tubules in a patient with history of Peutz-Jeghers syndrome and multiple malignancies. Eur J Gynaecol Oncol. 2011;32:452–4.
59. Lele SM, Sawh RN, Zaharopoulos P, et al. Malignant ovarian sex cord tumor with annular tubules in a patient with Peutz-Jeghers syndrome: a case report. Mod Pathol. 2000;13:466–70.
60. Young RH. Sex cord-stromal tumors of the ovary and testis: their similarities and differences with consideration of selected problems. Mod Pathol. 2005;18(Suppl 2):S81–98.
61. Goulvent T, Ray-Coquard I, Borel S, et al. DICER1 and FOXL2 mutations in ovarian sex cord-stromal tumours: a GINECO Group study. Histopathology. 2016;68:279–85.
62. Alsop K, Fereday S, Meldrum C, et al. BRCA mutation frequency and patterns of treatment response in BRCA mutation-positive women with ovarian cancer: a report from the Australian Ovarian Cancer Study Group. J Clin Oncol. 2012;30:2654–63.
63. Bolton KL, Chenevix-Trench G, Goh C, et al. Association between BRCA1 and BRCA2 mutations and survival in women with invasive epithelial ovarian cancer. JAMA. 2012;307:382–90.
64. Cass I, Baldwin RL, Varkey T, et al. Improved survival in women with BRCA-associated ovarian carcinoma. Cancer. 2003;97:2187–95.

65. Chetrit A, Hirsh-Yechezkel G, Ben-David Y, et al. Effect of BRCA1/2 mutations on long-term survival of patients with invasive ovarian cancer: the national Israeli study of ovarian cancer. J Clin Oncol. 2008;26:20–5.
66. Tan DS, Rothermundt C, Thomas K, et al. "BRCAness" syndrome in ovarian cancer: a case-control study describing the clinical features and outcome of patients with epithelial ovarian cancer associated with BRCA1 and BRCA2 mutations. J Clin Oncol. 2008;26:5530–6.
67. Yang D, Khan S, Sun Y, et al. Association of BRCA1 and BRCA2 mutations with survival, chemotherapy sensitivity, and gene mutator phenotype in patients with ovarian cancer. JAMA. 2011;306:1557–65.
68. Tan DS, Kaye SB. Chemotherapy for patients with BRCA1 and BRCA2-mutated ovarian cancer: same or different? Am Soc Clin Oncol Educ Book. 2015:114–21.
69. Pal T, Permuth-Wey J, Kapoor R, et al. Improved survival in BRCA2 carriers with ovarian cancer. Familial Cancer. 2007;6:113–9.
70. Vencken PM, Kriege M, Hoogwerf D, et al. Chemosensitivity and outcome of BRCA1- and BRCA2-associated ovarian cancer patients after first-line chemotherapy compared with sporadic ovarian cancer patients. Ann Oncol. 2011;22:1346–52.
71. Sun C, Li N, Ding D, et al. The role of BRCA status on the prognosis of patients with epithelial ovarian cancer: a systematic review of the literature with a meta-analysis. PLoS One. 2014;9:e95285.
72. Pennington KP, Walsh T, Harrell MI, et al. Germline and somatic mutations in homologous recombination genes predict platinum response and survival in ovarian, fallopian tube, and peritoneal carcinomas. Clin Cancer Res. 2014;20:764–75.
73. Evans DG, Gaarenstroom KN, Stirling D, et al. Screening for familial ovarian cancer: poor survival of BRCA1/2 related cancers. J Med Genet. 2009;46:593–7.
74. Woodward ER, Sleightholme HV, Considine AM, et al. Annual surveillance by CA125 and transvaginal ultrasound for ovarian cancer in both high-risk and population risk women is ineffective. BJOG. 2007;114:1500–9.
75. Jacobs IJ, Menon U, Ryan A, et al. Ovarian cancer screening and mortality in the UK Collaborative Trial of Ovarian Cancer Screening (UKCTOCS): a randomised controlled trial. Lancet. 2016;387:945–56.
76. Menon U, Gentry-Maharaj A, Hallett R, et al. Sensitivity and specificity of multimodal and ultrasound screening for ovarian cancer, and stage distribution of detected cancers: results of the prevalence screen of the UK Collaborative Trial of Ovarian Cancer Screening (UKCTOCS). Lancet Oncol. 2009;10:327–40.
77. Sherman ME, Piedmonte M, Mai PL, et al. Pathologic findings at risk-reducing salpingo-oophorectomy: primary results from Gynecologic Oncology Group trial GOG-0199. J Clin Oncol. 2014;32:3275–83.
78. Finch AP, Lubinski J, Moller P, et al. Impact of oophorectomy on cancer incidence and mortality in women with a BRCA1 or BRCA2 mutation. J Clin Oncol. 2014;32:1547–53.
79. Domchek SM, Friebel TM, Singer CF, Evans DG, Lynch HT, Isaacs C, Garber JE, Neuhausen SL, Matloff E, Eeles R, Pichert G, Van t'veer L, Tung N, Weitzel JN, Couch FJ, Rubinstein WS, Ganz PA, Daly MB, Olopade OI, Tomlinson G, Schildkraut J, Blum JL, Rebbeck TR. Association of risk-reducing surgery in BRCA1 or BRCA2 mutation carriers with cancer risk and mortality. JAMA. 2010;304:967–75.
80. Rebbeck TR, Kauff ND, Domchek SM. Meta-analysis of risk reduction estimates associated with risk-reducing salpingooophorectomy in BRCA1 or BRCA2 mutation carriers. J Natl Cancer Inst. 2009;101:80–7.
81. Rebbeck TR, Lynch HT, Neuhausen SL, et al. Prophylactic oophorectomy in carriers of BRCA1 or BRCA2 mutations. N Engl J Med. 2002;346:1616–22.
82. Kauff ND, Satagopan JM, Robson ME, et al. Risk-reducing salpingo-oophorectomy in women with a BRCA1 or BRCA2 mutation. N Engl J Med. 2002;346:1609–15.
83. Rebbeck TR, Levin AM, Eisen A, et al. Breast cancer risk after bilateral prophylactic oophorectomy in BRCA1 mutation carriers. J Natl Cancer Inst. 1999;91:1475–9.

84. Finch A, Shaw P, Rosen B, et al. Clinical and pathologic findings of prophylactic salpingo-oophorectomies in 159 BRCA1 and BRCA2 carriers. Gynecol Oncol. 2006;100:58–64.
85. Li X, You R, Wang X, et al. Effectiveness of prophylactic surgeries in BRCA1 or BRCA2 mutation carriers: a meta-analysis and systematic review. Clin Cancer Res. 2016;22:3971–81.
86. Eisen A, Lubinski J, Klijn J, et al. Breast cancer risk following bilateral oophorectomy in BRCA1 and BRCA2 mutation carriers: an international case-control study. J Clin Oncol. 2005;23:7491–6.
87. Kauff ND, Domchek SM, Friebel TM, et al. Risk-reducing salpingooophorectomy for the prevention of BRCA1- and BRCA2-associated breast and gynecologic cancer: a multicenter, prospective study. J Clin Oncol. 2008;26:1331–7.
88. Metcalfe K, Lynch HT, Foulkes WD, et al. Effect of oophorectomy on survival after breast cancer in BRCA1 and BRCA2 mutation carriers. JAMA Oncol. 2015;1:306–13.
89. Callahan MJ, Crum CP, Medeiros F, et al. Primary fallopian tube malignancies in BRCA-positive women undergoing surgery for ovarian cancer risk reduction. J Clin Oncol. 2007;25:3985–90.
90. Powell CB, Chen LM, McLennan J, et al. Risk-reducing salpingooophorectomy (RRSO) in BRCA mutation carriers: experience with a consecutive series of 111 patients using a standardized surgicalpathological protocol. Int J Gynecol Cancer. 2011;21:846–51.
91. Powell CB, Kenley E, Chen LM, et al. Risk-reducing salpingooophorectomy in BRCA mutation carriers: role of serial sectioning in the detection of occult malignancy. J Clin Oncol. 2005;23:127–32.
92. Shaw PA, Rouzbahman M, Pizer ES, et al. Candidate serous cancer precursors in fallopian tube epithelium of BRCA1/2 mutation carriers. Mod Pathol. 2009;22:1133–8.
93. Medeiros F, Muto MG, Lee Y, et al. The tubal fimbria is a preferred site for early adenocarcinoma in women with familial ovarian cancer syndrome. Am J Surg Pathol. 2006;30:230–6.
94. Rebbeck TR, Friebel T, Wagner T, et al. Effect of short-term hormone replacement therapy on breast cancer risk reduction after bilateral prophylactic oophorectomy in BRCA1 and BRCA2 mutation carriers: the PROSE Study Group. J Clin Oncol. 2005;23:7804–10.
95. Eisen A, Lubinski J, Gronwald J, et al. Hormone therapy and the risk of breast cancer in BRCA1 mutation carriers. J Natl Cancer Inst. 2008;100:1361–7.
96. Chlebowski RT, Prentice RL. Menopausal hormone therapy in BRCA1 mutation carriers: uncertainty and caution. J Natl Cancer Inst. 2008;100:1341–3.
97. Garber JE, Hartman AR. Prophylactic oophorectomy and hormone replacement therapy: protection at what price? J Clin Oncol. 2004;22:978–80.
98. McAlpine JN, Hanley GE, Woo MM, et al. Opportunistic salpingectomy: uptake, risks, and complications of a regional initiative for ovarian cancer prevention. Am J Obstet Gynecol. 2014;210:471. e471–411
99. Findley AD, Siedhoff MT, Hobbs KA, et al. Short-term effects of salpingectomy during laparoscopic hysterectomy on ovarian reserve: a pilot randomized controlled trial. Fertil Steril. 2013;100:1704–8.
100. Hartmann LC, Lindor NM. The role of risk-reducing surgery in hereditary breast and ovarian cancer. N Engl J Med. 2016;374:454–68.
101. Daly MB, Dresher CW, Yates MS, et al. Salpingectomy as a means to reduce ovarian cancer risk. Cancer Prev Res (Phila). 2015;8:342–8.
102. NCCN Clinical Practice Guidelines in Oncology (NCCN Guidelines) Ovarian Cancer Including Fallopian Tube Cancer and Primary Peritoneal Cancer Version 1.2016.
103. Mingels MJ, van Ham MA, de Kievit IM, et al. Müllerian precursor lesions in serous ovarian cancer patients: using the SEE-Fim and SEE-End protocol. Mod Pathol. 2014;27:1002–13.
104. Komiyama S, Katabuchi H, Mikami M, et al. Japan Society of Gynecologic Oncology guidelines 2015 for the treatment of ovarian cancer including primary peritoneal cancer and fallopian tube cancer. Int J Clin Oncol. 2016;21:435–46.
105. Suzuki N, Katabuchi H. The requirement of RRSO for BRCA1/2 mutation carriers. J Jpn Soc Obstet Gynecol. 2016;68:1332–4.

106. Iodice S, Barile M, Rotmensz N, et al. Oral contraceptive use and breast or ovarian cancer risk in BRCA1/2 carriers: a meta-analysis. Eur J Cancer. 2010;46:2275–84.
107. Narod SA, Risch H, Moslehi R, et al. Oral contraceptives and the risk of hereditary ovarian cancer. Hereditary Ovarian Cancer Clinical Study Group. N Engl J Med. 1998;339:424–8.
108. Moorman PG, Havrilesky LJ, Gierisch JM, et al. Oral contraceptives and risk of ovarian cancer and breast cancer among high-risk women: a systematic review and meta-analysis. J Clin Oncol. 2013;31:4188–98.
109. Lynch HT, Casey MJ, Snyder CL, et al. Hereditary ovarian carcinoma: heterogeneity, molecular genetics, pathology, and management. Mol Oncol. 2009;3:97–137.
110. Bonadona V, Bonaiti B, Olschwang S, et al. Cancer risks associated with germline mutations in MLH1, MSH2, and MSH6 genes in Lynch syndrome. JAMA. 2011;305:2304–10.
111. Kohlmann W, Gruber S. Lynch syndrome. Gene reviews at gene tests: medical genetics information resource. 2014.
112. Lindor NM, Petersen GM, Hadley DW, et al. Recommendations for the care of individuals with an inherited predisposition to Lynch syndrome: a systematic review. JAMA. 2006;296:1507–17.
113. Watson P, Vasen HF, Mecklin JP, et al. The risk of extra-colonic, extra-endometrial cancer in the Lynch syndrome. Int J Cancer. 2008;123:444–9.
114. Guillotin D, Martin SA. Exploiting DNA mismatch repair deficiency as a therapeutic strategy. Exp Cell Res. 2014;329:110–5.
115. Souza RF, Appel R, Yin J, et al. Microsatellite instability in theinsulin-like growth factor II receptor gene in gastrointestinal tumours. Nat Genet. 1996;14:255–7.
116. Rampino N, Yamamoto H, Ionovetal Y. Somatic frameshift mutations in the BAX gene in colon cancers of the microsatellite mutator phenotype. Science. 1997;275:967–9.
117. Ketabi Z, Bartuma K, Bernsteinetal I. Ovarian cancer linked to lynch syndrome typically presents as early-onset, non-serous epithelialtumors. Gynecol Oncol. 2011;121:462–5.
118. Ferreira AM, Westers H, Sousaetal S. Mono nucleotide precedes dinucleotide repeat instability during colorectal tumour development in Lynch syndrome patients. J Pathol. 2009;219:96–102.
119. Chui MH, Gilks CB, Cooper K, Clarke BA. Identifying Lynch syndrome in patients with ovarian carcinoma: the significance of tumor subtype. Adv Anat Pathol. 2013;20:378–86.
120. Cai KQ, Albarracin C, Rosen D, et al. Microsatellite instability and alteration of the expression of hMLH1 and hMSH2 in ovarian clea rcell carcinoma. Hum Pathol. 2004;35:552–9.
121. Liu J, Albarracin CT, Chang K-H, et al. Microsatellite instability and expression of hMLH1 and hMSH2 proteins in ovarian endometrioid cancer. Mod Pathol. 2004;17:75–80.
122. Pal T, Permuth-Wey J, Kumar A, Sellers TA. Systematic review and meta-analysis of ovarian cancers: estimation of microsatellite-high frequency and characterization no mismatch repair deficient tumor histology. Clin Cancer Res. 2008;14:6847–54.
123. Chui MH, Ryan P, Radigan J, et al. The histomorphology of Lynch syndrome-associated ovarian carcinomas: toward a subtype-specific screening strategy. Am J Surg Pathol. 2014;38:1173–81.
124. Watson P, utzow RB¨, Lynch HT, et al. The clinical features of ovarian cancer in hereditary nonpolyposis colorectal cancer. Gynecol Oncol. 2001;82:223–8.
125. Vasen HFA, Stormorken A, Menko FH, et al. MSH2 mutation carriers are at higher risk of cancer than MLH1 mutation carriers: a study of hereditary nonpolyposis colorectal cancer families. J Clin Oncol. 2001;19:4074–80.
126. Grindedal EM, Renkonen-Sinisalo L, Vasen H, et al. Survival in women with MMR mutations and ovarian cancer: a multi center study in Lynch syndrome kindreds. J Med Genet. 2010;47:99–102.
127. Baldwin LA, Huang B, Milleretal RW. Ten-year relative survival for epithelial ovarian cancer. Obstet Gynecol. 2012;120:612–8.
128. Chen LM, Yang KY, Little SE, et al. Gynecologic cancer prevention in Lynch syndrome/hereditary nonpolyposis colorectal cancer families. Obstet Gynecol. 2007;110:18–25.

129. Schmeler KM, Lynch HT, Chen LM, et al. Prophylactic surgery to reduce the risk of gynecologic cancers in the Lynch syndrome. N Engl J Med. 2006;354:261–9.
130. Stuckless S, Green J, Dawson L, et al. Impact of gynecological screening in Lynch syndrome carriers with an MSH2 mutation. Clin Genet. 2013;83:359–64.
131. Syngal S, Brand RE, Church JM, et al. ACG clinical guideline: genetic testing and management of hereditary gastrointestinal cancer syndromes. Am J Gastroenterol. 2015;110:223–62. quiz 263
132. Stoffel EM, Mangu PB, Gruber SB, et al. Hereditary colorectal cancer syndromes: American Society of Clinical Oncology Clinical Practice Guideline endorsement of the familial risk-colorectal cancer: European Society for Medical Oncology Clinical Practice Guidelines. J Clin Oncol. 2015;33:209–17.
133. Auranen A, Joutsiniemi T. A systematic review of gynecological cancer surveillance in women belonging to hereditary nonpolyposis colorectal cancer (Lynch syndrome) families. Acta Obstet Gynecol Scand. 2011;90:437–44.
134. Jarvinen HJ, Renkonen-Sinisalo L, Aktan-Collan K, et al. Ten years after mutation testing for Lynch syndrome: cancer incidence and outcome in mutation-positive and mutation-negative family members. J Clin Oncol. 2009;27:4793–7.
135. Renkonen-Sinisalo L, Butzow R, Leminen A, et al. Surveillance for endometrial cancer in hereditary nonpolyposis colorectal cancer syndrome. Int J Cancer. 2007;120:821–4.
136. Rijcken FE, Mourits MJ, Kleibeuker JH, et al. Gynecologic screening in hereditary nonpolyposis colorectal cancer. Gynecol Oncol. 2003;91:74–80.
137. Dove-Edwin I, Boks D, Goff S, et al. The outcome of endometrial carcinoma surveillance by ultrasound scan in women at risk of hereditary nonpolyposis colorectal carcinoma and familial colorectal carcinoma. Cancer. 2002;94:1708–12.
138. Veronica R, Hirshfield KM, Ganesan S, Rodriguez-Rodriguez L. Molecular characterization of epithelial ovarian cancer: implications for diagnosis and treatment. Int J Mol Sci. 2016;17:2113.
139. Cancer Genome Atlas Research Network. Integrated genomic analyses of ovarian carcinoma. Nature. 2011;474:609–15.
140. Konstantinopoulos PA, Ceccaldi R, Shapiro GI, D'Andrea AD. Homologous recombination deficiency: exploiting the fundamental vulnerability of ovarian cancer. Cancer Discov. 2015;5:1137–54.
141. Meindl A, Hellebrand H, Wiek C, et al. Germline mutations in breast and ovarian cancer pedigrees establish RAD51C as a human cancer susceptibility gene. Nat Genet. 2010;42:410–4.
142. Loveday C, Turnbull C, Ramsay E, et al. Germline mutations in RAD51D confer susceptibility to ovarian cancer. Nat Genet. 2011;43:879–82.
143. Loveday C, Turnbull C, Ruark E, et al. Germline RAD51C mutations confer susceptibility to ovarian cancer. Nat Genet. 2012;44:475–6. author reply 476
144. Song H, Dicks E, Ramus SJ, et al. Contribution of germline mutations in the RAD51B, RAD51C, and RAD51D genes to ovarian cancer in the population. J Clin Oncol. 2015;33:2901–7.
145. Rafnar T, Gudbjartsson DF, Sulem P, et al. Mutations in BRIP1 confer high risk of ovarian cancer. Nat Genet. 2011;43:1104–7.
146. Ramus SJ, Song H, Dicks E, et al. Germline mutations in the BRIP1, BARD1, PALB2, and NBN genes in women with ovarian cancer. J Natl Cancer Inst. 2015;107.
147. Sy SM, Huen MS, Chen J. PALB2 is an integral component of the BRCA complex required for homologous recombination repair. Proc Natl Acad Sci U S A. 2009;106:7155–60.
148. Poumpouridou N, Kroupis C. Hereditary breast cancer: beyond BRCA genetic analysis; PALB2 emerges. Clin Chem Lab Med. 2012;50:423–34.
149. Butler T, Maravent S, Boisselle J, et al. A review of 2014 cancer drug approvals, with a look at 2015 and beyond. P T. 2015;40:191–205.
150. Deeks ED. Olaparib: first global approval. Drugs. 2015;75:231–40.
151. Elit L, Hirte H. Palliative systemic therapy for women with recurrent epithelial ovarian cancer: current options. Onco Targets Ther. 2013;6:107–18.

152. Suh DH, Lee KH, Kim K, et al. Major clinical research advances in gynecologic cancer in 2014. J Gynecol Oncol. 2015;26:156–67.
153. Gelmon KA, Tischkowitz M, Mackay H, et al. Olaparib in patients with recurrent high-grade serous or poorly differentiated ovarian carcinoma or triple-negative breast cancer: a phase 2, multicentre, open-label, non-randomised study. Lancet Oncol. 2011;12:852–61.
154. Audeh MW, Carmichael J, Penson RT, et al. Oral poly(ADP-ribose) polymerase inhibitor olaparib in patients with BRCA1 or BRCA2 mutations and recurrent ovarian cancer: a proof-of-concept trial. Lancet. 2010;376:245–51.
155. Fong PC, Yap TA, Boss DS, et al. Poly(ADP)-ribose polymerase inhibition: frequent durable responses in BRCA carrier ovarian cancer correlating with platinum-free interval. J Clin Oncol. 2010;28:2512–9.
156. Ledermann J, Harter P, Gourley C, et al. Olaparib maintenance therapy in platinum-sensitive relapsed ovarian cancer. N Engl J Med. 2012;366:1382–92.
157. Ledermann J, Harter P, Gourley C, Friedlander M, Vergote I, Rustin G, Scott CL, Meier W, Shapira-Frommer R, Safra T, Matei D, Fielding A, Spencer S, Dougherty B, Orr M, Hodgson D, Barrett JC, Matulonis U. Olaparib maintenance therapy in patients with platinum-sensitive relapsed serous ovarian cancer: a preplanned retrospective analysis of outcomes by BRCA status in a randomised phase 2 trial. Lancet Oncol. 2014;15:852–61.
158. Kaufman B, Shapira-Frommer R, Schmutzler RK, et al. Olaparib monotherapy in patients with advanced cancer and a germline BRCA1/2 mutation. J Clin Oncol. 2015;33:244–50.
159. Oza AM, Cibula D, Benzaquen AO, Poole C, Mathijssen RH, Sonke GS, Colombo N, Špaček J, Vuylsteke P, Hirte H, Mahner S, Plante M, Schmalfeldt B, Mackay H, Rowbottom J, Lowe ES, Dougherty B, Barrett JC, Friedlander M. Olaparib combined with chemotherapy for recurrent platinum-sensitive ovarian cancer: a randomised phase 2 trial. Lancet Oncol. 2015;16:87–97.
160. Walsh CS. Two decades beyond BRCA1/2: homologous recombination, hereditary cancer risk and a target for ovarian cancer therapy. Gynecol Oncol. 2015;137:343–50.
161. Lee JM, Ledermann JA, Kohn EC. PARP inhibitors for BRCA1/2 mutation-associated and BRCA-like malignancies. Ann Oncol. 2014;25:32–40.

Morphological and Molecular Pathogenesis of Epithelial Ovarian Tumors

3

Hironori Tashiro, Yuko Imamura, Takeshi Motohara, Isao Sakaguchi, and Hidetaka Katabuchi

Abstract

Epithelial ovarian tumors (EOTs) are associated with a variety of distinct morphological characteristics that include serous, endometrioid, clear cell, and mucinous features and have a spectrum of biological behavior that ranges from benign to malignant. Traditionally, EOTs were believed to originate from the ovarian surface epithelium (OSE), but the latest research supports the concept that some subtypes of EOTs originate from extra-ovarian sites. Although a couple of paradigms in regard to the morphological and molecular pathogenesis of EOTs have dramatically changed in recent years, the delineation between old and new concepts remains confused. This chapter summarizes those concepts and the morphological and molecular alterations associated with each major subtype of EOT, to improve our understanding of the pathogenesis of EOTs.

Keywords

Epithelial ovarian tumor • Serous tumor • Endometrioid tumor • Clear cell tumor • Secondary Müllerian system • Imported disease • Two-tiered classification • Type I • Type II

H. Tashiro, M.D., Ph.D. (✉)
Department of Mother-Child Nursing, Faculty of Life Sciences, Kumamoto University, 4-24-1 Kuhonji, Chuo-ku, Kumamoto City, Kumamoto 862-0976, Japan
e-mail: htashiro@kumamoto-u.ac.jp

Y. Imamura, M.D. • T. Motohara, M.D., Ph.D. • I. Sakaguchi, M.D., Ph.D.
H. Katabuchi, M.D., Ph.D.
Department of Obstetrics and Gynecology, Faculty of Life Sciences, Kumamoto University, 1-1-1 Honjo, Chuo-ku, Kumamoto City, Kumamoto 860-8556, Japan

H. Katabuchi (ed.), *Frontiers in Ovarian Cancer Science*, Comprehensive Gynecology and Obstetrics, DOI 10.1007/978-981-10-4160-0_3

3.1 Introduction

Epithelial ovarian tumors (EOTs) represent a complex family of neoplasms, each with different morphologies that do not necessarily reflect that of the ovary. The major morphological types of EOTs (serous, endometrioid, clear cell, and mucinous) may variously resemble the epithelia of the adnexal (fallopian tube) and uterine regions (proliferative endometrium, endometrium with Arias-Stella reaction, and endocervix) but also the intestinal epithelium (Fig. 3.1). In regard to clinical behavior, EOTs can be further subdivided into benign and malignant tumors, with intermediate tumors of borderline malignancy. Malignant EOTs are generally known as "ovarian carcinomas."

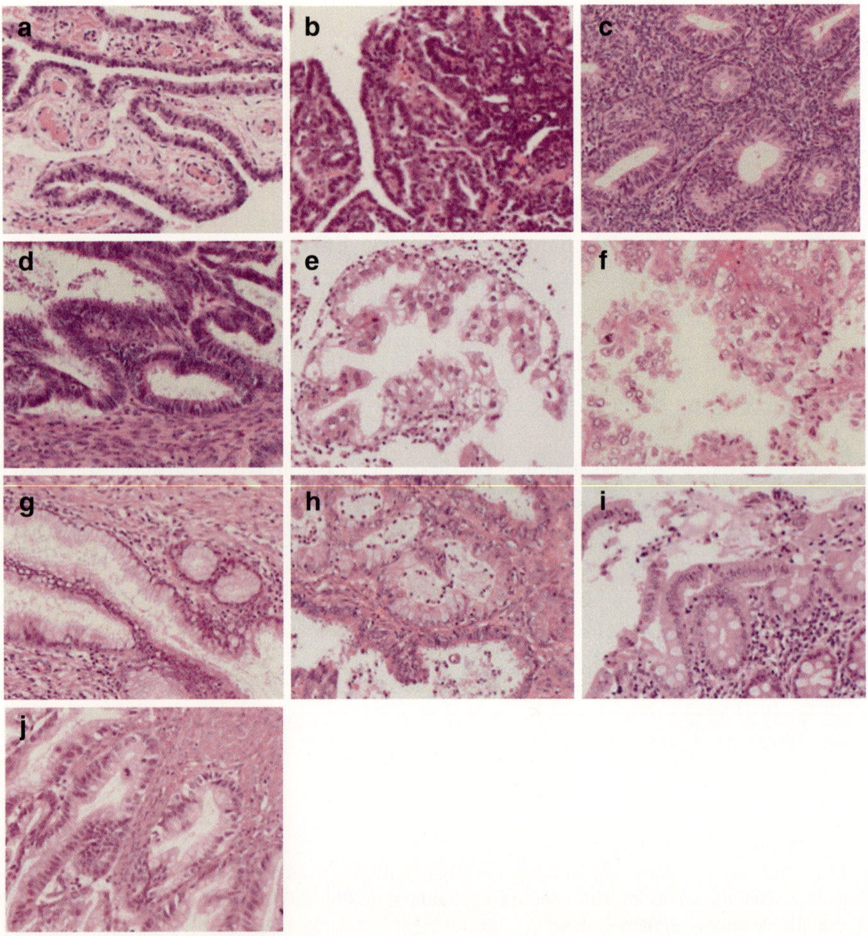

Fig. 3.1 The major morphological types of epithelial ovarian tumors and the mimic normal epithelia; (**a** and **b**) fallopian tubal epithelium (**a**) and serous carcinoma (**b**); (**c** and **d**) endometrium in proliferative phase (**c**) and endometrioid carcinoma (**d**); (**e** and **f**) gestational endometrium with Arias-Stella reaction (**e**) and clear cell carcinoma (**f**); (**g** and **h**) endocervical epithelium (**g**) and mucinous carcinoma which recently is classified in seromucinous carcinoma (**h**); (**i** and **j**) intestinal epithelium (**i**) and mucinous carcinoma (**j**) [(**a**–**j**) hematoxylin and eosin staining; (**a**–**j**) ×200]

The source of EOTs has been a recent topic of debate [1, 2]. The past and current paradigm is that EOTs arise from the ovarian surface epithelium (OSE) covering the ovary and lining inclusion cysts which are derived from surface invaginations. OSE originating developmentally from the coelomic epithelium is composed of flat, nondescript cells morphologically similar to the mesothelium lining of the peritoneal cavity. The OSE is thought to be capable of metaplasia to a Müllerian phenotype resembling oviductal, endometrial, or endocervical epithelia, known as a secondary Müllerian system [3–5]. Thus, the OSE is suspected to carry pluripotent cells, i.e., putative stem cells. The recent identification of such stem cells implicates the OSE in the pathogenesis of EOTs [6, 7].

Other recent studies have indicated that a considerable number of EOTs originate in the fallopian tube and the endometrium, before migrating to the ovary. This theory, one of "imported disease", is thought to be an influential paradigm shift in the morphological theory of EOTs. According to this theory, serous tumors arise from the implantation of epithelium from the oviduct, and endometrioid and clear cell tumors are associated with endometriosis that mainly develops from retrograde menstruation [4].

Clinical, morphological, and molecular studies have provided a model for malignant EOTs, with two broad categories designated as Type I and Type II. Type I carcinomas progress in an indolent course, are usually confined to the ovary at diagnosis, and are relatively genetically stable. Type I carcinomas exhibit a shared lineage with their corresponding benign and borderline-malignant tumors, supporting the concept of a morphological sequence of tumor progression. In contrast, Type II carcinomas are highly aggressive, progress rapidly, and are usually in an advanced stage at diagnosis. Type II carcinomas do not exhibit the shared lineage and are genetically unstable [8].

In the first section of this chapter, these important theories of ovarian tumorigenesis and the two-tiered system of classification are introduced and organized. Finally, the morphological and molecular details of four representative malignant EOTs, namely, serous carcinoma (high grade, low grade), endometrioid carcinoma, clear cell carcinoma, and mucinous carcinoma, will be presented and discussed.

3.2 Representative Theories Related to the Morphological Pathogenesis of EOTs

3.2.1 The Theory of the Secondary Müllerian System

In the first half of the twentieth century, it was believed that the OSE, which was also referred to as the germinal epithelium, carried pluripotent stem cells which differentiate to germ cells and follicular cells [9, 10]. Even now, it is thought that the OSE is derived from a common embryonic origin in the pluripotent coelomic epithelium which gives rise to the Müllerian ducts, i.e., the epithelia of the fallopian tubes, endometrium, uterine cervix, and upper part of the vagina. According to this theory, a subset of pluripotent OSE cells and cells lining the inclusion cysts have the propensity to differentiate along the lineage of the Müllerian epithelium [11], with this therefore being referred to as a secondary Müllerian system [12–14]. For example, serous metaplasia of OSE inclusion cysts is characterized by a cuboidal epithelium with cilia,

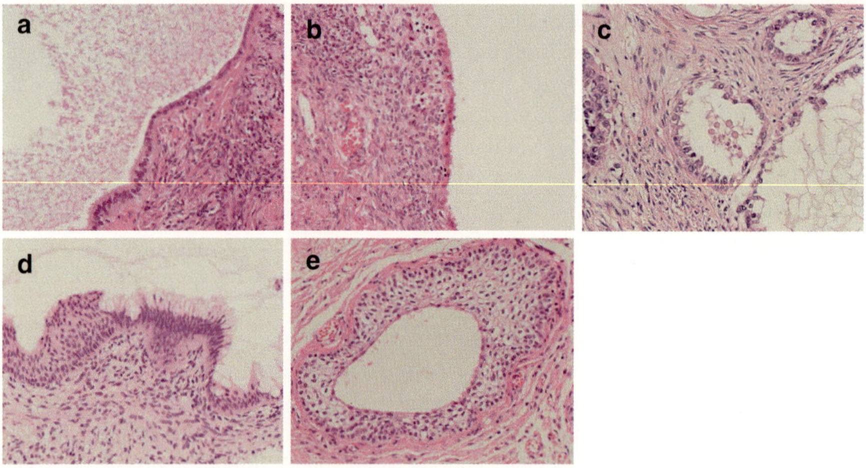

Fig. 3.2 Putative or possible sources of the major types of epithelial ovarian tumors. (**a**) inclusion cyst (cuboidal epithelium partially with cilia); (**b**) endometriosis; (**c**) adenofibroma (clear cell type); (**d**) teratoma (squamous cell and mucinous epithelia); (**e**) transitional cell (Walthard) nests [(**a–e**) hematoxylin and eosin staining; (**a–e**) ×200]

which mimics the endosalpingeal epithelium [15] (Fig. 3.2a). With this in mind, the morphological alteration of the OSE and its inclusion cysts has been suggested as a potential site of origin for the development of EOTs [5] (see also Sect. 5.3 in Chap. 5).

In regard to EOT tumorigenesis, the "incessant ovulation" hypothesis for ovarian cancer, which postulates that follicular rupture [16] and repair trauma increases OSE cell proliferation and risk of transformation, was proposed more than 40 years ago [17]. Besides primary endocrinological functions, gonadotropin hormones, such as follicle-stimulating hormone (FSH), luteinizing hormone (LH), and human chorionic gonadotropin (hCG), are thought to be involved in OSE cell proliferation and the repair of OSE following ovulatory trauma [18, 19]. Invagination and inclusion cysts form in the ovarian cortex as a result of the repair, and exposure of the entrapped cyst-lined OSE cells to foreign micro-substances within the cystic lumen, which come from the outside environment via the fallopian tube, causes their transformation [5]. In this process, stemlike cells undergo metaplasia and transformation to acquire a highly complex morphology resembling either the Müllerian duct-derived fallopian tube (serous type), the endometrium (endometrioid type), the endometrium with Arias-Stella reaction (clear cell type), or the endocervix (seromucinous or previously mucinous type) [20] (Fig. 3.1a–h).

Initially, the "incessant ovulation" hypothesis proposed for the stemlike cells of OSE was not widely accepted. The first scientific evidence for the existence of putative stem cells on the ovarian surface came in 2008, with a subset of stemlike cells experimentally identified by a stemness assay [6]. Subsequently, a subset of OSE cells expressing a common hematopoietic stem cell marker (Ly6a+) were identified in adult mouse ovaries [21], and more recent in vivo studies have used fate-mapping methodologies to provide direct evidence for the existence and location of self-renewing epithelial stem cells in the ovary [7, 22]. Stemlike OSE cells that display high aldehyde dehydrogenase (ALDH) activity [22] and high ALDH activity with expression of LGR5 (leucine-rich repeat-containing G protein-coupled receptor 5) [7] have been located in both the murine and human ovary hilum [20]. In view of such findings, it has been suggested that OSE stem cells might participate in post-ovulatory wound closure, as well as the tumorigenesis of EOTs [18, 23, 24].

3.2.2 The Theory of Imported Disease

Recent investigations have revealed that high-grade serous carcinomas are derived from the fimbriae of the fallopian tube. The theory of tubal involvement in the tumorigenesis of high-grade serous carcinoma proposes that serous tubal intraepithelial carcinomas (STICs) (Fig. 3.3a, b), which are known to occur in the fimbriae, are ectopically implanted into the ovarian stroma as cortical inclusion cysts, and that the exposure of these cells to the ovarian stromal microenvironment, which produces abundant growth factors designed for folliculogenesis, leads to "ovarian cancer" consisting of high-grade serous carcinoma [4, 8].

In endometrioid and clear cell carcinoma, it has been well recognized that malignant transformation can occur at epithelial components of endometriosis in endometriotic cysts of the ovary. A follow-up program for endometriotic cysts confirmed

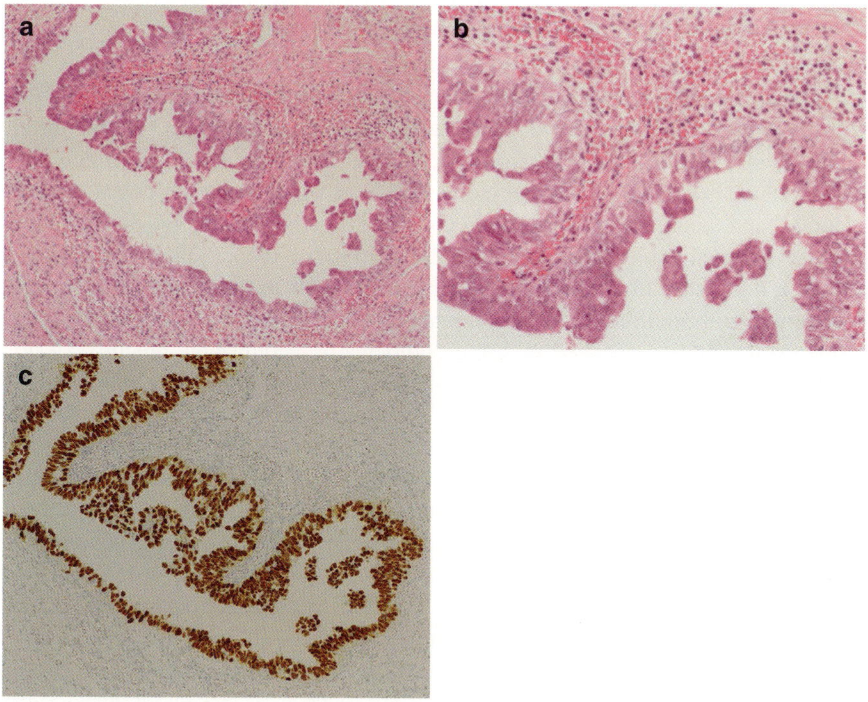

Fig. 3.3 Serous tubal intraepithelial carcinoma [(**a** and **b**) hematoxylin and eosin staining; (**c**) p53 immunostaining; (**a** and **c**) ×100; (**b**) ×200]

the risk of malignant transformation resulting from endometriosis [25]. Endometriosis is thought to occur via retrograde menstruation, where endometrial epithelial cells and stromal cells move from the uterus through the fallopian tubes and subsequently become established as an endometriotic cyst [26, 27]. It is also known that retrograde stromal cells from the endometrium can implant to the ovary during menstruation, inducing a metaplastic change in the OSE and resulting in endometriosis [28]. This creates a unique microenvironment where menstruation-like blood are trapped within the cyst, resulting in high concentrations of iron in a confined space, subsequent oxidative stress, and a hypoxic environment that promotes DNA damage and the accumulation of mutations [29–32].

Such studies suggest that the fallopian tube epithelium (benign or malignant) can implant onto the ovary to give rise to both low-grade and high-grade serous carcinomas and that similarly, endometrial tissue can implant onto the ovary with resulting endometriosis, then undergoing malignant transformation into endometrioid and clear cell carcinoma. According to the theory of "imported disease", these EOTs are not ovarian in origin therefore but rather represent "imported disease", and it is logical to conclude that the only true primary ovarian neoplasms are germ cell and gonadal stromal tumors, analogous to the situation in the testis which does not have epithelial tumors [4] (see also Sect. 5.3 in Chap. 5).

3.3 Two-Tiered Classification for Clinical, Morphological, and Molecular Pathogenesis

EOTs can be classified into Types I and II, which correspond to two distinct models of clinical, morphological, and molecular pathogenesis [33]. Type I tumors develop slowly, in a stepwise manner, from premalignant conditions or borderline tumors, and include low-grade serous carcinomas, endometrioid carcinomas, clear cell carcinomas, and mucinous carcinomas. In contrast, Type II tumors grow rapidly and are typically found to have spread beyond the ovaries at presentation. The predominate Type II tumors are high-grade serous carcinomas, with the remainder being carcinosarcomas and undifferentiated carcinomas. It was originally thought, since these tumors are rarely associated with morphologically recognizable precursor lesions, that they develop *de novo* from ovarian inclusion cysts or the surface epithelium [34, 35]. More recently, however, it has been recognized that Type II tumors with pelvic dissemination include carcinomas arising from the epithelium of the fimbriae.

Molecular studies have revealed that distinct biological signatures, compatible with the Type I and Type II classification system, exist among EOT subtypes. Although Type I carcinomas lack mutations in the *TP53* gene and have a stable genome, each morphological subtype exhibits a distinctive molecular profile. Moreover, Type I carcinomas typically exhibit a shared lineage with their corresponding benign and borderline-malignant tumors, supporting the concept of a morphological sequence of tumor progression. Type II carcinomas display *TP53* mutations in 80% or more of cases and rarely harbor the mutations that are found in Type I carcinomas. Type II carcinomas are typically associated with chromosome aneuploidy or chromosomal copy number abnormality resulting from an inherent chromosomal instability [8].

3.4 Morphological and Molecular Pathogenesis in Four Representative Malignant EOTs

3.4.1 Serous Carcinoma

3.4.1.1 High-Grade Serous Carcinoma

High-grade serous carcinoma is the most common type of malignant EOT and is classified as Type II. Morphologically, the tumor cells of high-grade serous carcinoma resemble the secretory cells of three distinct cell types from the fallopian tube epithelium, namely, secretary cells, ciliated cells, and peg cells [36–38]. Almost all of these tumors express the transcription factor PAX8 that is a marker of the secretory cell lineage in the fallopian tube epithelium. Until recently, all high-grade serous carcinomas were presumed to arise *de novo* in ovarian inclusion cysts or the OSE, although identification of putative precursors in these tissues had previously been difficult. Since the discovery of the tumor suppressor genes *BRCA1* [39] and *BRCA2* [40] (*BRCA1/2*) in 1994 and 1995, respectively, the use of mutation analysis in healthy women with a family history of hereditary breast and ovarian cancer (HBOC) syndrome has increased rates of prophylactic bilateral salpingo-oophorectomy. These surgical specimens have revealed that a subset of the fimbrial epithelium of the fallopian tube have lesions of occult carcinoma and STIC without any lesions in the ovary [41, 42]. It has also been reported that STIC of the fimbriae is concomitant with high-grade serous carcinoma of the ovary in sporadic but not only germline types and that STIC lesions have the same *TP53* mutations as the ovarian lesions. The *TP53* mutation findings indicate that there is clonal expansion between STIC and high-grade serous carcinoma of the ovary [43]. In fact, p53 immunopositivity by *TP53* mutation in STIC is occasionally found in cases with high-grade serous carcinoma (Fig. 3.3). Furthermore, it has been revealed that small foci of p53-immunoreactive cells exist in largely histologically normal fallopian tube epithelium [36]. These foci, which predominate in the distal portion of the fallopian tube, have been designated "p53 signatures". These p53 signatures probably represent early clonal expansion [44] and are found at the same frequency in women with or without *BRCA1/2* mutation [36]. *TP53* mutation is thus one of the earliest events in the genesis of high-grade serous carcinoma and may occur first in the discrete foci that lead to STIC in the distal fallopian tube. Extensive investigations have now examined the role of the fallopian tube in pathogenesis of the serous type of EOTs [36, 43, 45–47], yet it is clear that at least a subset of ovarian high-grade serous carcinomas do not have STIC involvement. Therefore, it is still considered that OSE may be a candidate as the site of origin for high-grade serous carcinoma without STIC. The exact proportion of tumors of ovarian and tubal derivation in cases of high-grade serous carcinoma could be revealed with the widespread implementation of an established pathology protocol for sectioning and examination of the fimbriae [46].

In high-grade serous carcinomas of the ovary including sporadic and hereditary types, *TP53* gene mutations are found in 95% or more of cases [48, 49]. Mutations in several other tumor suppressor genes and oncogenes, such as *NF1*, *RB1*, and *CDK12*, have been reported, but their mutation frequency is low [49–51]. As somatic mutations in *BRCA1/2* are known to be uncommon in sporadic serous tumors, it is possible that these genes are inactivated by mechanisms (loss of heterozygosity and/or methylation) other than mutation [52–54]. The proposed model is that loss of p53 and BRCA1/2 are early events that lead to a deficiency in homologous recombination repair of DNA double-strand breaks, triggering chromosomal instability and widespread copy number changes [34, 44, 49, 55–61]. The most common amplifications affect the genes *MYC*, *CCNE*, and *MECOM*, each of which is highly amplified in more than 20% of high-grade serous carcinomas [49], but it is the *MYC* gene that is the most often amplified and overexpressed [62]. In regard to other cancer-associated pathways harboring mutations, copy number changes, or changes in gene expression, the RB and phosphoinositide 3-kinase (PI3K)/RAS pathways are deregulated in 67% and 45% of high-grade serous carcinomas, respectively [49]. Various experimental models using OSE cells or tubal epithelial cells have supported the concept that molecular pathways based on *TP53* mutation play an important role for the carcinogenesis of high-grade serous carcinomas or Type II tumors [23, 63, 64] (Fig. 3.4a) (see also Sect. 7.2.2 in Chap. 7).

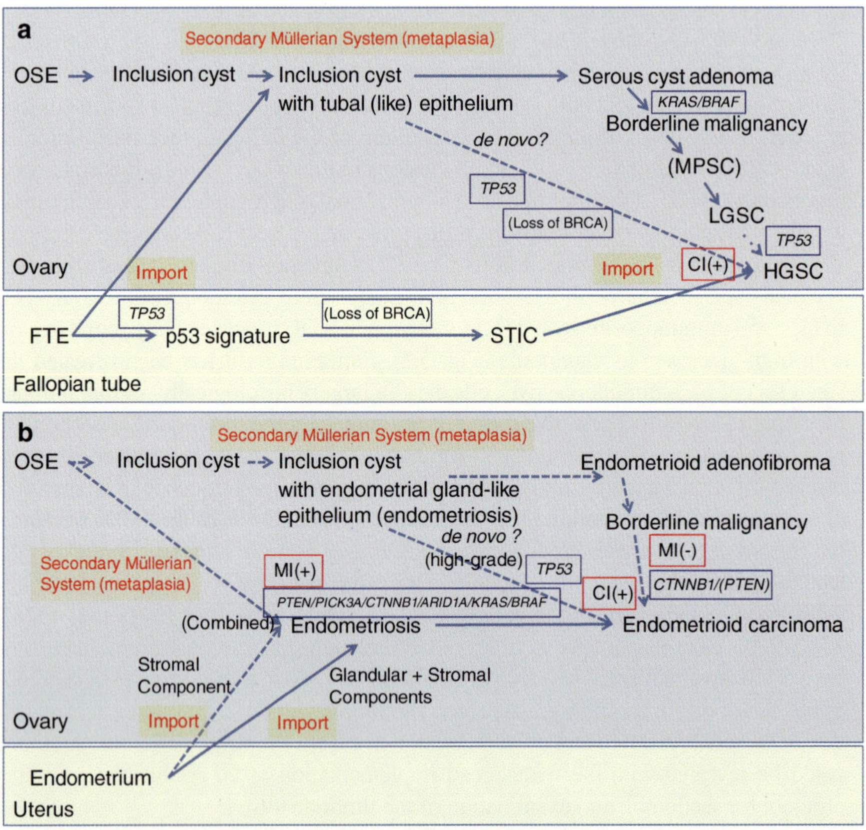

Fig. 3.4 Schematic diagram of morphological and molecular pathogenesis for ovarian carcinogenesis (**a**) serous tumors; (**b**) endometrioid tumors; (**c**) clear cell tumors; (**d**) mucinous tumors. *Solid lines*, major pathways; broken lines, minor or putative pathways; *blue frames*, gene mutations; *red frames*, genomic status. OSE, ovarian surface epithelium; FTE, fallopian tubal epithelium; STIC, serous tubal intraepithelial carcinomas; CI, chromosomal instability; MI, microsatellite instability; +, positive; –, negative

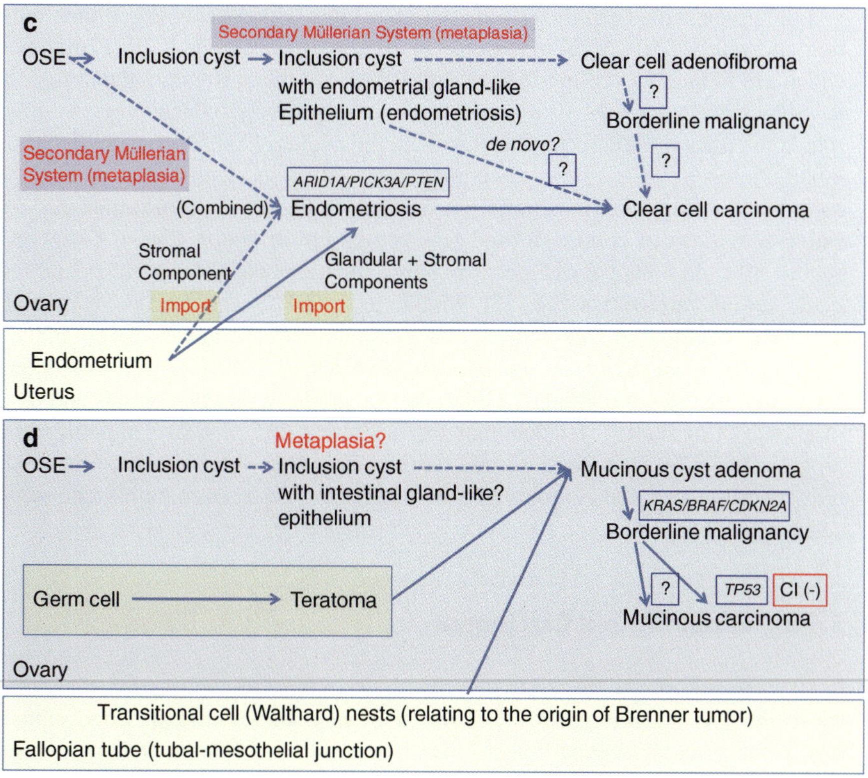

Fig. 3.4 (continued)

3.4.1.2 Low-Grade Serous Carcinoma

Low-grade serous carcinoma is much less common than high-grade carcinoma and is classified as a Type I tumor. These carcinomas frequently have a component of serous borderline tumor (SBT) or micropapillary serous carcinoma [65] and are thought to evolve in a stepwise fashion from benign serous cystadenoma through to SBT and finally to carcinoma. Morphologically, low-grade serous carcinomas also resemble tubal secretary cells and show small papillae of tumor cells exhibiting uniform nuclei within variable amounts of hyalinized stroma, which often contains psammoma bodies [66]. Low-grade serous carcinomas, like high-grade serous carcinomas, typically express the transcription factors PAX8 [67–69].

Low-grade serous carcinomas arise via the transformation of benign and SBTs, thought to be derived either from inclusion cysts originating from the OSE or from tubal epithelium that is shed and implanted onto the ovary and gives rise to inclusion cysts and subsequent serous neoplasms (Fig. 3.2a). An immunohistochemical study has shown that 80% of ovarian cortical inclusions express PAX8, a Müllerian marker, but not calretinin, a mesothelial marker, findings that support the concept of a tubal phenotype [70]. Recently, it has also been suggested that papillary tubal hyperplasia may be a putative precursor lesion for SBTs [71, 72].

Low-grade serous carcinomas are not associated with *BRCA1/2* germline mutation and rarely have *TP53* mutations, in contrast to *KRAS* and *BRAF* mutations which are frequently present. KRAS and BRAF are the upstream regulators in the RAS/RAF/MEK/ERK/MAP signal transduction pathway, which plays a critical role in the transmission of growth signals to the nucleus [73]. Oncogenic mutations in *BRAF* and *KRAS* result in the constitutive activation of this pathway and thus contribute to neoplastic transformation. Several studies have demonstrated that activating mutations in codon 12 (and less commonly in codon 13) of *KRAS* or in codons 599 and 600 of *BRAF* occur in approximately two thirds of SBTs and low-grade serous carcinomas [74, 75]. Mutations in *KRAS* and *BRAF* are mutually exclusive, such that tumors with mutant *KRAS* do not have mutant *BRAF* and vice versa. It has been suggested that mutations of *KRAS* and *BRAF* are early events associated with the initiation of SBTs and low-grade serous carcinomas and that a small subset of serous cystadenomas that acquire *KRAS* or *BRAF* mutations may progress to SBTs. Low-grade serous carcinomas do not show chromosomal instability and thus lack the complex genomic abnormalities seen in high-grade serous carcinomas (Fig. 3.4a) (see also Sect. 7.6 in Chap. 7).

3.4.2 Endometrioid Carcinoma

In 1927, Sampson was the first to describe the malignant transformation of endometriosis to ovarian carcinoma [76]. Thereafter, many studies have provided supporting evidence that malignant transformation can occur in ovarian endometriosis or the endometriotic cyst [77, 78] (Fig. 3.2b). The observation of a morphological transition from endometriosis to carcinoma in over one third of endometrioid carcinomas has led to endometriosis being considered its likely cause. It has thus been accepted that atypical endometriosis at the transition site is the precursor lesion for endometrioid carcinoma associated with endometriosis, and common genetic alterations have been documented in adjacent endometriosis, atypical endometriosis, and carcinoma [79]. Besides endometriosis, the coexistence of benign endometrioid neoplasms, such as adenofibromas or borderline tumors, with endometrioid carcinomas has been also recognized [80].

Endometriosis is thought to occur via retrograde menstruation, whereby epithelial and stromal cells of the endometrium are carried from the uterus through the fallopian tubes and can establish as an endometriotic cyst within the ovary [81]. Recent investigations suggest that the endometriotic cyst, in which chocolate-like blood is trapped for long time, maintains high concentrations of iron in the cystic fluid and that the iron-rich environment causes oxidative stress and hypoxia leading to DNA damage and accumulation of mutations [30, 32].

Like endometrial cancers, ovarian endometrioid carcinoma is commonly encountered in patients with Lynch syndrome. Microsatellite instability has been also observed in 13–20% of endometrioid carcinomas. Mutations in the *PTEN* tumor suppressor gene, resulting in the activation of PI3K signaling and inhibition of apoptosis, have been reported in a fifth or less of endometrioid carcinomas and are rare in other types of malignant EOT [82, 83]. Mutations in *PIK3CA*, which encodes the p110 catalytic subunit of PI3K, have also been identified in a fifth of endometrioid carcinomas and similarly result in activation of PI3K signaling [84, 85]. *PTEN* and *PIK3CA* mutations co-occur in a subset of endometrioid carcinomas [86, 87]. The Wnt/β-catenin signaling pathway is involved in the regulation of several important cellular processes, including cell fate determination, proliferation, motility, and survival. Mutations in *CTNNB1*, which encodes β-catenin, are typically found in endometrioid carcinomas but are uncommon in the other types of ovarian carcinoma [88], and several studies have noted the association of *CTNNB1* mutation with squamous differentiation.

The tumor suppressor gene *ARID1A*, which encodes BAF250a, plays a crucial role in chromatin remodeling as a member of the SWI/SNF chromatin remodeling complex. *ARID1A* mutation induces changes in the expression of multiple genes (*CDKN1A*, *SMAD3*, *MLH1*, and *PIK3IP1*) as the result of chromatin remodeling dysfunction and has been shown to contribute to molecular pathogenesis and cellular transformation in cooperation with the PI3K pathway [82, 83, 86, 89–92]. *KRAS* and *BRAF* mutations have been identified in endometrioid carcinomas, but the frequency of these mutations is rather low, being 7% or less [92–96]. The fact that *PTEN*, *KRAS*, and *ARID1A* mutations are also found in the epithelial components of endometriosis adjacent to endometrioid carcinomas provides additional evidence for the precursor role of endometriosis in the molecular pathogenesis of ovarian endometrioid carcinomas [29, 97, 98]. In regard to *TP53*, mutations have been reported in poorly differentiated or high-grade endometrioid carcinomas. *TP53* mutations are uncommon in tumors with Wnt/β-catenin and/or PI3K/PTEN signaling defects [96].

Using genetically engineered mice, experimental models of endometrioid tumor have now been developed. In one approach, simultaneous activation of *KRAS* and inactivation of *PTEN* in the OSE resulted in the development of ovarian tumors resembling human endometrioid carcinomas associated with endometriosis [99]. In another approach, conditional bi-allelic inactivation of *APC* and *PTEN* in the OSE promoted ovarian endometrioid tumors harboring Wnt and PI3K pathway defects comparable to human endometrioid carcinomas [92]. Furthermore, conditional inactivation of one or both *ARID1A* alleles in the OSE concurrently with *APC* and *PTEN* inactivation in these mice induced endometrioid tumors with morphological features similar to those of human endometrioid carcinoma [100] (Fig. 3.4b) (see also Sect. 7.4.1 in Chap. 7).

3.4.3 Clear Cell Carcinoma

The morphological characteristics of clear cell carcinoma are multiple complex papillae, densely hyaline basement membrane material expanding the cores of these papillae, and hyaline bodies. Mitotic figures are less frequent than in other types of ovarian carcinoma. As is the case for endometrioid carcinoma, there is a close association between endometriosis and clear cell carcinoma [101, 102]. The coexistence of adenofibromas or borderline tumors, with clear cell carcinomas, has been also recognized, being distinct from those arising from endometriosis [103, 104] (Fig. 3.2c).

Hepatocyte nuclear factor-1β (HNF-1β) is upregulated in clear cell tumors, including benign tumors, borderline tumors, and carcinomas [105], and thus most clear cell carcinomas are positive for HNF1-β [106, 107]. This transcription factor is expressed in the mid-to-late secretory and gestational endometrium with Arias-Stella reaction, atypical and inflammatory endometriosis, and clear cell carcinoma [105]. HNF-1β regulates several genes such as dipeptidyl peptidase IV (involved in the control of glycogen synthesis [108]), glutathione peroxidase 3, and annexin A4 [109]. The fact that HNF-1β is important in controlling multiple genes involved in glucose and glycogen metabolism suggests that upregulation of this factor may be responsible for the characteristic morphological feature of clear cell carcinoma, namely, a glycogen-rich cytoplasm with clear appearance [108, 110].

Mutations involving PI3K/PTEN signaling are common in clear cell carcinomas, with *PIK3CA* mutations reported in 20–25% of tumors and *PTEN* mutations in 8% of tumors [84, 86, 98]. Recently, it has been found that nearly half of clear cell carcinomas carry *ARID1A* mutations and lack BAF250 protein [97]. The occurrence of somatic mutations of *PTEN* and *ARID1A* in a subset of ovarian endometriotic cysts, within both tumor tissue and adjacent endometriosis, but not in distant endometriosis sites, suggests shared molecular alterations between clear cell and endometrioid carcinomas of the ovary and their putative precursor lesion [98]. This finding also suggests that *PTEN* and *ARID1A* inactivation occurs early during the malignant transformation of endometriosis [97].

Clear cell carcinomas do not appear to share other genetic changes with endometrioid carcinomas. Wnt signaling pathway defects and microsatellite instability, for example, have not been observed with significant frequency in these tumors [86, 111, 112] (Fig. 3.4c) (see also Sects. 7.3.3 and 7.3.4 in Chap. 7).

3.4.4 Mucinous Carcinoma

Although mucinous tumors account for 10–15% of EOTs, almost all are benign, with the remainder being of borderline malignancy. The tumors usually show cystic and multilocular features; those that are large and unilateral are likely to be primary lesions, while metastatic tumors are typically smaller and bilateral. Primary ovarian mucinous carcinomas are usually confined to the ovary however, and if external metastases to the ovary, particularly from the gastrointestinal tract, are carefully excluded, only 3–4% of ovarian carcinomas are typically found to be of the mucinous type. The cells of mucinous tumors may resemble those of the gastric pylorus, intestine, or endocervix (Fig. 3.1g–j). Recently, mucinous tumors with cells resembling those of the endocervical epithelium have been classified as separate category of seromucinous tumor that is associated with endometriosis or low-grade serous carcinoma [113]. The origin of mucinous tumors, which includes inclusion cyst or OSE, is not well characterized, but the association of some mucinous tumors with teratoma indicates that some may be of germ cell origin [114] (Fig. 3.2d). More recent data suggest that transitional cell (Walthard) nests, which relate to Brenner tumors, present at the tubal-mesothelial junction may also be a possible origin for these tumors [72, 115] (Fig. 3.2e) (see also Sect. 5.3 in Chap. 5 and Sect. 7.5.1 in Chap. 7). Mucinous carcinomas are often heterogeneous. Benign, borderline, noninvasive, and invasive features may all coexist within an individual tumor, suggesting that tumor progression proceeds from benign to borderline and from borderline to carcinoma [116].

KRAS mutations are frequent in mucinous carcinomas and are considered to be an early tumorigenic event [117]. Ovarian mucinous tumors are generally immunoreactive for cytokeratin 7 (CK7), whereas metastatic tumors from colorectal adenocarcinoma sites are usually CK7 negative but positive for CK20 [118]. Mucinous tumors express several mucin genes (*MUC2*, *MUC3*, and *MUC17*) irrespective of their tissue origins, as well as additional genes that are markers of intestinal differentiation, such as the caudal-type homeobox transcription factors *CDX1* and *CDX2* and *LGALS4*. LGALS4 is an intestinal cell surface adhesion molecule overexpressed in a spectrum of mucinous tumors, including intestinal carcinomas, but is not detectable in normal OSE. It is overexpressed in all ovarian mucinous tumors, however, including benign, borderline, and malignant tumors, indicating that LGALS4 overexpression is associated with a very early step in the molecular pathogenesis of this cancer type [119].

KRAS, *BRAF*, and *CDKN2A* (which encodes p16/INK4a) are often mutated in mucinous tumors, with the RAS/RAF pathway and p16/INK4a thought to be important contributors to molecular pathogenesis [120–122]. A recent study has suggested that a high percentage of mucinous carcinomas may have a *TP53* mutation (50–70%). While there is a similar, but lower (10–20%), frequency of *TP53* mutation in benign and borderline tumors, the high prevalence of *TP53* mutation in mucinous carcinomas suggests that aberrant p53 contributes to the invasive phenotype as a late event in the tumorigenic process [120, 123]. Interestingly, mucinous carcinomas do not share the widespread genomic instability seen in high-grade serous carcinomas that carry *TP53* mutations, suggesting that the effect of p53 mutation is distinct in these two kinds of malignant EOTs [120] (Fig. 3.4d) (see also Sect. 7.5.2 in Chap. 7).

Conclusion

Historically, the early morphological and molecular alterations in ovarian tumorigenesis have been a black box. While it is relatively easy to biopsy early lesions in cervical and endometrial carcinomas, this is difficult in ovarian carcinomas because of the location within the pelvic cavity. Since the introduction in 1995 of prophylactic salpingo-oophorectomy for carriers of *BRCA1/2* mutations, early lesions of high-grade serous carcinomas in HBOC have become readily identifiable. However, the identification of extra-ovarian STIC as a precursor lesion in such cases has led to a paradigm shift from the theory of the secondary Müllerian system of OSE to one of "imported disease". Despite this, many secrets of the black box remain, including the cellular origins of especially high-grade serous carcinoma without STIC, low-grade serous carcinoma, and mucinous carcinoma and the biological basis for the observed morphological diversity in these diseases. Further molecular studies are required to answer these remaining questions in regard to the pathogenesis of EOTs.

References

1. Banet N, Kurman RJ. Two types of ovarian cortical inclusion cysts: proposed origin and possible role in ovarian serous carcinogenesis. Int J Gynecol Pathol. 2015;34:3–8.
2. Auersperg N. Article by Natalie Banet and Robert J. Kurman: Two types of ovarian cortical inclusion cysts: proposed origin and possible role in ovarian serous carcinogenesis; Int. J. Gynecol. Pathol. 2015;34:3-8. Int J Gynecol Pathol. 2015;34:303-4.
3. Auersperg N. Ovarian surface epithelium as a source of ovarian cancers: unwarranted speculation or evidence-based hypothesis? Gynecol Oncol. 2013;130:246–51.
4. Kuhn E, Kurman RJ, Shih IM. Ovarian cancer is an imported disease: fact or fiction? Curr Obstet Gynecol Rep. 2012;1:1–9.
5. Okamura H, Katabuchi H. Pathophysiological dynamics of human ovarian surface epithelial cells in epithelial ovarian carcinogenesis. Int Rev Cytol. 2005;242:1–54.
6. Szotek PP, Chang HL, Brennand K, Fujino A, Pieretti-Vanmarcke R, Lo Celso C, et al. Normal ovarian surface epithelial label-retaining cells exhibit stem/progenitor cell characteristics. Proc Natl Acad Sci U S A. 2008;105:12469–73.
7. Ng A, Tan S, Singh G, Rizk P, Swathi Y, Tan TZ, et al. Lgr5 marks stem/progenitor cells in ovary and tubal epithelia. Nat Cell Biol. 2014;16:745–57.
8. Kurman RJ, Shih IM. The origin and pathogenesis of epithelial ovarian cancer: a proposed unifying theory. Am J Surg Pathol. 2010;34:433–43.
9. Dubeau L. The cell of origin of ovarian epithelial tumours. Lancet Oncol. 2008;9:1191–7.
10. Allen BM. The embrionic development of the ovary and testes of the mammals. Am J Anat. 1904;3:89–153.
11. Auersperg N, Wong AS, Choi KC, Kang SK, Leung PC. Ovarian surface epithelium: biology, endocrinology, and pathology. Endocr Rev. 2001;22:255–88.
12. Lauchlan SC. The secondary Mullerian system. Obstet Gynecol Surv. 1972;27:133–46.
13. Okamura H, Katabuchi H. Detailed morphology of human ovarian surface epithelium focusing on its metaplastic and neoplastic capability. Ital J Anat Embryol. 2001;106:263–76.
14. Okamura H, Katabuchi H, Ohba T. What we have learned from isolated cells from human ovary? Mol Cell Endocrinol. 2003;202:37–45.
15. Katabuchi H, Okamura H. Cell biology of human ovarian surface epithelial cells and ovarian carcinogenesis. Med Electron Microsc. 2003;36:74–86.
16. Okamura H, Katabuchi H, Nagai R. Ultrastructure of human ovulation: histofunctional parameters. In: Motta PM, editor. Microscopy of reproduction and development: a dynamic approach. Rome: Antonio Delfino Editore; 1997. p. 155–61.
17. Fathalla MF. Incessant ovulation--a factor in ovarian neoplasia? Lancet. 1971;2:163.
18. Tashiro H, Katabuchi H, Begum M, Li X, Nitta M, Ohtake H, et al. Roles of luteinizing hormone/chorionic gonadotropin receptor in anchorage-dependent and -independent growth in human ovarian surface epithelial cell lines. Cancer Sci. 2003;94:953–9.
19. Ji Q, Liu PI, Chen PK, Aoyama C. Follicle stimulating hormone-induced growth promotion and gene expression profiles on ovarian surface epithelial cells. Int J Cancer. 2004;112:803–14.
20. Ng A, Barker N. Ovary and fimbrial stem cells: biology, niche and cancer origins. Nat Rev Mol Cell Biol. 2015;16:625–38.
21. Gamwell LF, Collins O, Vanderhyden BC. The mouse ovarian surface epithelium contains a population of LY6A (SCA-1) expressing progenitor cells that are regulated by ovulation-associated factors. Biol Reprod. 2012;87:80.

22. Flesken-Nikitin A, Hwang CI, Cheng CY, Michurina TV, Enikolopov G, Nikitin AY. Ovarian surface epithelium at the junction area contains a cancer-prone stem cell niche. Nature. 2013;495:241–5.
23. Motohara T, Masuko S, Ishimoto T, Yae T, Onishi N, Muraguchi T, et al. Transient depletion of p53 followed by transduction of c-Myc and K-Ras converts ovarian stem-like cells into tumor-initiating cells. Carcinogenesis. 2011;32:1597–606.
24. Bhartiya D, Singh J. FSH-FSHR3-stem cells in ovary surface epithelium: basis for adult ovarian biology, failure, aging, and cancer. Reproduction. 2015;149:R35–48.
25. Kobayashi H, Sumimoto K, Moniwa N, Imai M, Takakura K, Kuromaki T, et al. Risk of developing ovarian cancer among women with ovarian endometrioma: a cohort study in Shizuoka, Japan. Int J Gynecol Cancer. 2007;17:37–43.
26. Giudice LC. Clinical practice. Endometriosis. N Engl J Med. 2010;362:2389–98.
27. Giudice LC, Kao LC. Endometriosis. Lancet. 2004;364:1789–99.
28. Ohtake H, Katabuchi H, Matsuura K, Okamura H. A novel in vitro experimental model for ovarian endometriosis: the three-dimensional culture of human ovarian surface epithelial cells in collagen gels. Fertil Steril. 1999;71:50–5.
29. McConechy MK, Ding J, Senz J, Yang W, Melnyk N, Tone AA, et al. Ovarian and endometrial endometrioid carcinomas have distinct CTNNB1 and PTEN mutation profiles. Mod Pathol. 2014;27:128–34.
30. Yamaguchi K, Mandai M, Toyokuni S, Hamanishi J, Higuchi T, Takakura K, et al. Contents of endometriotic cysts, especially the high concentration of free iron, are a possible cause of carcinogenesis in the cysts through the iron-induced persistent oxidative stress. Clin Cancer Res. 2008;14:32–40.
31. Van Langendonckt A, Casanas-Roux F, Dolmans MM, Donnez J. Potential involvement of hemoglobin and heme in the pathogenesis of peritoneal endometriosis. Fertil Steril. 2002;77:561–70.
32. Kobayashi H, Kajiwara H, Kanayama S, Yamada Y, Furukawa N, Noguchi T, et al. Molecular pathogenesis of endometriosis-associated clear cell carcinoma of the ovary (review). Oncol Rep. 2009;22:233–40.
33. Kurman RJ, Shih IM. Pathogenesis of ovarian cancer: lessons from morphology and molecular biology and their clinical implications. Int J Gynecol Pathol. 2008;27:151–60.
34. Cho KR, Shih IM. Ovarian cancer. Annu Rev Pathol. 2009;4:287–313.
35. Eddy JA, Hood L, Price ND, Geman D. Identifying tightly regulated and variably expressed networks by differential rank conservation (DIRAC). PLoS Comput Biol. 2010;6:e1000792.
36. Lee Y, Miron A, Drapkin R, Nucci MR, Medeiros F, Saleemuddin A, et al. A candidate precursor to serous carcinoma that originates in the distal fallopian tube. J Pathol. 2007;211:26–35.
37. Jarboe E, Folkins A, Nucci MR, Kindelberger D, Drapkin R, Miron A, et al. Serous carcinogenesis in the fallopian tube: a descriptive classification. Int J Gynecol Pathol. 2008;27:1–9.
38. Paik DY, Janzen DM, Schafenacker AM, Velasco VS, Shung MS, Cheng D, et al. Stem-like epithelial cells are concentrated in the distal end of the fallopian tube: a site for injury and serous cancer initiation. Stem Cells. 2012;30:2487–97.
39. Miki Y, Swensen J, Shattuck-Eidens D, Futreal PA, Harshman K, Tavtigian S, et al. A strong candidate for the breast and ovarian cancer susceptibility gene BRCA1. Science. 1994;266:66–71.
40. Wooster R, Bignell G, Lancaster J, Swift S, Seal S, Mangion J, et al. Identification of the breast cancer susceptibility gene BRCA2. Nature. 1995;378:789–92.
41. Paley PJ, Swisher EM, Garcia RL, Agoff SN, Greer BE, Peters KL, et al. Occult cancer of the fallopian tube in BRCA-1 germline mutation carriers at prophylactic oophorectomy: a case for recommending hysterectomy at surgical prophylaxis. Gynecol Oncol. 2001;80:176–80.
42. Carcangiu ML, Peissel B, Pasini B, Spatti G, Radice P, Manoukian S. Incidental carcinomas in prophylactic specimens in BRCA1 and BRCA2 germ-line mutation carriers, with emphasis on fallopian tube lesions: report of 6 cases and review of the literature. Am J Surg Pathol. 2006;30:1222–30.

43. Kindelberger DW, Lee Y, Miron A, Hirsch MS, Feltmate C, Medeiros F, et al. Intraepithelial carcinoma of the fimbria and pelvic serous carcinoma: evidence for a causal relationship. Am J Surg Pathol. 2007;31:161–9.
44. Bowtell DD. The genesis and evolution of high-grade serous ovarian cancer. Nat Rev Cancer. 2010;10:803–8.
45. Piek JM, van Diest PJ, Zweemer RP, Jansen JW, Poort-Keesom RJ, Menko FH, et al. Dysplastic changes in prophylactically removed fallopian tubes of women predisposed to developing ovarian cancer. J Pathol. 2001;195:451–6.
46. Medeiros F, Muto MG, Lee Y, Elvin JA, Callahan MJ, Feltmate C, et al. The tubal fimbria is a preferred site for early adenocarcinoma in women with familial ovarian cancer syndrome. Am J Surg Pathol. 2006;30:230–6.
47. Folkins AK, Jarboe EA, Saleemuddin A, Lee Y, Callahan MJ, Drapkin R, et al. A candidate precursor to pelvic serous cancer (p53 signature) and its prevalence in ovaries and fallopian tubes from women with BRCA mutations. Gynecol Oncol. 2008;109:168–73.
48. Salani R, Kurman RJ, Giuntoli R 2nd, Gardner G, Bristow R, Wang TL, et al. Assessment of TP53 mutation using purified tissue samples of ovarian serous carcinomas reveals a higher mutation rate than previously reported and does not correlate with drug resistance. Int J Gynecol Cancer. 2008;18:487–91.
49. Network CGAR. Integrated genomic analyses of ovarian carcinoma. Nature. 2011;474:609–15.
50. Merajver SD, Pham TM, Caduff RF, Chen M, Poy EL, Cooney KA, et al. Somatic mutations in the BRCA1 gene in sporadic ovarian tumours. Nat Genet. 1995;9:439–43.
51. Sangha N, Wu R, Kuick R, Powers S, Mu D, Fiander D, et al. Neurofibromin 1 (NF1) defects are common in human ovarian serous carcinomas and co-occur with TP53 mutations. Neoplasia. 2008;10:1362–72.
52. Cannistra SA. BRCA-1 in sporadic epithelial ovarian cancer: lessons learned from the genetics of hereditary disease. Clin Cancer Res. 2007;13:7225–7.
53. Wang C, Horiuchi A, Imai T, Ohira S, Itoh K, Nikaido T, et al. Expression of BRCA1 protein in benign, borderline, and malignant epithelial ovarian neoplasms and its relationship to methylation and allelic loss of the BRCA1 gene. J Pathol. 2004;202:215–23.
54. Baldwin RL, Nemeth E, Tran H, Shvartsman H, Cass I, Narod S, et al. BRCA1 promoter region hypermethylation in ovarian carcinoma: a population-based study. Cancer Res. 2000;60:5329–33.
55. Venkitaraman AR. Linking the cellular functions of BRCA genes to cancer pathogenesis and treatment. Annu Rev Pathol. 2009;4:461–87.
56. Pothuri B, Leitao MM, Levine DA, Viale A, Olshen AB, Arroyo C, et al. Genetic analysis of the early natural history of epithelial ovarian carcinoma. PLoS One. 2010;5:e10358.
57. Norquist BM, Garcia RL, Allison KH, Jokinen CH, Kernochan LE, Pizzi CC, et al. The molecular pathogenesis of hereditary ovarian carcinoma: alterations in the tubal epithelium of women with BRCA1 and BRCA2 mutations. Cancer. 2010;116:5261–71.
58. Schraml P, Schwerdtfeger G, Burkhalter F, Raggi A, Schmidt D, Ruffalo T, et al. Combined array comparative genomic hybridization and tissue microarray analysis suggest PAK1 at 11q13.5-q14 as a critical oncogene target in ovarian carcinoma. Am J Pathol. 2003;163:985–92.
59. Meinhold-Heerlein I, Bauerschlag D, Hilpert F, Dimitrov P, Sapinoso LM, Orlowska-Volk M, et al. Molecular and prognostic distinction between serous ovarian carcinomas of varying grade and malignant potential. Oncogene. 2005;24:1053–65.
60. Mayr D, Kanitz V, Anderegg B, Luthardt B, Engel J, Lohrs U, et al. Analysis of gene amplification and prognostic markers in ovarian cancer using comparative genomic hybridization for microarrays and immunohistochemical analysis for tissue microarrays. Am J Clin Pathol. 2006;126:101–9.
61. Nowee ME, Snijders AM, Rockx DA, de Wit RM, Kosma VM, Hamalainen K, et al. DNA profiling of primary serous ovarian and fallopian tube carcinomas with array comparative genomic hybridization and multiplex ligation-dependent probe amplification. J Pathol. 2007;213:46–55.

62. Tashiro H, Miyazaki K, Okamura H, Iwai A, Fukumoto M. C-myc over-expression in human primary ovarian tumours: its relevance to tumour progression. Int J Cancer. 1992;50:828–33.
63. Sasaki R, Narisawa-Saito M, Yugawa T, Fujita M, Tashiro H, Katabuchi H, et al. Oncogenic transformation of human ovarian surface epithelial cells with defined cellular oncogenes. Carcinogenesis. 2009;30:423–31.
64. Jazaeri AA, Bryant JL, Park H, Li H, Dahiya N, Stoler MH, et al. Molecular requirements for transformation of fallopian tube epithelial cells into serous carcinoma. Neoplasia. 2011;13:899–911.
65. Katabuchi H, Tashiro H, Cho KR, Kurman RJ, Hedrick EL. Micropapillary serous carcinoma of the ovary: an immunohistochemical and mutational analysis of p53. Int J Gynecol Pathol. 1998;17:54–60.
66. Motohara T, Tashiro H, Miyahara Y, Sakaguchi I, Ohtake H, Katabuchi H. Long-term oncological outcomes of ovarian serous carcinomas with psammoma bodies: a novel insight into the molecular pathogenesis of ovarian epithelial carcinoma. Cancer Sci. 2010;101:1550–6.
67. O'Neill CJ, Deavers MT, Malpica A, Foster H, McCluggage WG. An immunohistochemical comparison between low-grade and high-grade ovarian serous carcinomas: significantly higher expression of p53, MIB1, BCL2, HER-2/neu, and C-KIT in high-grade neoplasms. Am J Surg Pathol. 2005;29:1034–41.
68. Shimizu M, Toki T, Takagi Y, Konishi I, Fujii S. Immunohistochemical detection of the Wilms' tumor gene (WT1) in epithelial ovarian tumors. Int J Gynecol Pathol. 2000;19:158–63.
69. Liliac L, Carcangiu ML, Canevari S, Caruntu ID, Ciobanu Apostol DG, Danciu M, et al. The value of PAX8 and WT1 molecules in ovarian cancer diagnosis. Romanian J Morphol Embryol. 2013;54:17–27.
70. Li J, Abushahin N, Pang S, Xiang L, Chambers SK, Fadare O, et al. Tubal origin of 'ovarian' low-grade serous carcinoma. Mod Pathol. 2011;24:1488–99.
71. Kurman RJ, Vang R, Junge J, Hannibal CG, Kjaer SK, Shih IM. Papillary tubal hyperplasia: the putative precursor of ovarian atypical proliferative (borderline) serous tumors, noninvasive implants, and endosalpingiosis. Am J Surg Pathol. 2011;35:1605–14.
72. Lim D, Oliva E. Precursors and pathogenesis of ovarian carcinoma. Pathology. 2013;45:229–42.
73. Peyssonnaux C, Eychene A. The Raf/MEK/ERK pathway: new concepts of activation. Biol Cell. 2001;93:53–62.
74. Singer G, Oldt R 3rd, Cohen Y, Wang BG, Sidransky D, Kurman RJ, et al. Mutations in BRAF and KRAS characterize the development of low-grade ovarian serous carcinoma. J Natl Cancer Inst. 2003;95:484–6.
75. Jones S, Wang TL, Kurman RJ, Nakayama K, Velculescu VE, Vogelstein B, et al. Low-grade serous carcinomas of the ovary contain very few point mutations. J Pathol. 2012;226:413–20.
76. Sampson JA. Metastatic or embolic endometriosis, due to the menstrual dissemination of endometrial tissue into the venous circulation. Am J Pathol. 1927;3:93–110.43.
77. Scully RE, Richardson GS, Barlow JF. The development of malignancy in endometriosis. Clin Obstet Gynecol. 1966;9:384–411.
78. Sainz de la Cuesta R, Eichhorn JH, Rice LW, Fuller AF Jr, Nikrui N, Goff BA. Histologic transformation of benign endometriosis to early epithelial ovarian cancer. Gynecol Oncol. 1996;60:238–44.
79. Jiang X, Morland SJ, Hitchcock A, Thomas EJ, Campbell IG. Allelotyping of endometriosis with adjacent ovarian carcinoma reveals evidence of a common lineage. Cancer Res. 1998;58:1707–12.
80. Bell KA, Kurman RJ. A clinicopathologic analysis of atypical proliferative (borderline) tumors and well-differentiated endometrioid adenocarcinomas of the ovary. Am J Surg Pathol. 2000;24:1465–79.
81. Fukunaga M, Nomura K, Ishikawa E, Ushigome S. Ovarian atypical endometriosis: its close association with malignant epithelial tumours. Histopathology. 1997;30:249–55.
82. Obata K, Morland SJ, Watson RH, Hitchcock A, Chenevix-Trench G, Thomas EJ, et al. Frequent PTEN/MMAC mutations in endometrioid but not serous or mucinous epithelial ovarian tumors. Cancer Res. 1998;58:2095–7.
83. Catasus L, Bussaglia E, Rodrguez I, Gallardo A, Pons C, Irving JA, et al. Molecular genetic alterations in endometrioid carcinomas of the ovary: similar frequency of beta-catenin

abnormalities but lower rate of microsatellite instability and PTEN alterations than in uterine endometrioid carcinomas. Hum Pathol. 2004;35:1360–8.
84. Campbell IG, Russell SE, Choong DY, Montgomery KG, Ciavarella ML, Hooi CS, et al. Mutation of the PIK3CA gene in ovarian and breast cancer. Cancer Res. 2004;64:7678–81.
85. Nakayama K, Nakayama N, Kurman RJ, Cope L, Pohl G, Samuels Y, et al. Sequence mutations and amplification of PIK3CA and AKT2 genes in purified ovarian serous neoplasms. Cancer Biol Ther. 2006;5:779–85.
86. Willner J, Wurz K, Allison KH, Galic V, Garcia RL, Goff BA, et al. Alternate molecular genetic pathways in ovarian carcinomas of common histological types. Hum Pathol. 2007;38:607–13.
87. Catasus L, Gallardo A, Cuatrecasas M, Prat J. PIK3CA mutations in the kinase domain (exon 20) of uterine endometrial adenocarcinomas are associated with adverse prognostic parameters. Mod Pathol. 2008;21:131–9.
88. Wright K, Wilson P, Morland S, Campbell I, Walsh M, Hurst T, et al. Beta-catenin mutation and expression analysis in ovarian cancer: exon 3 mutations and nuclear translocation in 16% of endometrioid tumours. Int J Cancer. 1999;82:625–9.
89. Palacios J, Gamallo C. Mutations in the beta-catenin gene (CTNNB1) in endometrioid ovarian carcinomas. Cancer Res. 1998;58:1344–7.
90. Gamallo C, Palacios J, Moreno G. Calvo de Mora J, Suarez a, Armas a. Beta-catenin expression pattern in stage I and II ovarian carcinomas : relationship with beta-catenin gene mutations, clinicopathological features, and clinical outcome. Am J Pathol. 1999;155:527–36.
91. Saegusa M, Okayasu I. Frequent nuclear beta-catenin accumulation and associated mutations in endometrioid-type endometrial and ovarian carcinomas with squamous differentiation. J Pathol. 2001;194:59–67.
92. Wu R, Hendrix-Lucas N, Kuick R, Zhai Y, Schwartz DR, Akyol A, et al. Mouse model of human ovarian endometrioid adenocarcinoma based on somatic defects in the Wnt/beta-catenin and PI3K/Pten signaling pathways. Cancer Cell. 2007;11:321–33.
93. Enomoto T, Weghorst CM, Inoue M, Tanizawa O, Rice JM. K-ras activation occurs frequently in mucinous adenocarcinomas and rarely in other common epithelial tumors of the human ovary. Am J Pathol. 1991;139:777–85.
94. Caduff RF, Svoboda-Newman SM, Bartos RE, Ferguson AW, Frank TS. Comparative analysis of histologic homologues of endometrial and ovarian carcinoma. Am J Surg Pathol. 1998;22:319–26.
95. Amemiya S, Sekizawa A, Otsuka J, Tachikawa T, Saito H, Okai T. Malignant transformation of endometriosis and genetic alterations of K-ras and microsatellite instability. Int J Gynaecol Obstet. 2004;86:371–6.
96. Mayr D, Hirschmann A, Lohrs U, Diebold J. KRAS and BRAF mutations in ovarian tumors: a comprehensive study of invasive carcinomas, borderline tumors and extraovarian implants. Gynecol Oncol. 2006;103:883–7.
97. Wiegand KC, Shah SP, Al-Agha OM, Zhao Y, Tse K, Zeng T, et al. ARID1A mutations in endometriosis-associated ovarian carcinomas. N Engl J Med. 2010;363:1532–43.
98. Sato N, Tsunoda H, Nishida M, Morishita Y, Takimoto Y, Kubo T, et al. Loss of heterozygosity on 10q23.3 and mutation of the tumor suppressor gene PTEN in benign endometrial cyst of the ovary: possible sequence progression from benign endometrial cyst to endometrioid carcinoma and clear cell carcinoma of the ovary. Cancer Res. 2000;60:7052–6.
99. Dinulescu DM, Ince TA, Quade BJ, Shafer SA, Crowley D, Jacks T. Role of K-ras and Pten in the development of mouse models of endometriosis and endometrioid ovarian cancer. Nat Med. 2005;11:63–70.
100. Zhai Y, Kuick R, Tipton C, Wu R, Sessine M, Wang Z, et al. Arid1a inactivation in an Apc- and Pten-defective mouse ovarian cancer model enhances epithelial differentiation and prolongs survival. J Pathol. 2016;238:21–30.
101. Komiyama S, Aoki D, Tominaga E, Susumu N, Udagawa Y, Nozawa S. Prognosis of Japanese patients with ovarian clear cell carcinoma associated with pelvic endometriosis: clinicopathologic evaluation. Gynecol Oncol. 1999;72:342–6.

102. Matsuo Y, Tashiro H, Yanai H, Moriya T, Katabuchi H. Clinicopathological heterogeneity in ovarian clear cell adenocarcinoma: a study on individual therapy practice. Med Mol Morphol. 2015;48:146–54.
103. Yamamoto S, Tsuda H, Yoshikawa T, Kudoh K, Kita T, Furuya K, et al. Clear cell adenocarcinoma associated with clear cell adenofibromatous components: a subgroup of ovarian clear cell adenocarcinoma with distinct clinicopathologic characteristics. Am J Surg Pathol. 2007;31:999–1006.
104. Veras E, Mao TL, Ayhan A, Ueda S, Lai H, Hayran M, et al. Cystic and adenofibromatous clear cell carcinomas of the ovary: distinctive tumors that differ in their pathogenesis and behavior: a clinicopathologic analysis of 122 cases. Am J Surg Pathol. 2009;33:844–53.
105. Kato N, Sasou S, Motoyama T. Expression of hepatocyte nuclear factor-1beta (HNF-1beta) in clear cell tumors and endometriosis of the ovary. Mod Pathol. 2006;19:83–9.
106. Kobel M, Kalloger SE, Carrick J, Huntsman D, Asad H, Oliva E, et al. A limited panel of immunomarkers can reliably distinguish between clear cell and high-grade serous carcinoma of the ovary. Am J Surg Pathol. 2009;33:14–21.
107. Kobel M, Kalloger SE, Boyd N, McKinney S, Mehl E, Palmer C, et al. Ovarian carcinoma subtypes are different diseases: implications for biomarker studies. PLoS Med. 2008;5:e232.
108. Senkel S, Lucas B, Klein-Hitpass L, Ryffel GU. Identification of target genes of the transcription factor HNF1beta and HNF1alpha in a human embryonic kidney cell line. Biochim Biophys Acta. 1731;2005:179–90.
109. Kobayashi H, Yamada Y, Kanayama S, Furukawa N, Noguchi T, Haruta S, et al. The role of hepatocyte nuclear factor-1beta in the pathogenesis of clear cell carcinoma of the ovary. Int J Gynecol Cancer. 2009;19:471–9.
110. Tanaka T, Tomaru Y, Nomura Y, Miura H, Suzuki M, Hayashizaki Y. Comprehensive search for HNF-1beta-regulated genes in mouse hepatoma cells perturbed by transcription regulatory factor-targeted RNAi. Nucleic Acids Res. 2004;32:2740–50.
111. Fujita M, Enomoto T, Yoshino K, Nomura T, Buzard GS, Inoue M, et al. Microsatellite instability and alterations in the hMSH2 gene in human ovarian cancer. Int J Cancer. 1995;64:361–6.
112. King BL, Carcangiu ML, Carter D, Kiechle M, Pfisterer J, Pfleiderer A, et al. Microsatellite instability in ovarian neoplasms. Br J Cancer. 1995;72:376–82.
113. Kobel M, Bell DA, Carcangiu ML, Oliva E, Prat J, Shih IM, et al. Seromucinous tumours. In: Kurman RJ, Carcangiu ML, Herrington CS, Young RH, editors. WHO classification of tumours of female reproductive organs. 4th ed. IARC: Lyon; 2014.
114. Vang R, Gown AM, Zhao C, Barry TS, Isacson C, Richardson MS, et al. Ovarian mucinous tumors associated with mature cystic teratomas: morphologic and immunohistochemical analysis identifies a subset of potential teratomatous origin that shares features of lower gastrointestinal tract mucinous tumors more commonly encountered as secondary tumors in the ovary. Am J Surg Pathol. 2007;31:854–69.
115. Seidman JD, Khedmati F. Exploring the histogenesis of ovarian mucinous and transitional cell (Brenner) neoplasms and their relationship with Walthard cell nests: a study of 120 tumors. Arch Pathol Lab Med. 2008;132:1753–60.
116. Rodriguez IM, Prat J. Mucinous tumors of the ovary: a clinicopathologic analysis of 75 borderline tumors (of intestinal type) and carcinomas. Am J Surg Pathol. 2002;26:139–52.
117. Cuatrecasas M, Villanueva A, Matias-Guiu X, Prat J. K-ras mutations in mucinous ovarian tumors: a clinicopathologic and molecular study of 95 cases. Cancer. 1997;79:1581–6.
118. Park SY, Kim HS, Hong EK, Kim WH. Expression of cytokeratins 7 and 20 in primary carcinomas of the stomach and colorectum and their value in the differential diagnosis of metastatic carcinomas to the ovary. Hum Pathol. 2002;33:1078–85.
119. Heinzelmann-Schwarz VA, Gardiner-Garden M, Henshall SM, Scurry JP, Scolyer RA, Smith AN, et al. A distinct molecular profile associated with mucinous epithelial ovarian cancer. Br J Cancer. 2006;94:904–13.
120. Ryland GL, Hunter SM, Doyle MA, Caramia F, Li J, Rowley SM, et al. Mutational landscape of mucinous ovarian carcinoma and its neoplastic precursors. Genome Med. 2015;7:87.

121. Anglesio MS, Kommoss S, Tolcher MC, Clarke B, Galletta L, Porter H, et al. Molecular characterization of mucinous ovarian tumours supports a stratified treatment approach with HER2 targeting in 19% of carcinomas. J Pathol. 2013;229:111–20.
122. Hunter SM, Gorringe KL, Christie M, Rowley SM, Bowtell DD, Campbell IG. Pre-invasive ovarian mucinous tumors are characterized by CDKN2A and RAS pathway aberrations. Clin Cancer Res. 2012;18:5267–77.
123. Mackenzie R, Kommoss S, Winterhoff BJ, Kipp BR, Garcia JJ, Voss J, et al. Targeted deep sequencing of mucinous ovarian tumors reveals multiple overlapping RAS-pathway activating mutations in borderline and cancerous neoplasms. BMC Cancer. 2015;15:415.

Screening and Prevention of Ovarian Cancer

4

Hiroshi Kobayashi

Abstract

The aim of this study is to review clinical studies for organizing a screening and prevention program for ovarian cancer. A search of the relevant English-language literature published between 1986 and 2016 was conducted using the MEDLINE online database. Several reviews have dealt with ovarian cancer screening in the general populations and specific high-risk groups. The results from the medical literature showed that a variety of screening of ovarian cancer were unable to provide the impact on clinical survival benefit. Although the survival data from the UK study provided a modest degree of hope, at present there is no effective screening test for ovarian cancer. Since ovarian cancer is not a uniform entity, it is unlikely that a single approach to screening will be appropriate for all patients. Clinical guidelines are available for HBOC, which include breast and ovarian cancer screening (surveillance) and risk-reducing interventions (risk-reducing surgical and medical options). Surgical and pharmacological options are available. Prophylactic RRSO and RRM reduced cancer incidence compared to chemoprevention or surveillance, but many women who are at risk for BRCA1/2 mutations delay or decline prophylactic surgery. Oral contraceptives are proposed as a chemoprevention agent for ovarian cancer. Chemoprevention contributes to reducing ovarian cancer deaths, with a special attention on the breast cancer risk. Importantly, a recent meta-analysis demonstrated a significant ovarian cancer risk reduction and no increased breast cancer risk with oral contraceptive use by BRCA mutation carriers. Breast cancer risk may vary by age at first oral contraceptive use, duration of use, intervals

H. Kobayashi, M.D., Ph.D.
Department of Obstetrics and Gynecology, Nara Medical University,
840 Shijo-cho, Kashihara, 634-8522 Nara, Japan
e-mail: hirokoba@naramed-u.ac.jp

H. Katabuchi (ed.), *Frontiers in Ovarian Cancer Science*, Comprehensive Gynecology and Obstetrics, DOI 10.1007/978-981-10-4160-0_4

from the last use, and oral contraceptive formulation. At present, there is no effective screening for ovarian cancer. Clinicians are recommended to encourage high-risk women who delay or decline risk-reducing surgery to discuss risk-reducing pharmacologic options in order to prevent ovarian cancer progression without elevation of breast cancer risk.

Keywords
Screening • Prevention • Ovarian cancer • Breast cancer

4.1 Introduction

Epithelial ovarian cancer (EOC) is the leading cause of cancer death among all gynecological malignancies worldwide. More than 50% of patients have already reached to the advanced stages of disease in which 5-year survival rate is <40%. The incidence of sporadic and hereditary EOC increases with age. EOC, highly heterogeneous histological appearances, including serous, clear cell, endometrioid, and mucinous carcinomas, was divided into type I and type II tumors [1]. At least the type I tumors are mostly low-grade, low-growing, and well- or intermediately differentiated tumors of endometrioid or clear cell histological subtype. They demonstrate a stepwise progression from a benign precursor such as endometriosis to atypical endometriosis as an intermediate lesion and subsequently to endometriosis-associated ovarian cancer (EAOC). EAOC was frequently diagnosed at a younger age and an earlier stage of disease with favorable clinical outcome compared to high-grade serous carcinoma. A number of specific genetic alterations, like loss of heterozygosity (LOH), microsatellite instability, PTEN (phosphatase and tensin homolog), KRAS (KRAS proto-oncogene, GTPase), CTNNB1 (catenin beta 1), and ARID1A (AT-rich interaction domain 1A) mutations, have been found in EAOC. In contrast, type II tumors, including high-grade serous carcinoma (HGSC), are clinically aggressive, accompanied by rapid growth and present in advanced stage with unfavorable clinical outcome. Among EOC, HGSC accounts for 70–80% of cancer deaths. Deleterious point mutations in tumor suppressor genes, such as TP53 (tumor protein p53), BRCA1 (BRCA1, DNA repair associated), and BRCA2, are relatively common in HGSC. Mutations of BRCA1 and BRCA2, the most frequently affected genes, are associated with the hereditary breast and ovarian cancer (HBOC) syndrome. BRCA1/2 mutation carriers have an increased risk of developing breast cancer and gynecologic cancers including ovarian, fallopian, and peritoneal cancers. This type of ovarian cancers might originate from the distal end of the fallopian tube (fimbria), but not from the precursor cells in the ovarian surface epithelium as previously believed [2]. Morphologically transformed cells with p53 mutations cannot be detected in inclusion cysts of the ovary in a series of prophylactic oophorectomy specimens [3]. Widespread disease can be diagnosed <6 months after a negative surveillance using transvaginal sonography (TVS) and CA125 test [4].

Epidemiologic studies have identified that nulliparity, age at first pregnancy, early menarche, late menopause, a greater number of ovulatory cycles, cumulatively summed as lifetime number of ovulatory cycles, infertility, obesity, and hormone replacement therapy have been associated with definite risks of ovarian cancer. Protective factors have been identified, which include oral contraceptive use, multiparity, hysterectomy, tubal ligation, breastfeeding, prior oophorectomy, and NSAID and oral contraceptive use [5].

Interestingly, there is a significant difference by race in the histology of EOC [6]. Of Caucasians, 70–80% had HGSC and <10% had clear cell carcinoma. Of Asians (or Japanese), 40% had HGSC and 25% had clear cell lesions. Type II tumors are significantly common in Caucasians, and the rate of type I tumors is relatively higher in Japanese than in Caucasians. Japanese researchers have been trying to identify suitable or novel screening methods that enable stratification of patients with type I ovarian cancer for optimal screening (see Sect. 4.4.4).

Population-based cancer screening programs for breast, lung, gastric, colon, and cervical cancers allow an early diagnosis, even before the onset of symptoms. Effective screening methods have impacted on a cost-effective prevention and survival in these cancers. Ovarian cancer screening strategies are as follows: to identify women without symptoms in an early stage allowing curative treatment; to improve survival for the screeners versus non-screeners; to avoid false-positive findings, leading to unnecessary workup or surgery; to avoid causing harm to the women who do not have the disease; and routine screening or surveillance for early detection is not costly. An effective screening requires a sufficient time interval from initiation to the metastatic stage, namely, a sufficient window for early detection. Indeed, ovarian cancer cells rapidly spread in the peritoneum, and most diseases are diagnosed at an advanced stage. The endeavor may be hindered because of the lack of cost-effective screening strategies.

Several reviews have dealt with ovarian cancer screening in the general populations and specific high-risk groups. The ideal strategy for surveillance of high-risk ovarian cancer has become increasingly challenging. The purpose of this article is to critically review the published literature on the factors associated with ovarian cancer screening and prevention program. Since EOC is not a uniform entity, it is unlikely that a single approach to screening will be appropriate for all patients. The goal is to identify modifiable screening methods for the Japanese population.

4.2 Materials and Methods

4.2.1 Search Strategy and Selection Criteria

A literature review was conducted to identify screening and prevention program for ovarian cancer. MEDLINE search via PubMed, Scopus, and the Cochrane Central Register of Controlled Trials (CENTRAL) of the relevant literature published between January 1, 1986, and July 31, 2016, was systematically performed using the following keywords: "epithelial ovarian cancer," "breast cancer," "screening," "prevention," "general population," "high-risk population," "HBOC," "BRCA1," and "BRCA2." English-language publication search results from MEDLINE and references within the relevant articles were analyzed. Furthermore, references within the references were searched to identify additional relevant studies.

4.3 Results

4.3.1 The Systematic Literature Review

The systematic search resulted in the identification of 1617 citations, and 56 additional studies were identified through manual searches of accepted studies and published systematic reviews. Of the 1673 citations identified in the search, 1286 were further excluded following abstract screening. Of the 387 full-text articles retrieved and reviewed, we selected RCTs and prospective studies. Overall, 35 studies (17 for ovarian cancer screening and 18 for ovarian cancer prevention) were included in this review.

4.3.2 Ovarian Cancer Screening in the General Population

In the general populations, it is prudent to target an older population, especially postmenopausal women. The serum marker CA125 and transvaginal sonography (TVS) have received the most attention to date.

4.3.2.1 CA125

CA125 is a high molecular weight transmembrane mucin (MUC16). This marker, currently the most widely used tumor marker for EOC, was elevated in serum from 90% of patients with advanced EOC and released into blood from cancer cells, possibly through the tumor necrosis factor (TNF)-alpha and interferon (IFN)-gamma stimulation [7]. CA125 was originally developed to monitor patients previously diagnosed with ovarian cancer. To date, CA125 can help in the evaluation of an adnexal mass in appropriate patients. In most studies, CA125 was elevated in approximately 50–60% of stage I disease, demonstrating that this marker is not sufficiently sensitive to detect all cases of early-stage ovarian cancer [8]. In addition, a number of common benign conditions, including endometriosis, adenomyosis, ovarian cysts, uterine fibroids, renal dysfunction, hepatic disease, and inflammation, can cause elevation of CA125 levels. In ovarian cancer patients, an exponential rise is seen in CA125 level before clinical detection of diseases, which was documented in some studies [9]. Taken together, CA125 alone was not recommended as a screening test in asymptomatic women, because of its low sensitivity and limited specificity.

Table 4.1 A summary of the key findings of the two ovarian cancer screening trials using CA125

	St Bartholomew's Hospital trial	The Boston study
Ref.	[9]	[10]
Published	1996	2003
Design	Single arm prospective study	Single arm prospective study.
Subjects	The low-risk asymptomatic women > or = 45 years of age. 22,000 volunteers	33,621 CA125 results from 9233 low-risk women older than 45 years for whom two or more serial samples were available
Recruitment	Between June 1, 1986 and May 1, 1990, London	Between June 1, 1986, and May 1, 1990
Strategy	CA125 measured annually for 1–4 years and a positive CA125 was recalled for ultrasound	CA125 II levels
Interpretation	A CA125 concentration > or = 30 U/mL	Calculation based on serial CA125 II levels
Results	The relative risk of developing ovarian and fallopian cancers within 5 years was increased 14.3-fold (8.5–24.3) after a CA125 cut-off > or = 30 U/mL and 74.5-fold (31.1–178.3) after a cut-off > or = 100 U/mL	The risk calculation significantly improved the area under the curve from 84 to 93% compared with a fixed cutoff for CA125. CA125 achieved a sensitivity of 62%
Mortality	Serial CA125 elevation is associated with an increase in risk of an index cancer in asymptomatic women older than 45 years. The mortality effect has not been reported as yet	Serial CA125 elevation improved the ovarian cancer detection rate in asymptomatic women. The mortality effect has not been reported as yet

Although an effective strategy must meet the stringent requirement of screening, several studies have reported ovarian cancer screening trials that have been conducted using CA125 in postmenopausal women in the general population. Table 4.1 is a summary of the key findings of the two ovarian cancer screening trials using CA125. In the Boston study, serial CA125 elevation contributed more significantly to successfully predict the risk of ovarian cancer compared with a fixed cutoff in asymptomatic women older than 45 years [10]. However, the survival benefit has not been reported as yet. At present, CA125 alone cannot be recommended for screening for ovarian cancer in asymptomatic women [11]. Given the heterogeneity of EOC, a panel of biomarkers may be more effective than a single marker. CA125 is more often negative in clear cell carcinoma than in other subtypes of EOC. Recent study has demonstrated that a new marker TFPI2 may be useful for detection of clear cell carcinoma [12]. Current biomarkers including TFPI2 will be investigated in combination with CA125 in larger cohorts to improve ovarian cancer diagnosis.

4.3.2.2 Transvaginal Sonography

Transvaginal sonography (TVS) has been considered a primary imaging modality for diagnosing and evaluating adnexal masses. TVS has high specificity and sensitivity for detecting an adnexal mass based on a pattern recognition approach and morphological feature through gray-scale ultrasound. Table 4.2 is a summary of the findings of the four major ovarian cancer screening trials using TVS. These studies used gray-scale TVS as a primary screening modality [13, 14, 16, 17]. The percentage of the total number of stage I cases increased after the induction of screening (stage shift). It was not effective in detecting ovarian cancers in women who had normal ovarian volume. The use and role of Doppler ultrasonography as a screening technique are controversial. Color flow imaging for detection of ovarian cancer greatly improves specificity but at the expense of potential sensitivity in the triage of adnexal masses. Dr. van Nagell and his colleagues have reported some encouraging evidence of not only stage shift but also survival benefit by a single-arm prospective study, not a RCT [18]. A large-scale RCT is required for answering this question. Further, stringent quality control and quality assurance are necessary for TVS screening of asymptomatic postmenopausal women.

4.3.2.3 Two-Stage Strategies

Several studies have assessed the diagnostic value of combinations of CA125 and imaging concurrently or sequentially to augment the specificity and sensitivity for screening. Clinicians and public health informants were in consensus that the key issue is to reduce mortality. Table 4.3 is a summary of the key conclusions from the five major ovarian cancer screening trials using CA125 and TVS.

First, Jacobs and coworkers studied a group of 1010 asymptomatic postmenopausal women, comparing the specificities of individual evaluation or a combination of CA125, TVS, and pelvic examination (the first London study) [19]. Their study showed a specificity of 99.8% and 99.0% for CA125 plus TVS and CA125 plus pelvic examination, respectively, indicating that the combination of CA125 with TVS achieved acceptable specificity.

In the second study (a pilot randomized controlled trial in the second London study) conducted in the UK by Jacobs and coworkers, the specificity of CA125 alone or in combination with abdominal ultrasound was evaluated in postmenopausal women 45 years of age or above [20]. The subjects were divided into a control group (10,977) and a screened group (10,985). A total of 16 and 21 cancers were detected in the screened and control group, respectively, during the same interval. Median survival in the screened group (72.9 months) was significantly greater than in the control group (41.8 months) [20].

Third, the original intention in the Shizuoka study (RCT with one screening strategy in study group) conducted in Japan by Kobayashi and coworkers was to offer women in the intervention group annual screens by gynecological examination (sequential TVS and serum CA125 test) [21]. Women with abnormal TVS findings and/or elevated CA125 values were referred for surgical investigation by a gynecological oncologist. Twenty-seven index cancers were detected in the 41,688 screened women. Eight cancers were diagnosed outside the screening program. Among the 40,779 control women, 32 women developed ovarian cancer. The detection rate of early-stage ovarian cancer was elevated in the screened group compared with the controls, which did not reach statistical significance (63% vs 38%, $p = 0.2285$). Interestingly, sub-analysis assessment identified that the Shizuoka screening

Table 4.2 A summary of the findings of the four major ovarian cancer screening trials using TVS

	The London study	The First Kentucky study	The Hirosaki, Japan study	The Second Kentucky study	The Third Kentucky study
Ref.	[13]	[14, 15]	[16]	[15, 17]	[15, 18]
Published	1993	2000	2000	2007	2011
Design	Single arm prospective study	Single arm prospective study	Single arm prospective study	Single arm prospective study	Single arm prospective study, not a RCT
Subjects	1601 self referred asymptomatic women aged 17 to 79 (mean 47) years, with a family history of ovarian cancer, aged 17 to 79 (mean 47) years. 60% were premenopausal	14,469 asymptomatic women; women >/= 50 years of age in the general populations and women >/= 25 years of age with a family history of ovarian cancer	51,550 low-risk asymptomatic women who participated in annual uterine cervical carcinoma screening.	25,327 asymptomatic women aged > or = 50 years in the general populations and women aged > or = 25 years who had a family history of ovarian cancer	37,293 asymptomatic women aged > or = 50 years in the general populations and women aged > or = 25 years who had a family history of ovarian cancer
Recruitment		Between 1987 and 1999	Between 1989 and 1999	Between 1987 and 2005	Between 1987 and 2011
Strategy	Transvaginal ultrasonography with color blood flow imaging	Annual transvaginal sonography (TVS)	Annual transvaginal sonography (TVS)	Annual transvaginal sonography (TVS)	Annual transvaginal sonography (TVS). Women with abnormal screens underwent tumor morphology indexing, serum biomarker analysis, and surgery
Interpretation	Morphological score > or = 5 and pulsatility index <1.0	An abnormal sonogram	An abnormal sonogram (a mass > 30 mm in greatest dimension or a mass with a mixed pattern)	An abnormal sonogram	An abnormal sonogram

(continued)

Table 4.2 (continued)

	The London study	The First Kentucky study	The Hirosaki, Japan study	The Second Kentucky study	The Third Kentucky study
Results	61 women had a positive screening result (3.8%, 95% confidence interval 2.9 to 4.9%), six of whom had primary ovarian cancer detected at surgery (five stage Ia, one stage III)	180 patients with persisting TVS abnormalities underwent exploratory laparoscopy or laparotomy. 17 ovarian cancers were detected: 11 Stage I, 3 Stage II, and 3 Stage III. Four and four patients developed ovarian cancer within 12 months of a negative scan and more than 12 months following a normal screen, respectively. Statistical variables: sensitivity, 81%; specificity, 98.9%; positive predictive value, 9.4%; and negative predictive value, 99.97%	Secondary screening was required for 5309 participants (10.3%). Surgery was performed on 324 participants. Twenty-two primary tumors and 2 metastatic tumors were detected for a diagnostic rate of 0.047%. 77.3% were classified as Stage I carcinoma.	Among 364 patients (1.4%) with a persisting ovarian tumor, 35 primary invasive ovarian cancers, 9 serous ovarian tumors of low malignant potential, and 7 cancers metastatic to the ovary were detected. Nine women developed ovarian cancer within 12 months of a negative screen. A sensitivity of 85.0%, specificity of 98.7%, positive predictive value of 14.0%, and negative predictive value of 99.9%	Forty-seven invasive epithelial ovarian cancers and 15 epithelial ovarian tumors of low malignant potential were detected. Stage distribution: stage I, 47%; stage II, 23%; stage III, 30%, and stage IV, 0%. The 5-year survival rate for all women with invasive index cancer detected by screening as well as interval cancers was 74.8% compared with 53.7% for unscreened women with ovarian cancer ($P < 0.001$)

Mortality	TVU with color flow imaging can effectively detect early ovarian cancer in women with a family history of the disease. The mortality effect has not been reported as yet	A decrease in stage at detection (stage shift) and a possible decrease in case-specific ovarian cancer mortality	Stage shift may decrease the mortality of the disease. The mortality effect in comparison with the non-screening group has not been reported as yet	Stage shift. Although a significantly higher fraction of early-stage cancer was detected, they also had nine patients who developed ovarian cancer within 12 months of a normal scan. The mortality effect in comparison with the non-screening group has not been reported as yet. Although a significantly higher fraction of early-stage cancer was detected, they also had nine patients who developed ovarian cancer within 12 months of a normal scan	Some encouraging evidence of stage shift and survival benefit

Table 4.3 A summary of the key conclusions from the five major ovarian cancer screening trials using CA125 and TVS

	The First London study	The Second London study	Japanese Shizuoka Cohort Study of Ovarian Cancer Screening (SCSOCS)	Prostate, Lung, Colorectal and Ovarian (PLCO) Cancer Screening Trial in the United States of America (USA)	United Kingdom Collaborative Trial of Ovarian Cancer Screening (UKCTOCS)
Ref.	[19]	[20]	[15, 21]	[15, 22, 23]	[15, 24, 25]
Published	1988	1999	2008	2016	2016
Design	Single arm prospective study	A pilot randomized controlled trial	RCT with 1 screening strategy in study group	RCT with 1 screening strategy in study group	RCT with 2 screening strategies in study group
Subjects	1010 low-risk asymptomatic postmenopausal women	The low-risk postmenopausal women aged 45 years or older. Randomized to a screened group ($n = 10,958$) or control group ($n = 10,977$)	41,688 low-risk asymptomatic postmenopausal women. Either an intervention group ($n = 41,688$) or a control group ($n = 40,799$), with follow-up of mean 9.2 years	78,216 low risk asymptomatic women aged 55 to 74 of whom 39,105 underwent screening	An RCT of 202,638 low risk asymptomatic women aged 50–74 years from the general population randomized in 2001–2005 to no intervention (control: 101,359) or annual screening using either TVS alone (50,639) or serum CA125 interpreted by a 'Risk of Ovarian Cancer' algorithm (ROCA) with TVS as a second line test (multimodal screening, MMS; 50,640)

Recruitment	For an ovarian cancer screening programme	Between 1989 and 1998	Between 1985 and 1999	Between 1993 and 2007, at a median follow-up of 12.4 years (25th–75th centile 10.9–13.0)	Randomized in 2001–2005
Strategy	CA125 measurement and vaginal examination as initial tests and real-time ultrasonography as a secondary procedure in selected cases	Multimodal screening with sequential CA 125 and TVS to detect invasive epithelial cancers of the ovary or fallopian tube (index cancers). In the screened group, CA125 was measured annually for 3 years	Physical exam, ultrasound and CA125 concurrently	Ultrasound and CA125. The women were screened using serum CA125 and TVS for 4 years followed by CA125 alone for a further 2 years. The patients with pelvic lesions or an elevated CA125 level were referred to their local physicians for further management	Two screening arms (TVS) and CA125 followed by ultrasound (MMS)
Interpretation	The normal range for serum CA125 in postmenopausal women was established	CA 125 was 30 U/mL or more	CA125 using a 35 U/mL cutoff	CA125 using a 35 U/mL cutoff and/or an abnormal sonogram	CA125 interpreted using the Risk of Ovarian Cancer algorithm (ROCA). The ROCA is a statistical tool that considers current and past CA125 values to determine ovarian cancer risk

(continued)

Table 4.3 (continued)

	The First London study	The Second London study	Japanese Shizuoka Cohort Study of Ovarian Cancer Screening (SCSOCS)	Prostate, Lung, Colorectal and Ovarian (PLCO) Cancer Screening Trial in the United States of America (USA)	United Kingdom Collaborative Trial of Ovarian Cancer Screening (UKCTOCS)
Results	The combinations of serum CA125 measurement with ultrasound and vaginal examination with ultrasound achieved specificities of 99.8% and 99.0%, respectively. 100% specificity was achieved by serum CA125 measurement with vaginal examination and by the combination of all three tests	Of 468 women in the screened group with a raised CA125, 29 were referred for a gynecological opinion; screening detected an index cancer in six and 23 had false-positive screening results. The positive predictive value was 20.7%. Median survival of women with index cancers in the screened group was 72.9 months and in the control group was 41.8 months ($p = 0.0112$). The number of deaths from an index cancer did not differ significantly between the control and screened groups (18 of 10,977 vs. nine of 10,958, relative risk 2.0 [95% CI 0.78–5.13])	Encouraging sensitivity (77.1%) for primary ovarian cancer. Stage shift: more Stage I ovarian cancers in the screened group (63%) compared to the control (38%), which did not reach statistical significance. The Japanese screening trial enables diagnosis of EAOC at an early stage of the disease.	Lower sensitivity (69.5%); only 28% were Stage I/II. Abnormal TVS and elevated CA125 were found in 4.7%, and 1.4% of the participants, respectively. The positive predictive value for detection of ovarian cancer for CA125 alone and for TVS alone was 3.7% was 1.0%, respectively. The PPV for both tests combined was 23.5%, but 60% of early-stage disease would have been missed [5]. 118 and 100 deaths were reported in the screening and control arm, respectively, with a mortality rate ratio of 1.18 (95%CI 0.91–1.54)	Encouraging sensitivity (89.4% MMS/84.9% TVS) for primary index cancer; 84.9% MMS/75.0% TVS for primary invasive index cancer (47% MMS/50% TVS were Stage I/II). Superior sensitivity (88.6% vs 65.8%) and PPV (21.7% vs 5.8%) of MMS compared to the TVS arm for detection of primary invasive index cancers during incidence screening, with 40.3% in the MMS and 51.5% in the TVS arm detected at early stage

Mortality	The combination of CA125 with ultrasound achieved acceptable specificity. The mortality effect has not been reported as yet	A larger randomized trial to see whether screening affects mortality	The mortality effect has not been reported as yet	No mortality benefit. Screening with concurrent CA 125 and TVS has no evidence of a mortality benefit	The stages at detection were relatively earlier (stage I/II: 44%) in the screening cohort. Although the mortality reduction was not significant in the primary analysis, researchers noted a significant mortality reduction with MMS when prevalent cases were excluded. MMS significantly reduced ovarian cancer mortality after excluding either deaths in the first 7 years after randomization or prevalent cancers. The large number of false positive surgeries (roughly 2100 surgeries) would be needed in order to prevent the small cancer deaths (about 40 deaths in each screening group)

favorably detected certain histotypes such as clear cell and endometrioid types that are more common, low-grade, and less aggressive tumors in Japan. Since the progression of endometriosis to cancer is usually slow, recognition of patients at early stages may improve survival.

Fourth, the prostate, lung, colon, and ovary (PLCO) screening trial in the USA aimed to conduct concurrent testing of CA125 and TVS in the low-risk asymptomatic women between 55 and 74 years of age to determine if screening could reduce mortality in these cancers [22]. This RCT of screening versus usual care was initiated in 1993 and has studied 78,216 women. Data from the PLCO trial has not shown mortality benefit [15, 22, 23].

Finally, the UK Collaborative Trial of Ovarian Cancer Screening (UKCTOCS) used the risk of ovarian cancer algorithm (ROCA) to interpret the impact of CA125, which has shown an encouraging sensitivity and specificity [15]. The mortality reduction was not significant in the primary analysis, but this trial may have the potential to make an impact on survival benefit when prevalent cases were excluded [24]. The survival data from the UKCTOCS study provide a modest degree of hope.

Given the paucity of randomized controlled trial data, at present there is no effective screening test for ovarian cancer. The previous RCT results are unable to provide the impact on clinical survival benefit. This allowed us to explore the impact of growing insights into disease etiology and biomarker discovery on future screening strategies. In an era of promising advances in ovarian cancer screening, researchers have to focus on detecting low-volume disease using cancer-specific markers and targeted imaging. More cost-effective approaches might utilize novel biomarkers alone or in combination with imaging modalities in a more limited number of women.

4.3.3 Ovarian Cancer Screening in the High-Risk Population

Hereditary breast and ovarian cancer (HBOC) syndrome accounts for 5%–10% of breast cancers and 15% of invasive ovarian cancers [26]. Mutations in two genes, BRCA1 and BRCA2, are associated with HBOC. The average lifetime risk of EOC in the general populations is 1.3%, but the risk is markedly increased in women who carry mutations of the BRCA1 or BRCA2 (40% and 18% risk, respectively, by age 70 years) or the mismatch repair genes of hereditary nonpolyposis colorectal cancer (Lynch) syndrome (12% lifetime risk) [27–29]. Women with BRCA mutations have a markedly increased risk of early-onset breast, ovarian, pancreatic, and other cancers when compared to the risks in the general population. EOC is a spectrum of several subtypes, with different clinicopathological characteristics, possibly separate pathways of progression, and different sets of genetic and epigenetic characteristic of familial versus sporadic tumors. Since the molecular biology of the known hereditary disease may differ from that of sporadic cancer, separate trials and screening strategies may be required to detect hereditary and sporadic ovarian cancer. The overall occult gynecological carcinoma has been detected in 9.1% of BRCA mutation carriers [30]. Clinical guidelines are available for HBOC, such as those published by the National Comprehensive Cancer Network (NCCN), which include breast and ovarian cancer screening (surveillance) and risk-reducing interventions (risk-reducing surgical and medical options) [30, 31]. Published guidelines adopt standardized surveillance strategies that limit medication side effects, medical/surgical exposure without compromising cancer control and unnecessary cost, as well as enhance overall clinical and economic outcomes.

4.4 Prevention of Ovarian Cancer

Potential preventive strategies against breast and ovarian cancer are the mainstay of cancer risk management and for improving quality of life in BRCA mutation carriers. Surgical and pharmacological options are available.

4.4.1 Risk-Reducing Surgical Options

4.4.1.1 Risk-Reducing Salpingo-Oophorectomy (RRSO)

The prospective studies on the efficacy of RRSO in BRCA mutation carriers showed a significant reduction in the risk of breast and ovarian cancer-specific mortality (hazard ratio [HR] 0.44 and HR 0.21, respectively) [32]. The risk stratification data revealed that the risk of ovarian cancer is 10–21% by age 50 in BRCA1 mutation carriers, whereas BRCA2 mutation carriers have a 2–3% risk of ovarian cancer by age 50. Without any prophylactic therapeutic interventions, the likelihood ratio of survival to the age of 70 was 53% for BRCA1 and 71% for BRCA2 mutation carriers. The only effective and economical surgical strategy to control this disease was RRSO at age 40 plus RRM at age 25, which improves survival to 79% in BRCA1 and to 83% in BRCA2 mutation carriers. After RRSO at age 40, BRCA1 and BRCA2 mutation carriers had a 37% and 64% risk reduction for breast cancer, respectively. Delay in RRSO from age 40 to age 50 decreased the survival gain from 15 to 8% in BRCA1 mutation carriers and from 6 to 4% in BRCA2 mutation carriers. This analysis revealed that delaying RRSO until the early 40s for the BRCA2 mutation carrier appears safe [33] but does not provide breast cancer risk reduction [32]. Furthermore, delaying RRM until age 40 or replacing RRM with breast cancer screening decreased survival gain [32, 34]. In BRCA mutation carriers with a history of breast cancer, RRSO reduced breast cancers in the ipsilateral and contralateral breast, but other study showed that RRSO did not alter the risk of a second primary breast cancer [35, 36]. Taken together, the NCCN recommends RRSO between 35 and 40 years of age, upon completion of childbearing and based on the age of the youngest affected relative with an ovarian cancer diagnosis, regardless of the type of BRCA mutation [31]. Since changes in sexual function, body image, menopause quality of life, and psychological functions are common outcomes following RRSO, long-term follow-up will be needed and critical to a full understanding of the late medical impact of RRSO. Actually, many women do not undergo prophylactic surgery because of stress and anxiety [37, 38]. Rates of the surgery vary depending on balance between anxiety reduction and complications of surgery.

4.4.1.2 Risk-Reducing Oophorectomy (RRO)

BRCA germline mutation carriers are not only at risk for ovarian and breast cancer but also for primary fallopian tube carcinoma and peritoneal carcinoma. Some articles have compared the efficacy of patients with prophylactic bilateral risk-reducing oophorectomy (RRO) in the risk of fallopian tube carcinoma and peritoneal carcinoma to those of RRSO [39–41]. RRO has been chosen by some women with BRCA1 or BRCA2 mutation carriers as an alternative for RRSO. RRO reduces the risk of coelomic epithelial cancer (HR, 0.04; 95 percent confidence interval, 0.01–0.16) and breast cancer (HR, 0.47; 95 percent confidence interval, 0.29–0.77) in women at high-risk ovarian cancer due to inherited predisposition. Among the women with BRCA1 or BRCA2 mutations who chose RRSO, peritoneal cancer was not diagnosed in this group [41]. In contrast, primary peritoneal carcinoma has developed in 1.9% [40], 10.7% [39], and 11.5% [41] of women after RRO. Taken together, RRO may be ineffective in preventing papillary serous peritoneal cancer.

4.4.1.3 Risk-Reducing Salpingectomy (RRS)

Risk-reducing salpingectomy (RRS) with ovarian retention has been proposed as a bridge to RRO, due to evidence that ovarian cancer precursor lesions (e.g., serous tubal intraepithelial carcinoma, STIC) in BRCA mutation carriers may originate in the distal fimbrial end of the fallopian tubes [42]. RRS has the net clinical benefit, including sparing the ovaries until future oophorectomy (longer maintenance of ovarian function), offering delay of surgical menopause (delaying negative effects of early surgical menopause) and allowing for preservation of some reproductive options [43]. RRS has been suggested as a risk-reducing strategy for BRCA1/2 mutation carriers [44], but delay in RRO theoretically could reduce the protective effect against breast cancer. Although RRS should be considered an investigational risk management option, the application of prophylactic surgeries may reduce the incidence of ovarian cancer (65% risk reduction by RRS and 96% by RRSO) [45]. Prophylactic RRSO may provide greater benefits with the view of reducing the risk for ovarian cancer compared to RRS.

It has been reported that majority of cases with ovarian HGSC arise in the fallopian tube fimbria [46]. Furthermore, in the BRCA1/2 mutation carriers, the microscopic cancers were confined to not only the fallopian tubes but also ovaries only or peritoneal washings only, suggesting that the site of origin may be in the fallopian tube, ovary, or peritoneum [47]. This suggests that cancer initiation may occur in the fallopian tube fimbriae, but tumor growth and progression are favored in the ovary. Quite a lot of information may exist in favor of a cancer progression role of ovarian surface epithelium or inclusion cyst. Ovulation-induced inflammation and oxidative stress may induce genotoxic damage leading to ovarian carcinogenesis. Currently, RRS is not included in the NCCN guidelines as strategies for risk reduction in BRCA mutation carriers. Additional evidence is needed regarding the effectiveness of the surgical options such as RRS and RRO for cancer risk reduction. It remains unclear whether oral contraceptives would be useful in a decreased risk of ovarian cancer after RRS in BRCA mutation carriers.

4.4.1.4 Tubal Ligation

Tubal ligation has been associated with the risk reduction of ovarian cancer, particularly in the type II ovarian cancer, in the general populations [5]. There are a few small studies of ovarian cancer risk reduction with tubal ligation in BRCA mutation carriers. In a case-control study, a history of tubal ligation was associated with a decrease in risk for ovarian cancer in BRCA mutation carriers [48]. In contrast, tubal ligation may not be protective against ovarian cancer for BRCA mutation carriers [49]. It remained controversial that tubal ligation has the clinical benefit in the high-risk groups.

4.4.2 Risk-Reducing Pharmacologic Options

The NCCN guidelines recommend that BRCA mutation carriers could be followed with pelvic examinations, transvaginal ultrasounds, and serum CA125 levels every 6 months beginning at age 30 or 5–10 years earlier than the youngest diagnosed relative with ovarian cancer, whichever comes first [31]. Published data clearly indicated that in women at increased risk due to a family history or confirmed mutations in high-penetrance genes such as BRCA1/2, annual screening with CA125 and TVS concurrently or sequentially did not detect early-stage cancers [50, 51]. It is also important to recognize that these surveillance methods have not been shown to reduce ovarian cancer mortality [51]. Therefore, screening at present cannot be considered as a safe alternative strategy to risk-reducing surgery.

In the general populations, low parity, infertility, early menarche, and late menopause have all been associated with an increased risk of ovarian cancer. A meta-analysis of case-control and cohort studies showed that use of oral contraceptives is associated with a 40–50% lifetime risk reduction of ovarian cancer [52, 53]. The risk reduction does not differ between the use of the current low-dose oral contraceptives and the high-dose formulations used in the past (OR, 0.5; 95% CI, 0.3–0.7). A survival benefit from oral contraceptives was achieved with longer use. A 36% risk reduction occurred with an additional 10 years of use (summary relative risk [SRR], 0.64; 95% CI, 0.53–0.78), and the benefit can last for 15 years after discontinuation of use.

In the high-risk populations, a meta-analysis of 18 case-control and retrospective cohort studies in BRCA1/2 mutation carriers who used oral contraceptives identified a significant reduction in the risk of ovarian cancer (SRR, 0.50; 95% CI, 0.33–0.75) [54] and by as much as 44%–60% [55, 56]. There is a positive correlation between the duration of oral contraceptive use (regardless of the continuous and discontinuous use) and the degree of ovarian cancer protection, quantified as a 5%–13% risk reduction per year [57–59]. Therefore, in the general populations and the BRCA mutation carriers, women might consider taking oral contraceptives to reduce their ovarian cancer risk in clinical decision-making. Since risk-reducing pharmacologic options provide improved prevention strategies for high-risk women who delay or decline RRSO, alternative ovarian cancer risk-reduction strategies should be discussed.

In addition, a systematic review on a correlation between the use of oral contraceptives and breast cancer risk in the general population has been carried out and concluded that there may be a small increased risk of breast cancer (OR, 1.08; 95% CI, 1.00–1.17) and thrombosis [60]. The results indicated that the risk of breast cancer may vary considerably based on several factors: age at which oral contraceptive commenced (under the age of 30), the length of oral contraceptive use (an increased risk with use beyond 5 years and the current recommendation of short-term use), time since cessation of oral contraceptives, and formulation of oral contraceptives (an increased risk occurred with formulations used before 1975, but this risk was not found for the more recent formulations) [61–65]. There was no significant association between modern oral contraceptive use and breast cancer risk (SRR, 1.13; 95% CI, 0.88–1.45). There have been conflicting data demonstrating the efficacy of oral contraceptive use on the risk of breast cancer in BRCA mutation carriers [56, 61, 65]. Importantly, a recent meta-analysis demonstrated a significant ovarian cancer risk reduction and no increased breast cancer risk with oral contraceptive use by BRCA mutation carriers [63]. The management guidelines for cancer screening and risk-reducing options will continue to be updated.

4.5 Prevention of Breast Cancer

4.5.1 Risk-Reducing Surgical Options

Risk-reducing bilateral mastectomy (RRM) decreases breast cancer risk by up to 95% in BRCA mutation carriers [66]. A significant impact on life expectancy gain is derived from RRM in the fourth decade of life. In clinical practice, individualized recommendations should be made based on the critical role for pretest genetic counseling, the age at which family members developed breast cancer, and addressing psychosocial concerns after surgery.

4.5.2 Risk-Reducing Pharmacologic Options

Although limited data exist on their efficacy in BRCA mutation carriers, chemoprevention with selective estrogen-receptor modulators (tamoxifen and raloxifene) and aromatase inhibitors (e.g., exemestane) reduced breast cancer incidence [67]. In contrast, a case-control study of BRCA1/2 mutation carriers with breast cancer demonstrated a strong protective effect of tamoxifen against contralateral breast cancer in both BRCA1 (OR, 0.5) and BRCA2 (OR, 0.4) mutation carriers, irrespective of estrogen-receptor status of the initial breast cancer [68]. In a subset analysis of another study showed that tamoxifen reduced invasive breast cancer by 62% in

BRCA2 mutation carriers, but not in BRCA1 mutation carriers [67]. Tamoxifen also increased the risks of endometrial cancer, thromboembolic events, stroke, cataracts, and others (vasomotor symptoms, leg cramps, vaginal discharge, and irritation) [69]. The use of tamoxifen should be approached with caution.

4.6 Ovarian Cancer Screening in the Japanese Population

Japanese patients presented with higher incidence of ovarian clear cell carcinoma that is the second-most common type of EOC in Asia. Endometriosis serves as a precursor of EAOC, especially of the clear cell and endometrioid subtypes. More than half of the EOC were attributable to EAOC in Japan. The ovarian cancer screening program in Japan would be to predict malignant transformation of endometriosis and identify women with EAOC in an early stage, which may improve survival.

Recent studies have indicated the clinical utility of measurement of cyst fluid iron, hemoglobin (Hb) species, and their concentrations for the early prediction of malignant transformation of endometriosis [70]. EAOC cyst fluids had much lower levels of total iron, heme iron, and free iron compared with endometriotic cyst samples. Iron-related compounds may serve as predictive biomarkers for early diagnosis of malignant transformation for women with endometriosis. Possible biomarkers have also been extensively investigated in EAOC and endometriosis: methemoglobin (metHb) and oxyhemoglobin (oxyHb) are one of the most abundant Hb species in benign endometriotic cysts and EAOC cysts, respectively [71]. The metHb/oxyHb ratio had a sensitivity, specificity, positive predictive value, and negative predictive value of 62.5%, 100.0%, 100.0%, and 92.1%, respectively, and may predict subsequent malignant transformation from endometriosis to EAOC. Iron concentration and Hb species in the cyst are the central diagnostic indicators for malignant transformation of endometriosis. Therefore, they can be helpful in the delineation of malignant tissue from nonneoplastic tissue.

Several imaging technologies have evolved into a clinically translatable platform to measure the cyst fluid concentrations of iron and Hb species: the potential techniques include conductance methods using electrical admittance plethysmography, combination near-infrared (NIR) vascular imaging/spectrophotometry, NIR transmission spectroscopy, steady-state visible and NIR diffuse reflectance spectrophotometry, or optoacoustic spectroscopy based on pulse-echo ultrasound [72]. The Hb values may be estimated by the portable devices across a wide Hb spectrum, including the Rad-87™ pulse CO-Oximeter with Rainbow Set technology (Masimo), Haemospect® (MBR Optical Systems), or a transcutaneous spectroscopic device (Mediscan 2000, MBR Optical Systems, Wuppertal, Germany) by noninvasive and contact procedures [73, 74]. A truly noninvasive device with the miniaturization and simplification of actuators has to be adopted as a standard of care in a clinical practice. These devices' performance would provide adequate potential for screening purposes in malignant transformation of endometriosis, more than half of the patients diagnosed with ovarian cancer in Japan.

4.7 Discussion

This review focused on the screening and prevention of ovarian cancer. It is a general consensus that at present no population-based screening test is recommended for ovarian cancer detection in the general populations and the high-risk groups. Although annual screening may be associated with the limited stage shift at ovarian cancer detection in the UK (the UKCTOCS study) [24, 25] but no stage shift in the USA (the PLCO study) [22, 23] and Japan (the Shizuoka study) [21], there are no established data in these randomized controlled trials that the mortality of ovarian cancer can be decreased by the screening arm. Interestingly, the results of the UKCTOCS study showed that annual multimodal screening significantly reduced ovarian cancer mortality after excluding either deaths in the first 7 years after randomization or prevalent cancers [24, 25]. However, exclusion of all deaths in years 0–7 is hard to understand: the impact of multimodal screening on ovarian cancer mortality may not be established. In the Shizuoka study, stage shift was found in the screening group, more stage I ovarian cancers in the screened group (63%) compared to the control (38%), but this did not reach statistical significance [21]. However, this screening mainly detected at an earlier stage the less aggressive and low-grade cancers, which include EAOC (clear cell [33%] and endometrioid [19%] subtypes) [21]. These data theoretically imply that ovarian cancer mortality may be lowered by annual screening of endometriosis in Japan [75].

This review also discussed the available data on the risk-reducing surgical options and chemoprevention strategies in ovarian cancer. Up to now, management of this condition relied mostly on surgical treatments. The use of preventive surgery can dramatically reduce ovarian and breast cancer risks and mortality in women who carry the BRCA1 and BRCA2 mutations. Although prophylactic RRSO and RRM reduced cancer incidence compared to chemoprevention or surveillance, many women who are at risk for BRCA1/2 mutations delay or decline prophylactic surgery [37, 38]. In general, 10%–50% opted for prophylactic surgeries in asymptomatic women with BRCA1/2 mutations. The factors that influence decisions to undergo or decline prophylactic surgery are age, having children, country, race, genetic testing itself, risk perceptions, cancer witnessed in family members, family obligations, concerns about fertility and menopause, psychological factors, and fear of surgical complications. Women must balance short- and long-term benefits of anxiety reduction against a series of potential complications of surgery.

Oral contraceptives are proposed as a chemoprevention agent for ovarian cancer. Chemoprevention is an attractive option to prevent the disease in the general populations and high-risk populations. Chemoprevention contributes to reducing ovarian cancer deaths, with a special attention on the breast cancer risk. Breast cancer risk may vary by age at first oral contraceptive use, duration of use, intervals from the last use, and oral contraceptive formulation.

We conclude that since there is no effective screening for ovarian cancer in the general population and high-risk groups, screening at present cannot be considered as a safe alternative strategy to risk-reducing surgery in the BRCA mutation carriers. Clinicians are recommended to encourage high-risk women who delay or decline risk-reducing surgery to discuss risk-reducing pharmacologic options in order to prevent ovarian cancer progression without elevation of breast cancer risk.

Conclusion

The aim of this study is to review clinical studies for organizing a screening and prevention program for ovarian cancer. At present, there is no effective screening for ovarian cancer. Clinicians are recommended to encourage high-risk women who delay or decline risk-reducing surgery to discuss risk-reducing pharmacologic options in order to prevent ovarian cancer progression without elevation of breast cancer risk.

Acknowledgments Grant support: Supported by Grant-in-aid for Scientific Research from the Ministry of Education, Science, and Culture of Japan to the Department of Obstetrics and Gynecology, Nara Medical University (H. Kobayashi).

Conflict of interest The author declares no conflict of interest.

References

1. Kurman RJ, Shih IM. The origin and pathogenesis of epithelial ovarian cancer: a proposed unifying theory. Am J Surg Pathol. 2010;34:433–43.
2. Kim J, Coffey DM, Ma L, Matzuk MM. The ovary is an alternative site of origin for high-grade serous ovarian cancer in mice. Endocrinology. 2015;156:1975–81.
3. Folkins AK, Jarboe EA, Saleemuddin A, Lee Y, Callahan MJ, Drapkin R, et al. A candidate precursor to pelvic serous cancer (p53 signature) and its prevalence in ovaries and fallopian tubes from women with BRCA mutations. Gynecol Oncol. 2008;109:168–73.
4. Badgwell D, Bast RC Jr. Early detection of ovarian cancer. Dis Markers. 2007;23:397–410.
5. Terada KY, Ahn HJ, Kessel B. Differences in risk for type 1 and type 2 ovarian cancer in a large cancer screening trial. J Gynecol Oncol. 2016;27:e25.
6. Kobayashi H, Ohno S, Sasaki Y, Matsuura M. Hereditary breast and ovarian cancer susceptibility genes. Oncol Rep. 2013;30:1019–29.
7. Morgado M, Sutton MN, Simmons M, Warren CR, Lu Z, Constantinou PE, et al. Tumor necrosis factor-α and interferon-γ stimulate MUC16 (CA125) expression in breast, endometrial and ovarian cancers through NFκB. Oncotarget. 2016;7:14871–84.
8. Jacobs I, Bast RC Jr. The CA 125 tumour-associated antigen: a review of the literature. Hum Reprod. 1989;4:1–12.
9. Jacobs IJ, Skates S, Davies AP, Woolas RP, Jeyerajah A, Weidemann P, et al. Risk of diagnosis of ovarian cancer after raised serum CA 125 concentration: a prospective cohort study. BMJ. 1996;313:1355–8.
10. Skates SJ, Menon U, MacDonald N, Rosenthal AN, Oram DH, Knapp RC, et al. Calculation of the risk of ovarian cancer from serial CA-125 values for preclinical detection in postmenopausal women. J Clin Oncol. 2003;21(10 Suppl):206s–10s.
11. Duffy MJ, Bonfrer JM, Kulpa J, Rustin GJ, Soletormos G, Torre GC, et al. CA125 in ovarian cancer: European group on tumor markers guidelines for clinical use. Int J Gynecol Cancer. 2005;15:679–91.
12. Arakawa N, Miyagi E, Nomura A, Morita E, Ino Y, Ohtake N, et al. Secretome-based identification of TFPI2, a novel serum biomarker for detection of ovarian clear cell adenocarcinoma. J Proteome Res. 2013;12:4340–50.

13. Bourne TH, Campbell S, Reynolds KM, Whitehead MI, Hampson J, Royston P, et al. Screening for early familial ovarian cancer with transvaginal ultrasonography and colour blood flow imaging. BMJ. 1993;306:1025–9.
14. van Nagell JR Jr, PD DP, Reedy MB, Gallion HH, Ueland FR, Pavlik EJ, et al. The efficacy of transvaginal sonographic screening in asymptomatic women at risk for ovarian cancer. Gynecol Oncol. 2000;77:350–6.
15. Menon U, Griffin M, Gentry-Maharaj A. Ovarian cancer screening--current status, future directions. Gynecol Oncol. 2014;132:490–5.
16. Sato S, Yokoyama Y, Sakamoto T, Futagami M, Saito Y. Usefulness of mass screening for ovarian carcinoma using transvaginal ultrasonography. Cancer. 2000;89:582–8.
17. van Nagell JR Jr, PD DP, Ueland FR, CP DS, Cooper AL, JM MD, et al. Ovarian cancer screening with annual transvaginal sonography: findings of 25,000 women screened. Cancer. 2007;109:1887–96.
18. van Nagell JR Jr, Miller RW, CP DS, Ueland FR, Podzielinski I, Goodrich ST, et al. Long-term survival of women with epithelial ovarian cancer detected by ultrasonographic screening. Obstet Gynecol. 2011;118:1212–21.
19. Jacobs I, Stabile I, Bridges J, Kemsley P, Reynolds C, Grudzinskas J, et al. Multimodal approach to screening for ovarian cancer. Lancet. 1988;1:268–71.
20. Jacobs IJ, Skates SJ, MacDonald N, Menon U, Rosenthal AN, Davies AP, et al. Screening for ovarian cancer: a pilot randomised controlled trial. Lancet. 1999;353:1207–10.
21. Kobayashi H, Yamada Y, Sado T, Sakata M, Yoshida S, Kawaguchi R, et al. A randomized study of screening for ovarian cancer: a multicenter study in Japan. Int J Gynecol Cancer. 2008;18:414–20.
22. Buys SS, Partridge E, Greene MH, Prorok PC, Reding D, Riley TL, et al. PLCO Project Team. Ovarian cancer screening in the Prostate, Lung, Colorectal and Ovarian (PLCO) cancer screening trial: findings from the initial screen of a randomized trial. Am J Obstet Gynecol. 2005;193:1630–9.
23. Buys SS, Partridge E, Black A, Johnson CC, Lamerato L, Isaacs C, et al. PLCO Project Team. Effect of screening on ovarian cancer mortality: the Prostate, Lung, Colorectal and Ovarian (PLCO) Cancer Screening Randomized Controlled Trial. JAMA. 2011;305:2295–303.
24. Jacobs IJ, Menon U, Ryan A, Gentry-Maharaj A, Burnell M, Kalsi JK, et al. Ovarian cancer screening and mortality in the UK Collaborative trial of ovarian cancer screening (UKCTOCS): a randomised controlled trial. Lancet. 2016;387:945–56.
25. Skates SJ, Xu FJ, Yu YH, Sjövall K, Einhorn N, Chang Y, et al. Toward an optimal algorithm for ovarian cancer screening with longitudinal tumor markers. Cancer. 1995;76:2004–10.
26. Campeau PM, Foulkes WD, Tischkowitz MD. Hereditary breast cancer: new genetic developments, new therapeutic avenues. Hum Genet. 2008;124:31–42.
27. Chen S, Parmigiani G. Meta-analysis of BRCA1 and BRCA2 penetrance. J Clin Oncol. 2007;25:1329–33.
28. Carlson KJ, Skates SJ, Singer DE. Screening for ovarian cancer. Ann Intern Med. 1994;121:124–32.
29. Kuznia AL, Roett MA. Genital cancers in women: ovarian cancer. FP Essent. 2015;438:24–30.
30. Stan DL, Shuster LT, Wick MJ, Swanson CL, Pruthi S, Bakkum-Gamez JN. Challenging and complex decisions in the management of the BRCA mutation carrier. J Womens Health (Larchmt). 2013;22:825–34.
31. National Comprehensive Cancer Network (NCCN) Clinical practice guidelines in oncology, genetic/familial high-risk assessment: Breast and ovarian. www.nccn.org. [5 Feb 2013]. www.nccn.org.
32. Domchek SM, Friebel TM, Singer CF, Evans DG, Lynch HT, Isaacs C, et al. Association of risk-reducing surgery in BRCA1 or BRCA2 mutation carriers with cancer risk and mortality. JAMA. 2010;304:967–75.
33. King MC, Marks JH, Mandell JB, New York Breast Cancer Study Group. Breast and ovarian cancer risks due to inherited mutations in BRCA1 and BRCA2. Science. 2003;302:643–6.
34. Kurian AW, Sigal BM, Plevritis SK. Survival analysis of cancer risk reduction strategies for BRCA1/2 mutation carriers. J Clin Oncol. 2010;28:222–31.

35. Metcalfe K, Gershman S, Lynch HT, Ghadirian P, Tung N, Kim-Sing C, et al. Predictors of contralateral breast cancer in BRCA1 and BRCA2 mutation carriers. Br J Cancer. 2011;104:1384–92.
36. Pierce LJ, Levin AM, Rebbeck TR, Ben-David MA, Friedman E, Solin LJ, et al. Ten-year multi-institutional results of breast-conserving surgery and radiotherapy in BRCA1/2-associated stage I/II breast cancer. J Clin Oncol. 2006;24:2437–43.
37. Klitzman R, Chung W. The process of deciding about prophylactic surgery for breast and ovarian cancer: patient questions, uncertainties, and communication. Am J Med Genet A. 2010;152A:52–66.
38. Bermejo-Pérez MJ, Márquez-Calderón S, Llanos-Méndez A. Effectiveness of preventive interventions in BRCA1/2 gene mutation carriers: a systematic review. Int J Cancer. 2007;121:225–31.
39. Tobacman JK, Greene MH, Tucker MA, Costa J, Kase R, Fraumeni JF Jr. Intra-abdominal carcinomatosis after prophylactic oophorectomy in ovarian-cancer-prone families. Lancet. 1982;2:795–7.
40. Piver MS, Jishi MF, Tsukada Y, Nava G. Primary peritoneal carcinoma after prophylactic oophorectomy in women with a family history of ovarian cancer. A report of the Gilda Radner familial ovarian cancer registry. Cancer. 1993;71:2751–5.
41. Olivier RI, van Beurden M, Lubsen MA, Rookus MA, Mooij TM, van de Vijver MJ, et al. Clinical outcome of prophylactic oophorectomy in BRCA1/BRCA2 mutation carriers and events during follow-up. Br J Cancer. 2004;90:1492–7.
42. Medeiros F, Muto MG, Lee Y, Elvin JA, Callahan MJ, Feltmate C, et al. The tubal fimbria is a preferred site for early adenocarcinoma in women with familial ovarian cancer syndrome. Am J Surg Pathol. 2006;30:230–6.
43. Kwon JS, Tinker A, Pansegrau G, McAlpine J, Housty M, McCullum M, et al. Prophylactic salpingectomy and delayed oophorectomy as an alternative for BRCA mutation carriers. Obstet Gynecol. 2013;121:14–24.
44. Leblanc E, Narducci F, Farre I, Peyrat JP, Taieb S, Adenis C, et al. Radical fimbriectomy: a reasonable temporary risk-reducing surgery for selected women with a germ line mutation of BRCA 1 or 2 genes? Rationale and preliminary development. Gynecol Oncol. 2011;121:472–6.
45. Harmsen MG, IntHout J, Arts-de Jong M, Hoogerbrugge N, Massuger LF, Hermens RP, et al. Salpingectomy with delayed oophorectomy in BRCA1/2 mutation carriers: estimating ovarian cancer risk. Obstet Gynecol. 2016;127:1054–63.
46. Gilks CB, Irving J, Köbel M, Lee C, Singh N, Wilkinson N, et al. Incidental nonuterine high-grade serous carcinomas arise in the fallopian tube in most cases: further evidence for the tubal origin of high-grade serous carcinomas. Am J Surg Pathol. 2015;39:357–64.
47. Yates MS, Meyer LA, Deavers MT, Daniels MS, Keeler ER, Mok SC, et al. Microscopic and early-stage ovarian cancers in BRCA1/2 mutation carriers: building a model for early BRCA-associated tumorigenesis. Cancer Prev Res (Phila). 2011;4:463–70.
48. McLaughlin JR, Risch HA, Lubinski J, Moller P, Ghadirian P, Lynch H, et al. Hereditary ovarian cancer clinical study group. Reproductive risk factors for ovarian cancer in carriers of BRCA1 or BRCA2 mutations: a case-control study. Lancet Oncol. 2007;8:26–34.
49. Vicus D, Finch A, Rosen B, Fan I, Bradley L, Cass I. Et al; hereditary ovarian cancer clinical study group. Risk factors for carcinoma of the fallopian tube in women with and without a germline BRCA mutation. Gynecol Oncol. 2010;118:155–9.
50. Hermsen BB, Olivier RI, Verheijen RH, van Beurden M, de Hullu JA, Massuger LF, et al. No efficacy of annual gynaecological screening in BRCA1/2 mutation carriers; an observational follow-up study. Br J Cancer. 2007;96:1335–42.
51. Stirling D, Evans DG, Pichert G, Shenton A, Kirk EN, Rimmer S, et al. Screening for familial ovarian cancer: failure of current protocols to detect ovarian cancer at an early stage according to the international federation of gynecology and obstetrics system. J Clin Oncol. 2005;23:5588–96.
52. Havrilesky LJ, Moorman PG, Lowery WJ, Gierisch JM, Coeytaux RR, Urrutia RP, et al. Oral contraceptive pills as primary prevention for ovarian cancer: a systematic review and meta-analysis. Obstet Gynecol. 2013;122:139–47.

53. Walker JL, Powell CB, Chen LM, Carter J, Bae Jump VL, Parker LP, et al. Society of Gynecologic Oncology recommendations for the prevention of ovarian cancer. Cancer. 2015;121:2108–20.
54. Iodice S, Barile M, Rotmensz N, Feroce I, Bonanni B, Radice P, et al. Oral contraceptive use and breast or ovarian cancer risk in BRCA1/2 carriers: a meta-analysis. Eur J Cancer. 2010;46:2275–84.
55. Narod SA, Risch H, Moslehi R, Dørum A, Neuhausen S, Olsson H, et al. Oral contraceptives and the risk of hereditary ovarian cancer. Hereditary Ovarian Cancer Clinical Study Group. N Engl J Med. 1998;339:424–8.
56. Vessey M, Painter R. Oral contraceptive use and cancer. Findings in a large cohort study, 1968-2004. Br J Cancer. 2006;95:385–9.
57. Whittemore AS, Balise RR, Pharoah PD, Dicioccio RA, Oakley-Girvan I, Ramus SJ, et al. Oral contraceptive use and ovarian cancer risk among carriers of BRCA1 or BRCA2 mutations. Br J Cancer. 2004;91:1911–5.
58. Antoniou AC, Rookus M, Andrieu N, Brohet R, Chang-Claude J, Peock S, et al. Reproductive and hormonal factors, and ovarian cancer risk for BRCA1 and BRCA2 mutation carriers: results from the international BRCA1/2 carrier cohort study. Cancer Epidemiol Biomark Prev. 2009;18:601–10.
59. McGuire V, Felberg A, Mills M, Ostrow KL, DiCioccio R, John EM, et al. Relation of contraceptive and reproductive history to ovarian cancer risk in carriers and noncarriers of BRCA1 gene mutations. Am J Epidemiol. 2004;160:613–8.
60. Gierisch JM, Coeytaux RR, Urrutia RP, Havrilesky LJ, Moorman PG, Lowery WJ, et al. Oral contraceptive use and risk of breast, cervical, colorectal, and endometrial cancers: a systematic review. Cancer Epidemiol Biomark Prev. 2013;22:1931–43.
61. Milne RL, Knight JA, John EM, Dite GS, Balbuena R, Ziogas A, et al. Oral contraceptive use and risk of early-onset breast cancer in carriers and noncarriers of BRCA1 and BRCA2 mutations. Cancer Epidemiol Biomark Prev. 2005;14:350–6.
62. Haile RW, Thomas DC, McGuire V, Felberg A, John EM, Milne RL, et al. BRCA1 and BRCA2 mutation carriers, oral contraceptive use, and breast cancer before age 50. Cancer Epidemiol Biomark Prev. 2006;15:1863–70.
63. Cibula D, Zikan M, Dusek L, Majek O. Oral contraceptives and risk of ovarian and breast cancers in BRCA mutation carriers: a meta-analysis. Expert Rev Anticancer Ther. 2011;11:1197–207.
64. Narod SA, Dubé MP, Klijn J, Lubinski J, Lynch HT, Ghadirian P, et al. Oral contraceptives and the risk of breast cancer in BRCA1 and BRCA2 mutation carriers. J Natl Cancer Inst. 2002;94:1773–9.
65. Lee E, Ma H, McKean-Cowdin R, Van Den Berg D, Bernstein L, Henderson BE, et al. Effect of reproductive factors and oral contraceptives on breast cancer risk in BRCA1/2 mutation carriers and noncarriers: results from a population-based study. Cancer Epidemiol Biomark Prev. 2008;17:3170–8.
66. Cortesi L, Razzaboni E, Toss A, De Matteis E, Marchi I, Medici V, et al. A rapid genetic counselling and testing in newly diagnosed breast cancer is associated with high rate of risk-reducing mastectomy in BRCA1/2-positive Italian women. Ann Oncol. 2014;25:57–63.
67. Vogel VG, Costantino JP, Wickerham DL, Cronin WM, Cecchini RS, Atkins JN. Et al; National Surgical Adjuvant Breast and Bowel Project. Update of the National Surgical Adjuvant Breast and Bowel Project study of Tamoxifen and Raloxifene (STAR) P-2 trial: preventing breast cancer. Cancer Prev Res (Phila). 2010;3:696–706.
68. Gronwald J, Tung N, Foulkes WD, Offit K, Gershoni R, Daly M, et al. Hereditary breast cancer clinical study group. Tamoxifen and contralateral breast cancer in BRCA1 and BRCA2 carriers: an update. Int J Cancer. 2006;118:2281–4.
69. Land SR, Wickerham DL, Costantino JP, Ritter MW, Vogel VG, Lee M, et al. Patient-reported symptoms and quality of life during treatment with tamoxifen or raloxifene for breast cancer prevention: the NSABP study of Tamoxifen and Raloxifene (STAR) P-2 trial. JAMA. 2006;295:2742–51.

70. Yoshimoto C, Iwabuchi T, Shigetomi H, Kobayashi H. Cyst fluid iron-related compounds as useful markers to distinguish malignant transformation from benign endometriotic cysts. Cancer Biomark. 2015;15:493–9.
71. Iwabuchi T, Yoshimoto C, Shigetomi H, Kobayashi H. Cyst fluid hemoglobin species in endometriosis and its malignant transformation: the role of metallobiology. Oncol Lett. 2016;11:3384–8. Epub 2016 Mar 29
72. McMurdy JW, Jay GD, Suner S, Crawford G. Noninvasive optical, electrical, and acoustic methods of total hemoglobin determination. Clin Chem. 2008;54:264–72.
73. Crowley C, Montenegro-Bethancourt G, Solomons NW, Schűmann K. Validity and correspondence of non-invasively determined hemoglobin concentrations by two trans-cutaneous digital measuring devices. Asia Pac J Clin Nutr. 2012;21:191–200.
74. Rabe H, Alvarez RF, Whitfield T, Lawson F, Jungmann H. Spectroscopic noninvasive measurement of hemoglobin compared with capillary and venous values in neonates. Neonatology. 2010;98:1–5.
75. Koshiyama M, Matsumura N, Konishi I. Clinical efficacy of ovarian cancer screening. J Cancer. 2016;7:1311–6.

Pathology of Epithelial Ovarian Tumors

5

Hiroyuki Yanai

Abstract

Various types of epithelial tumors occur in the ovary. They are classified according to the phenotype of the tumor cells, patterns of growth, and malignant potential. The major phenotypical categories are serous, mucinous, endometrioid, clear cell, Brenner, and seromucinous tumors. Tumors of each category are subclassified as benign, borderline malignancy/atypical proliferative tumor, or malignant (carcinoma). Phenotypically, tumor cells of serous tumors resemble the tubal epithelium. Tumor cells of mucinous tumors are similar to the gastrointestinal epithelium. Endometrioid and clear cell tumors have epithelium resembling endometrial glandular cells, with the latter recapitulating the morphology of the Arias-Stella reaction. Brenner tumors show characteristics of the urothelium. Seromucinous tumors show proliferation of various types of Müllerian epithelium. Recent studies have revealed the tumorigenesis of each type of ovarian epithelial tumor, thus establishing new concepts of ovarian carcinogenesis. These findings and concepts are reflected in the last (4th) edition of the World Health Organization classification of ovarian tumors. In this chapter, the clinicopathological features, etiology, gross and microscopic features, and certain molecular mechanisms of each type of ovarian epithelial tumor are discussed.

Keywords

Ovary • Borderline tumor • Atypical proliferative tumor • Carcinoma • Histopathology

H. Yanai, M.D., Ph.D.
Department of Pathology, Okayama University Hospital,
2-5-1 Shikata-cho, Kita-ku, Okayama 700-8558, Japan
e-mail: yanaih@md.okayama-u.ac.jp

H. Katabuchi (ed.), *Frontiers in Ovarian Cancer Science*, Comprehensive Gynecology and Obstetrics, DOI 10.1007/978-981-10-4160-0_5

5.1 Introduction

Epithelial tumors are one of the major categories of ovarian tumors, and they account for two thirds of ovarian tumors and 90% of ovarian malignant tumors. Ovarian epithelial tumors are traditionally classified according to morphological features of tumor cells. Recent clinicopathological and molecular studies reveal that morphologically different tumors associate with different origin and molecular mechanisms and support validity of the principle of classification. As each type of carcinoma shows different clinical behavior and response to therapy, correct histological diagnosis is essential to effective treatment. In this chapter, pathological features of each type of tumors are discussed.

5.2 Classification and Nomenclature of Epithelial Ovarian Tumors

Ovarian epithelial tumors are classified according to three aspects: tumor cell phenotype, pattern of growth, and malignant potential. In the 4th edition of the World Health Organization (WHO) classification of ovarian tumors, epithelial tumors are classified into serous, mucinous, endometrioid, clear cell, Brenner, seromucinous, and undifferentiated tumors according to the tumor cell types [1]. For a predominantly cystic ovarian epithelial tumor, the prefix "cysto" is applied, while tumors with prominent fibrous proliferation have the suffix "firoma." Tumors with both of cystic and fibrous components are described as "cystadenofibroma." Occasionally, serous tumors show surface exophytic proliferation, and such tumor is described as "surface papilloma" or with the term "surface papillary."

In view of malignant potential, each type of ovarian epithelial tumor is further subclassified as benign, borderline/atypical proliferative, and malignant (carcinoma). Principally, carcinomas are defined as epithelial tumors with destructive invasion, while borderline/atypical proliferative tumors have clinicopathological features that are intermediate between clearly benign tumors and clearly malignant tumors. Some pathologists prefer "atypical proliferative tumors" because of favorable prognosis after excluding tumors with special types of proliferation. Historically, various terms such as "tumor of low malignant potential" and "semimalignant tumor" have also been applied for this category; however, these terms are not recommended in modern practice.

Although several grading systems have been proposed for ovarian cancer, there is no unified grading system, which is applicable to all types of ovarian cancer. For ovarian endometrioid carcinoma, the grading system of endometrial endometrioid carcinoma, which is defined by proportion of solid growth, is applied. Since low-grade and high-grade serous carcinomas have their own precursor lesions and molecular abnormalities, these two tumors are different type of carcinomas rather than different grade of a single entity.

5.3 Origin of Ovarian Epithelial Tumors

Historically, it has been believed that most ovarian epithelial tumors are derived from ovarian surface epithelium (OSE), also known as surface epithelium or germinal epithelium. Congenital rests were also thought to be a possible origin of epithelial tumors.

Recently, thorough examination of prophylactically resected ovaries and fallopian tubes of women who have a germline mutation of *BRCA* genes revealed that early serous carcinomas are present in the fallopian tubes, not in the ovaries [2]. Some of these carcinomas are noninvasive and designated as "serous tubal intraepithelial carcinomas (STICs)" (Fig. 5.1). STICs have been shown to accompany ovarian or pelvic high-grade serous carcinoma in women without any BRCA mutation [3–6]. As STICs and accompanying serous carcinomas share the same *TP53* mutation, STICs are accepted as the precursor lesions of high-grade serous carcinoma [4]. An immunohistochemical study of the fallopian tubes revealed epithelial foci of p53 overexpression without cellular atypia and proliferative activities (Fig. 5.2). Such foci were designated as "p53 signature" and considered to be the earliest event of serous carcinogenesis. p53 signatures were also observed in women without *BRCA* mutations [3]. About 60% of p53 signature harbor mutation of *TP53* [3].

Ovarian inclusion cysts have previously been considered to be precursors of serous cystadenoma or serous borderline tumors. Recently, however, it has been suggested that some inclusion cysts are derived from implanted tubal epithelium, not from ovarian surface cells [7]. Since aneuploidy of inclusion cyst epithelium is frequently associated with serous borderline tumors, inclusion cysts could be precursor of serous borderline tumors [8]. Moreover, some investigators propose that high-grade serous carcinoma could also originate from inclusion cysts. Together, these observations and hypotheses suggest that at least some serous tumors are ultimately derived from tubal epithelium.

Abovementioned "tubal origin" theory of ovarian tumorigenesis cannot explain origin of all serous tumors because some of them lack tubal precursor lesions instead of exhaustive search. Some researchers have claimed that some ovarian epithelial tumors derived from OSE or inclusion cysts derived from invaginated OSE [9]. Since both OSE and Müllerian epithelium develop from coelomic epithelium, it is thought that OSE has the ability to differentiate Müllerian epithelium and transform to epithelial tumors. Some morphological and immunohistochemical observations support this metaplasia and transformation theory. In addition, animal models with genetic alterations showed induction of carcinoma from OSE.

Another possible origin of ovarian epithelial tumors is epithelium of endometriosis. Strong association between endometrioid, clear, and seromucinous tumors and endometriosis has been described, resulting in these tumors being designated as endometriosis-related ovarian neoplasms (ERONs) [10]. Endometriosis with cellular atypia (atypical endometriosis) is thought to be a precursor of ERONs. *ARID1A* mutation is frequently detected among ERONs in whole genome analysis; for

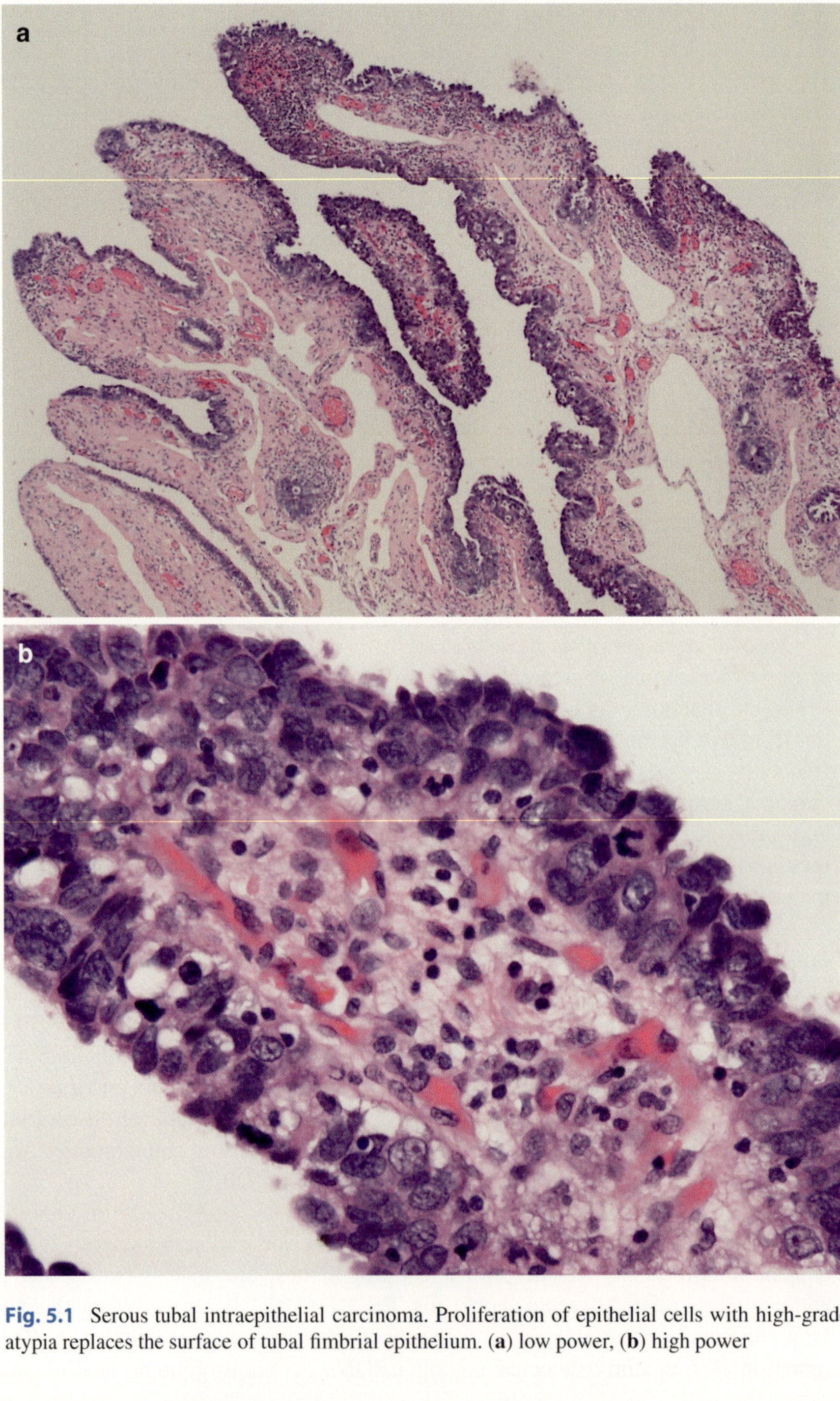

Fig. 5.1 Serous tubal intraepithelial carcinoma. Proliferation of epithelial cells with high-grade atypia replaces the surface of tubal fimbrial epithelium. (**a**) low power, (**b**) high power

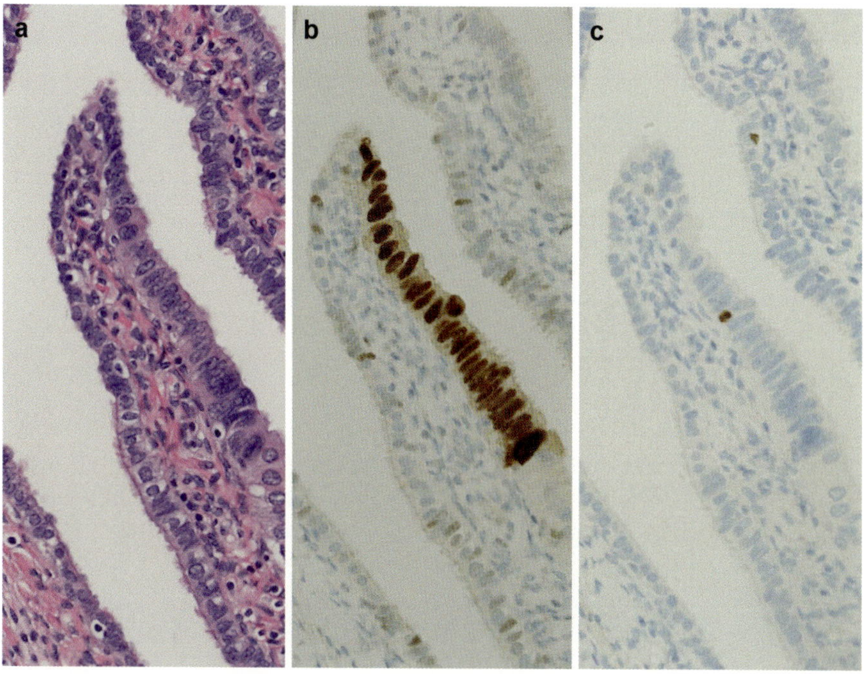

Fig. 5.2 p53 signature. The fimbrial epithelium without nuclear atypia (**a**) has focus of continuous p53 positivity (**b**). Ki-67 positive cells are not increased (**c**)

example, 50% of clear cell carcinomas (CCCs) and 40% of endometrioid carcinoma have this mutation [11, 12]. One immunohistochemical study showed that 33% of seromucinous borderline tumor might harbor an *ARID1A* mutation [13]. *ARID1A* encodes the protein BAF250a, a subunit of switch/sucrose non-fermentable (SWI/SNF) complex, which binds to AT-rich DNA sequences, and participates in chromatin remodeling and regulation of gene transcription. Mutation of *ARID1A* results in defective BAF250a and loss of function as tumor suppressor molecule. Since mutation of *ARID1A* is observed in epithelium of atypical or normal-appearing endometriosis adjacent to ERONs, it might be an early event of ERON tumorigenesis [12].

Although the histogenesis of mucinous tumors is uncertain, their association with teratomas and Brenner tumors sheds light on their origin. Fujii et al. conducted molecular study of mucinous tumors associated with teratomas and showed that these tumors are derived from germ cells [14]. Frequent coexistence of mucinous and Brenner tumors suggests a possible common origin. Some studies showed that Brenner tumors and associated mucinous tumor harbored identical gene mutations and suggested that some mucinous tumors developed from Brenner tumors [15–17] (see also Sects. 3.1.2 and 3.4.4 in Chap. 3).

5.4 Serous Tumors

Serous tumors are composed of an epithelium resembling the fallopian tube epithelium and often have psammoma bodies. Serous tumors are the most common ovarian epithelial tumors; in the Western world, approximately 60% are benign, 10% borderline, and 30% carcinoma [18]. Nakashima et al. reported the same distribution for patients in a Japanese institute [19].

5.4.1 Benign Serous Tumors

Serous adenomas occur in women of a wide age range. Most serous adenomas are uni- or oligolocular cystic tumors (serous cystadenoma). Sometimes, they show surface papillary growth (serous surface papilloma) or have a prominent solid fibrous component (serous adenofibroma). Usually, tumors are less than 10 cm in size. Inner surface of cysts is usually flat or shows low elevated nodules. Differentiation between ovarian inclusion cysts and serous cystadenomas is arbitrary, and cystic lesions with tubal-type epithelium larger than 1 cm are diagnosed as serous cystadenomas [1].

Microscopically, a single layer of cuboidal to low columnar epithelium lines the inner surface. Some tumor cells have cilia on their surface (Fig. 5.3). Papillary

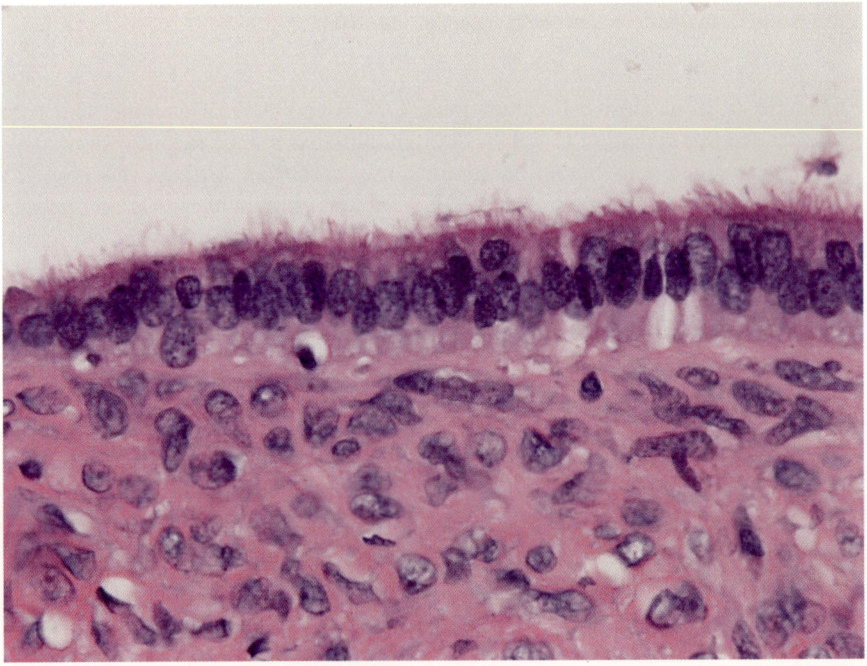

Fig. 5.3 Serous adenoma. The inner surface of cystic tumor is lined by single layer of ciliated epithelium

proliferation of less than 10% of the tumor area is compatible with benign serous tumors. The stromal component of adenofibroma is composed of spindle cells without remarkable cellular atypia.

Benign serous tumors present with characters of tubal epithelium. Like tubal epithelium, tumor cells are cytokeratin (CK) 7 positive and CK20 negative; they are also estrogen receptor (ER) and progesterone receptor (PR) positive in most cases. Like tubal epithelium, serous tumors express WT1.

Most serous adenomas are polyclonal and lack mutation of *KRAS* or *BRAF* genes. Large serous adenomas tend to be monoclonal [20].

5.4.2 Serous Borderline Tumor/Atypical Proliferative Serous Tumor

A serous borderline tumor/atypical proliferative tumor (SBT/APT) is characterized by proliferative activity between clearly benign and clearly malignant tumors and the absence of frank stromal invasion. The mean age of patients is 42 years [21]. SBT/APTs are histologically classified as either usual or micropapillary type. Since micropapillary SBTs are more frequently associated with extraovarian invasive implants and poorer outcome than usual SBT/APTs [22], some investigators have proposed that these tumors should be diagnosed as noninvasive serous carcinomas. On the other hand, others claim that a micropapillary pattern is not in itself an independent prognostic factor [21]. In the WHO classification 2014, the term noninvasive low-grade serous carcinoma (LGSC) is used as a synonym of micropapillary SBT.

5.4.2.1 Usual Serous Borderline Tumor/Atypical Proliferative Serous Tumor

Usual SBTs/APTs have papillary excrescence as intracystic or surface papillary pattern, or both. They have hierarchical papillary proliferation of cuboidal to low columnar cells with some ciliated cells resembling the fallopian tube epithelium and large cells with eosinophilic cytoplasm (Fig. 5.4). Atypia is mild to moderate and mitotic figures are rare.

Immunohistochemically, the tumor cells are positive for ER, PR, WT1, and PAX8. Unlike high-grade serous carcinomas (HGSCs), SBT/APTs do not harbor a *TP53* mutation, and p53 immunoreactivity of these tumors is weak and patchy (wild-type pattern). SBTs/APTs also show patchy or focal expression of p16 [23].

5.4.2.2 Micropapillary Variant Serous Borderline Tumor (Noninvasive Low-Grade Serous Carcinoma)

Micropapillary proliferation in SBTs is defined as long (fivefold longer than the width) non-hierarchical papillary growth directly arising from the thick stalks or inner surface of the cyst (Fig. 5.5). This pattern of growth is known as the filigree or medusa head pattern. Cribriform growth in a similar pattern also constitutes part of the micropapillary pattern. A micropapillary component larger than 5 mm in

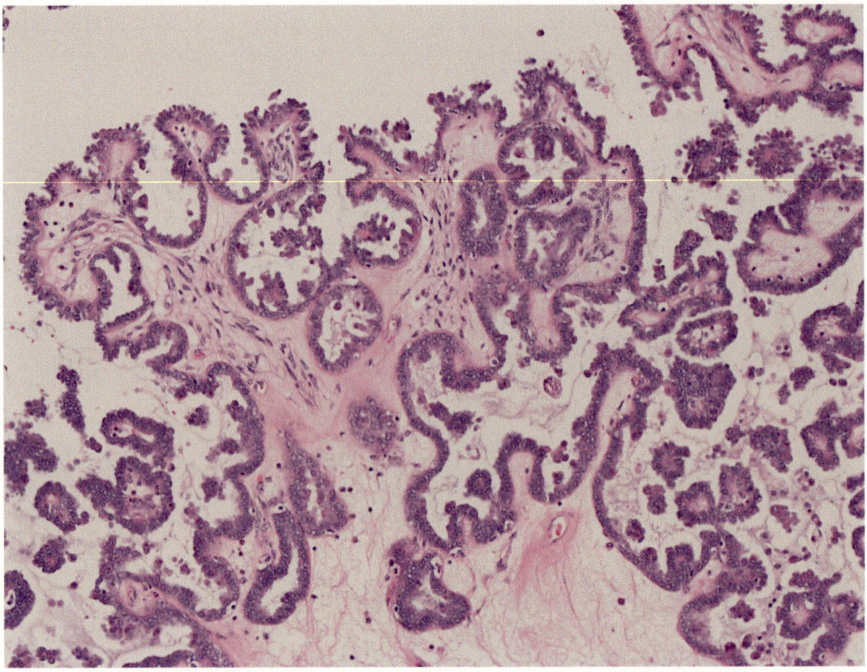

Fig. 5.4 Serous borderline tumor, usual type. The tumor shows hierarchical papillary growth

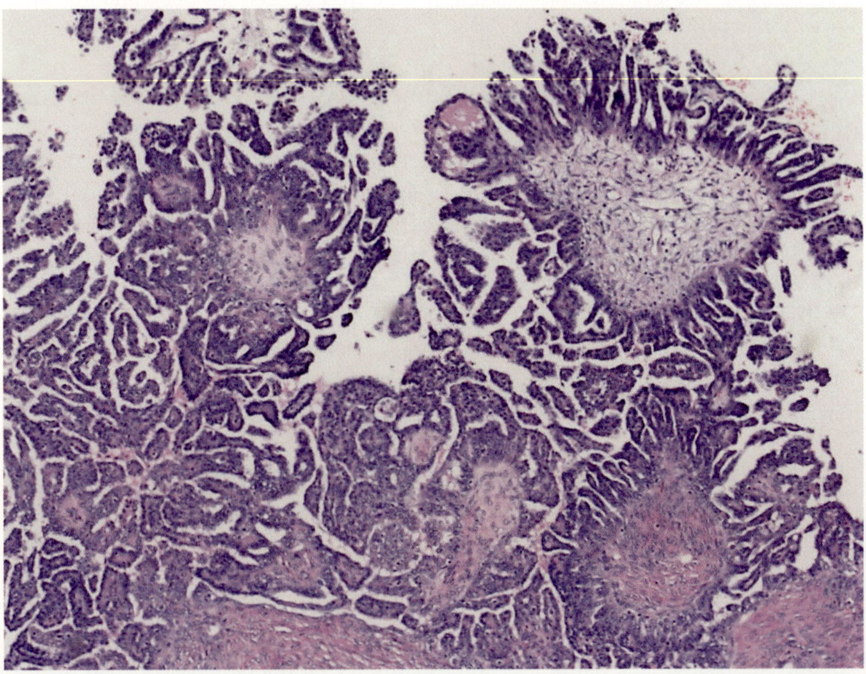

Fig. 5.5 Micropapillary variant of serous borderline tumor/noninvasive low-grade serous carcinoma. The tumor shows non-hierarchical, filigree pattern

one dimension warrants a diagnosis of micropapillary SBT. Micropapillary SBTs are composed of uniform small and cuboidal to low columnar cells, and ciliated cells are rare. Their immunohistochemical findings are almost identical to usual SBTs/APTs.

5.4.2.3 Serous Borderline Tumor with Microinvasive Components

About 10% of all SBTs/APTs have foci of minute stromal invasion. Microinvasion, that is, invasive lesions less than 5 mm in size, is acceptable with a diagnosis of SBT/APT. Microinvasive lesions are further subclassified into two categories according to histological findings [24]. The first is classical microinvasion, which is characterized by individual or a small cluster of eosinophilic cells in the stroma that are terminally differentiated or in senescence (Fig. 5.6) [25]. This pattern of microinvasion is not associated with an aggressive course, whereas the second pattern, which is characterized by complex, branching micropapillae embedded in the stroma and surrounded by a cleft, has an unfavorable prognosis. Histological similarity and unfavorable prognosis has led some pathologists to propose that the second pattern of microinvasion is a small LGSC component and should be diagnosed as an SBT/APT with microinvasive carcinoma [26].

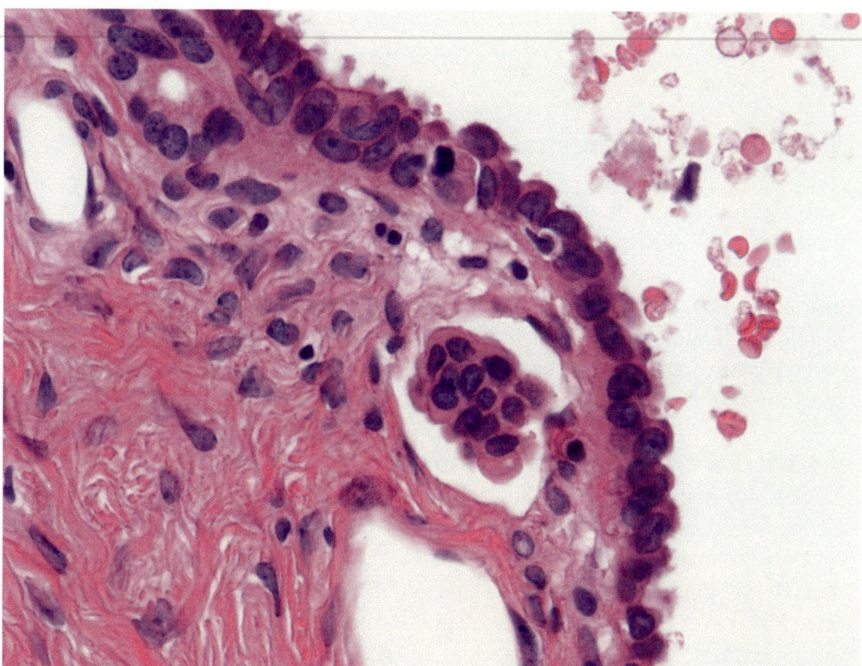

Fig. 5.6 Microinvasion of serous borderline tumor. A small cluster of eosinophilic cells is seen in the stroma

5.4.2.4 Extraovarian Spread of Serous Borderline Tumor

Peritoneal Implants

Peritoneal lesions of SBTs are found in 30–40% of ovarian SBT/APTs and have been called as implants. Histologically, implants are classified into noninvasive or invasive implants [27, 28]. Noninvasive implants show well-circumscribed proliferation of epithelium limited to the surface of peritoneum or septa of the omental adipose tissue. According to the absence or presence of the desmoplastic reaction, noninvasive implants are further classified into "epithelial-type" and "desmoplastic-type" implant. Invasive implants are characterized by haphazard, destructive infiltration of tumor cells into the underlying structure. Solid cell nests or papillae in the stroma with surrounding retraction artifacts and micropapillary proliferation are also considered to be invasive implants by some pathologists [27, 28]. SBTs/APTs with invasive implants should be diagnosed as LGSCs, since their clinical behaviors resemble each other.

Lymph Node Involvement

Lymph node involvement (LNI) has been reported in about 30% of SBT/APT patients who have undergone lymph node dissection. Mostly, LNI presents as isolated cells, cell clusters, small papillae, papillae, or cribriform glands. LNI as simple cysts composed of single layer of tubal type cells is termed endosalpingiosis. The presence of LNI does not affect the clinical course. Rarely, LGSC-like lesions replace nodal parenchyma, and such cases should be diagnosed as LGSCs.

5.4.3 Serous Carcinoma

Serous carcinoma is the most common type of ovarian carcinoma and accounts for more than 50% of ovarian cancers. According to Japanese statistics, 35% of ovarian malignancies are serous carcinoma. In the 4th edition of the WHO classification of ovarian tumors, serous carcinoma is subclassified as LGSC and HGSC. Since their histological features, molecular abnormalities, and precursor lesion are different, these two types of carcinoma are separated disease entities and not within the same disease spectrum. Rare cases of transformation of LGSCs to HGSC have been reported [29].

5.4.3.1 Low-Grade Serous Carcinoma

LGSCs are rare carcinomas that account for about 5% of all serous carcinomas. LGSCs are composed of tumor cells with low-grade atypia and low mitotic index (usually less than 12 per 10 high power fields). LGSC patients are typically younger than HGSC patients (mean, 41.7 years vs. 55 years) [30]. An association between 60 to 80% cases of LGSCs and usual and/or micropapillary SBT/APTs supports the theory that SBT/APTs are precursor of LGSCs [30–32].

LGSCs resemble SBTs/APSTs macroscopically. Histologically, LGSCs show characteristic invasive patterns such as micro- or macropapillae, or compact cell nests surrounded by clefts between the tumor cells and stroma. Less commonly, cribriform, glandular and/or cystic, solid sheets with slit-like spaces or single cells are seen.

Immunohistochemically, tumor cells are positive for ER, PR, WT1, and PAX8. Unlike HGSCs, LGSCs show wild-type p53 immunoreactivity and a negative/patch pattern of p16 expression [23].

Differential diagnosis of LGSCs includes SBT/APT with microinvasion and HGSC. Distinction between LGSCs and SBTs/APTs with microinvasion depends on the pattern and size of the invasive lesion. If each invasive focus shows LGSC-like invasive pattern and is less than 5 mm in size, a diagnosis of SBT/APT with microinvasive carcinoma should be made. It should be noted that some HGSCs show an invasive micropapillary pattern resembling LGSCs. In this situation, nuclear atypia and mitotic figure counts should be evaluated carefully. Immunohistochemical studies of p53 expression are useful since most HGSCs show an aberrant p53 expression pattern (see section of HGSCs), while LGSCs do not [23].

5.4.3.2 High-Grade Serous Carcinoma

HGSCs show a predilection for older patients and are detected at an advanced stage. Macroscopically, HGSCs are solid, cystic, or mixed. Histologically, they show proliferation of highly atypical tumor cells with various histological patterns including solid, papillary, glandular, and transitional cell-like patterns (Fig. 5.7). Nuclei have coarsely vesicular chromatin and prominent nucleoli. Many mitotic figures are observed.

Thorough examination of fimbria reveals that about half cases of HGSCs are accompanied with serous tubal intraepithelial carcinoma.

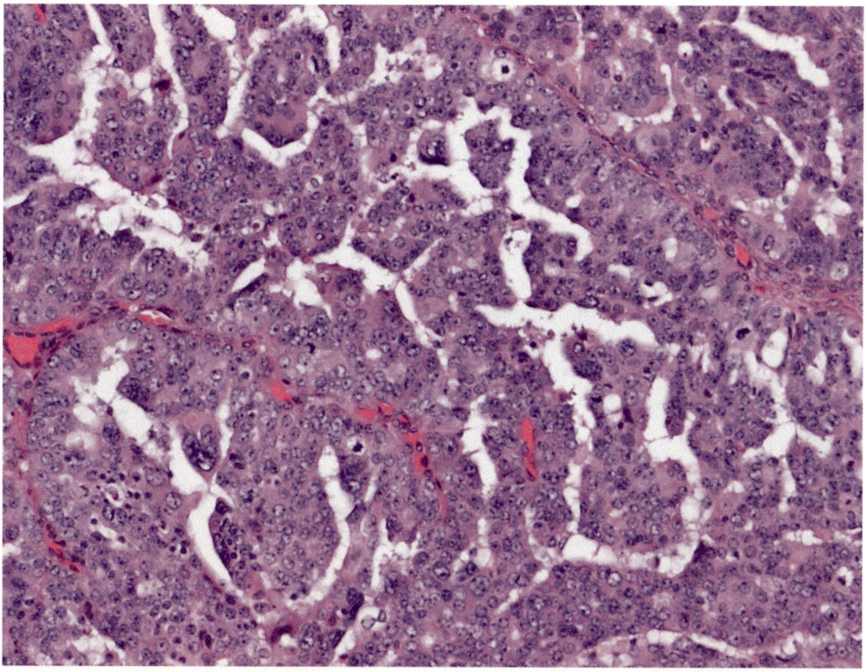

Fig. 5.7 High-grade serous carcinoma (HGSC). The tumor cells have highly atypical nucleus. Slit-like lumen is characteristic for HGSC

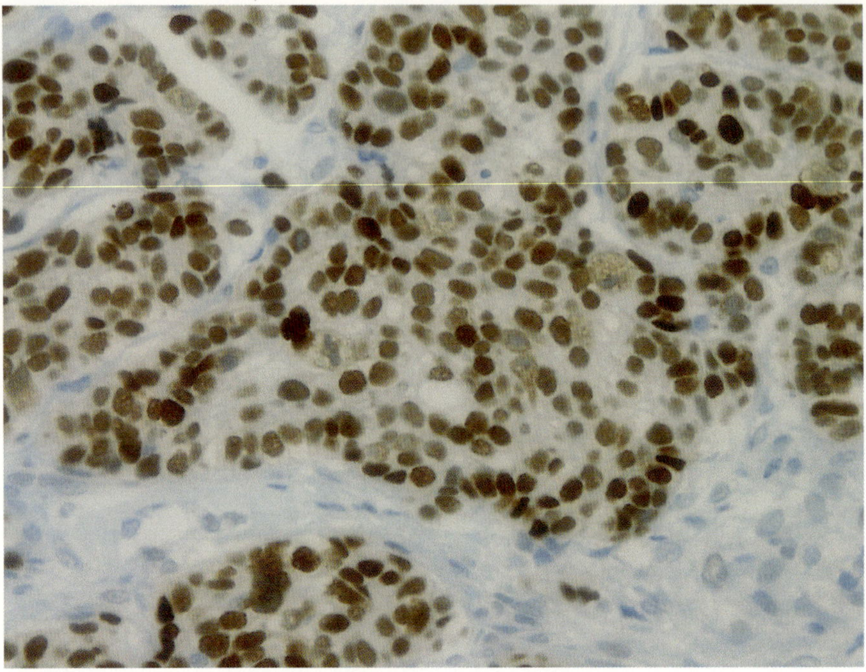

Fig. 5.8 Aberrant p53 expression in high-grade serous carcinoma (HGSC). Diffuse and strong positivity of p53 immunohistochemistry suggest mutation of *TP53*

Immunohistochemically, HGSCs are positive for CK7 but negative for CK20. Most cases are positive for WT1 and PAX8 and show variable positivity for ER and PR. As most HGSCs harbor the *TP53* mutation, the p53 protein expression pattern in HGSCs is diffuse and strongly positive (Fig. 5.8) or completely negative ("null") [23].

Other types of ovarian cancers should be distinguished from HGSC. Some HGSCs show glandular proliferation of columnar cells and resemble endometrioid carcinoma, but HGSCs usually have aberrant p53 expression and are positive for WT1, while endometrioid carcinomas show a wild-type p53 immunostaining pattern and are WT1 negative. Sometime, HGSCs show papillary growth of clear cells, and, hence, clear cell carcinoma has to be included in the differential diagnosis. Differential diagnosis between HGSCs with clear cells and clear cell carcinoma is discussed in the section of clear cell carcinoma (please see Sect. 5.7.2 of this chapter).

5.5 Mucinous Tumors

Mucinous tumors are epithelial tumors composed of gastrointestinal-type mucinous epithelium. Goblet cells, Paneth cells, and neuroendocrine cells also appear in mucinous tumors. Previously, tumors with mucinous epithelium resembling the endocervix have been included among mucinous tumors. However, in the 4th edition of WHO classification, these are designated as seromucinous tumors.

Although mucinous tumors are more frequent in older patients, they are also more common in children and adolescents than other types of ovarian epithelial tumors.

Usually, mucinous tumors are large, multilocular cystic tumors. Most cases are unilateral. The tumor size is not associated with the malignant potential. Since the coexistence of tumor components of different malignancy is not unusual in mucinous tumors, careful gross observation and adequate sampling are keys to accurate histological diagnosis. Mucinous tumors less than 10 cm in greatest dimension require one section per 1 cm, but larger tumors or those with microinvasion or intraepithelial carcinoma require two sections per cm [33]. As most malignant components tend to be small cystic or solid, such area should be extensively sampled at the time of dissection.

5.5.1 Mucinous Cystadenoma/Adenofibroma

These tumors are composed of cyst of various sizes or glands lined with a single layer of columnar epithelium containing intracytoplasmic mucin (Fig. 5.9). Goblet cells are often observed. Mucinous adenofibromas contain solid fibrous stroma. Tumors with papillary proliferation of epithelium, which occupy less than 10% of the tumor, are classified into this category.

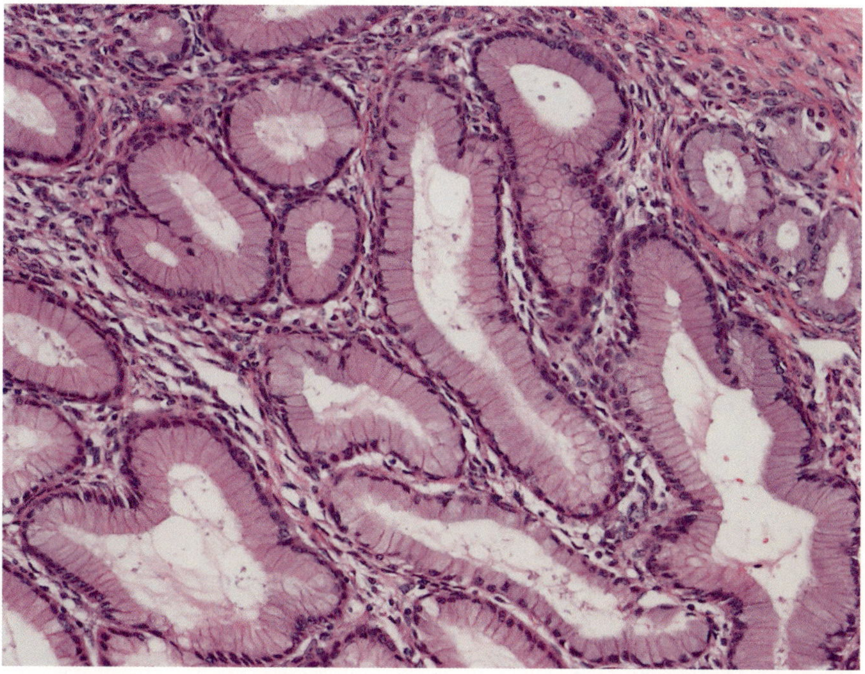

Fig. 5.9 Mucinous adenoma. Columnar epithelium with abundant intracytoplasmic mucin forms glands. Cellular atypia is mild

5.5.2 Mucinous Borderline Tumor/Atypical Proliferative Mucinous Tumor (MBT/APMT)

The characteristic feature of MBT/APMT is papillary proliferation of epithelium associated with mild to moderate nuclear atypia (Figs. 5.10 and 5.11). Foci of marked cellular atypia in MBT/APMT are designated as intraepithelial carcinoma. Stromal invasion of less than 5 mm in maximal linear dimension is defined as microinvasion, and tumors with this feature are designated as MBT/APMT with microinvasion. In these tumors, the microinvasive component with marked cellular atypia is classified as microinvasive carcinoma. A tumor stage ≥IC, intraepithelial carcinoma, microinvasion, and patient age of less than 45 years are associated with tumor recurrence [34].

5.5.3 Mucinous Carcinoma

Mucinous carcinoma is a malignant tumor, comprising of gastrointestinal-type mucinous epithelium. Mucinous carcinoma is usually unilateral, and advanced stage disease is rare [35].

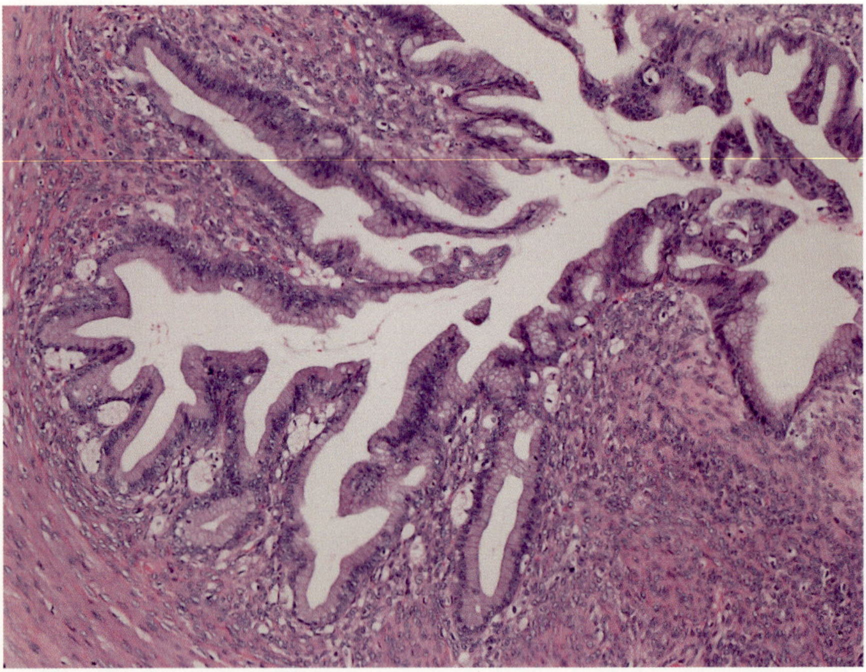

Fig. 5.10 Mucinous borderline tumor. The tumor shows complex papillary growth of mucinous epithelium

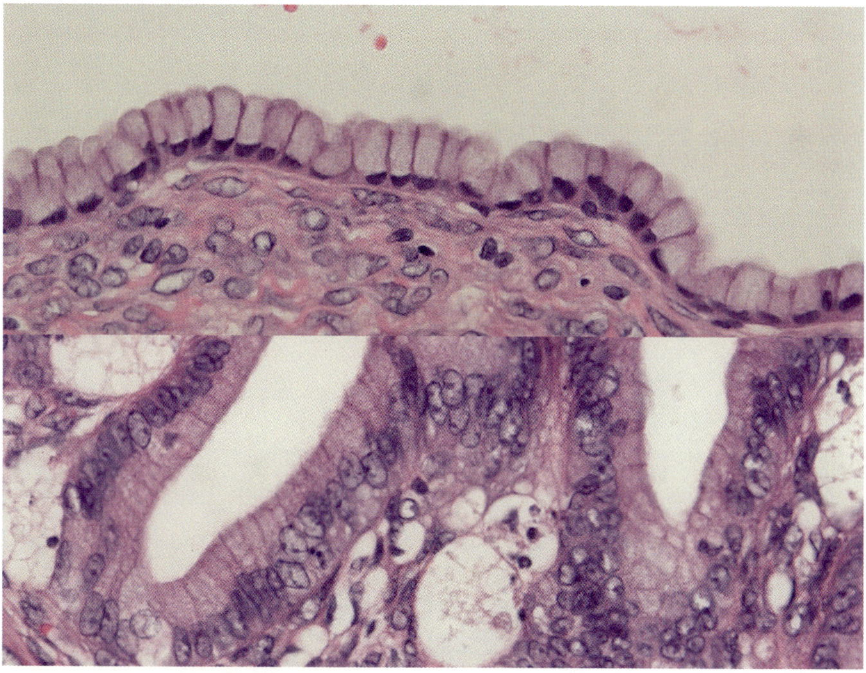

Fig. 5.11 Mucinous borderline tumor. In contrast to benign mucinous tumors (*upper*), tumor cells of borderline tumors (*lower*) show nuclear atypia that is short for diagnosis of carcinoma

Two types of stromal invasion are recognized for mucinous carcinoma: confluent invasion and destructive invasion. Confluent or expansile invasion (Fig. 5.12) is defined as marked glandular crowding or cribriform growth of mucinous epithelium with significant cellular atypia. Such an area should be larger than 5 mm to make a diagnosis of carcinoma. The destructive stromal invasive pattern (Fig. 5.13) is characterized by proliferation of glands with irregular shape in haphazard arrangement in usually desmoplastic stroma.

Mucinous tumor cells are diffusely positive for CK7 and show variable positivity for CK20. Positivity of CDX2 expression also varies [36], while ER and PR are usually negative. PAX8 is positive in about half the cases [37]. A recent study showed that the expression of SATB2, a transcription regulator expressed in colorectal normal epithelium and carcinoma, is negative in primary ovarian mucinous carcinoma [38].

The most critical differential diagnosis of mucinous carcinoma is metastatic adenocarcinoma, especially of colonic or pancreatobiliary origin. Some metastatic adenocarcinomas are similar to primary ovarian mucinous tumors both macroscopically and microscopically. Bilaterality, small size (<10 cm), multinodular growth, hilar involvement, and the International Federation of Gynecology and Obstetrics (FIGO) stage III or IV suggest metastatic carcinoma [39]. Although both histological and immunohistochemical findings may help differential diagnosis, there is overlapping immunoreactivity [40]. For accurate diagnosis, histological findings, as

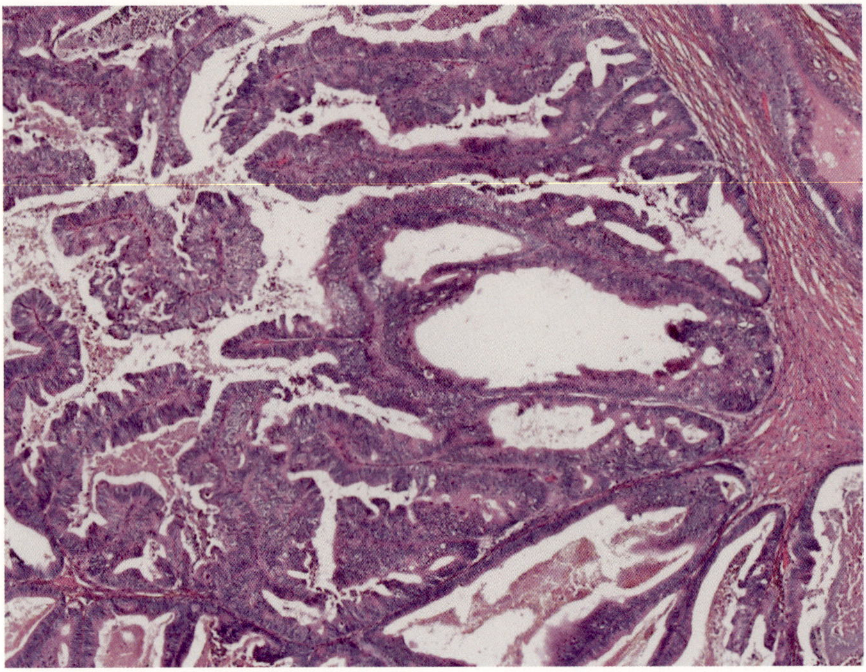

Fig. 5.12 Mucinous carcinoma with expansile invasion. Marked crowding of glands and severe nuclear atypia warrant the diagnosis of mucinous carcinoma

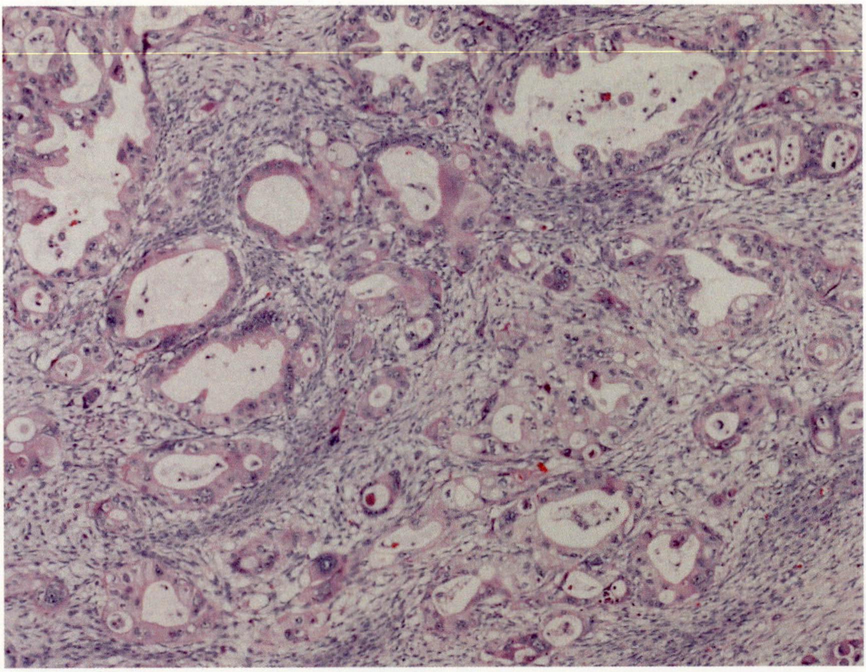

Fig. 5.13 Mucinous carcinoma with destructive invasion. Highly atypical mucinous glands proliferate haphazardly

well careful search of medical history, are essential. Even with no history of carcinoma, a systemic workup is highly recommended for patients whose tumor shows histological features characteristic of metastatic tumors.

5.5.4 Mucinous Tumor with Mural Nodule

MBTs/APMTs or mucinous carcinomas rarely have well-demarcated mural nodules. Histologically, three types of mural nodules have been described: reactive sarcoma-like mural nodules (SLMNs), anaplastic carcinoma, and sarcomatous nodules. Different types of mural nodules may be seen in a single tumor. SLMNs are composed of epulis-type giant cells, atypical spindle cells, and inflammatory cells. The SLMN cells are weakly/focally positive for cytokeratin and positive for vimentin and CD68. Mucinous tumors with SLMN are almost always detected in stage Ia, and the prognosis is favorable [41]. Anaplastic carcinomatous nodule shows sheet of highly atypical rhabdoid, spindle, or pleomorphic epithelial cells. In contrast to SLMN, anaplastic carcinoma cells are definitely positive for cytokeratin. Although the prognosis of mucinous tumors with anaplastic carcinomatous mural nodules is favorable in unruptured stage Ia cases, these tumors are often associated with extraovarian spreading, which usually predicts a poor prognosis [42]. Sarcomatous nodules may appear as fibrosarcomas, rhabdomyosarcomas, or undifferentiated sarcomas.

5.6 Endometrioid Tumors

Endometrioid tumors are defined as tumor with proliferation of endometrial-like epithelium. Most endometrioid tumors are malignant—benign and borderline endometrioid tumors are quite rare.

5.6.1 Benign Endometrioid Tumor

In the 4th edition of the WHO classification, endometriotic cysts are classified as benign endometrioid tumors. Endometrioid cystadenomas and adenofibromas show proliferation of endometrial-type epithelium without endometrial-type stroma.

5.6.2 Endometrioid Borderline Tumor/Atypical Proliferative Endometrioid Tumor

Endometrioid borderline tumors/atypical proliferative endometrioid tumors (EBTs/APETs) show intracystic or adenofibromatous growth. Tumor glands with mild to moderate cellular atypia show fused or confluent proliferation. Squamous differentiation or morula formation is not uncommon. By definition, borderline tumors lack more than 5 mm of confluent or infiltrative growth of the glands.

5.6.3 Endometrioid Carcinoma

Endometrioid carcinomas display proliferation of endometrial gland epithelium. Coexistence of endometriosis or endometriotic cysts has been reported in 9 to 70% of cases. Peak incidence is in the fifth and sixth decades of life. Uterine endometrial endometrioid carcinomas coexist in 15–20% of patients with ovarian endometrioid carcinoma [43].

A typical endometrioid carcinoma has confluent glandular, cribriform, and papillary proliferation of columnar cells (Fig. 5.14). Destructive infiltrative growth is also seen. Squamous differentiation is seen in 30–50% of cases. Squamous components are often in the form of morules (Fig. 5.15). The secretory variant of endometrioid carcinoma is characterized by cytoplasmic sub- and supranuclear vacuoles resembling early secretory phase endometrial glands. Ciliated variant is characterized by cilia on the luminal surface of the tumor cells. Oxyphilic variant has cells with abundant eosinophilic granular cytoplasm and centrally located nucleus. Spindle cell variants display proliferation of spindle-shaped epithelial cells. Occasionally, endometrioid carcinoma shows trabecular or small glandular

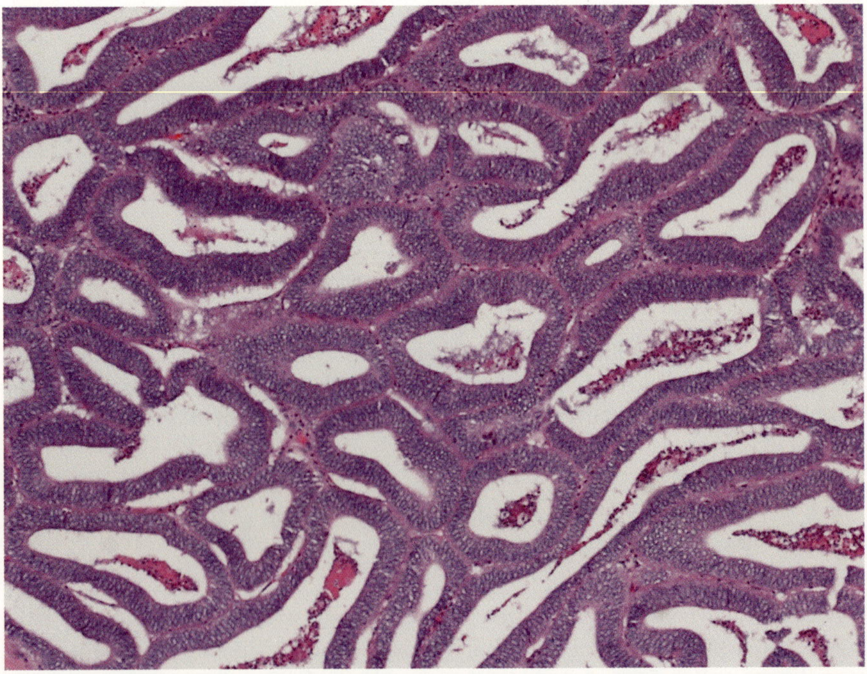

Fig. 5.14 Endometrioid carcinoma. Well-formed glands with columnar cells show confluent growth without intervening stroma

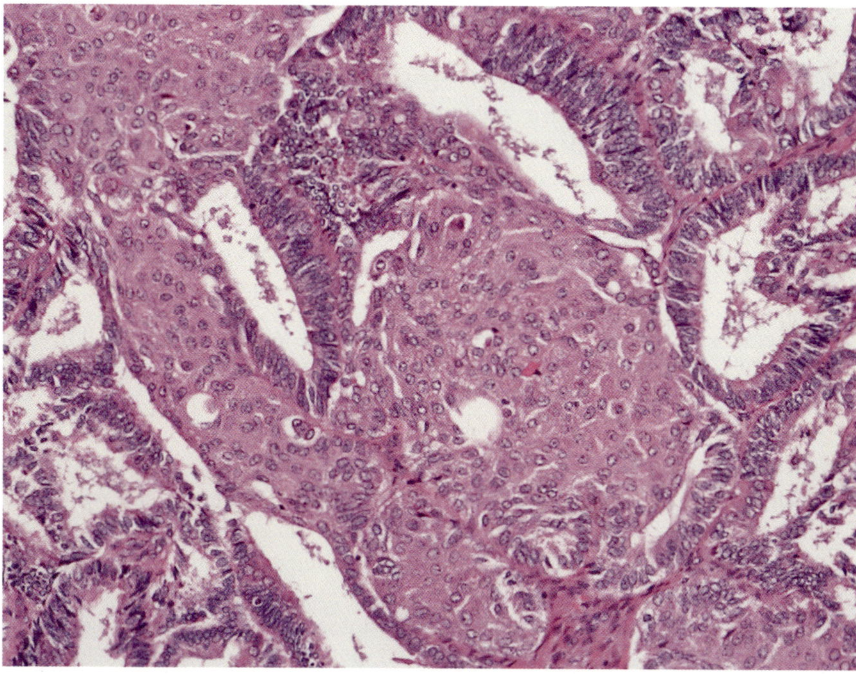

Fig. 5.15 Endometrioid carcinoma. Morula occupies the lumen of glands

pattern resembling sex cord tumors such as adult-type granulosa cell tumors or Sertoli cell tumors.

Endometrioid carcinoma cells express cytokeratin, vimentin, ER, and PR. Tumor with a *CTNNB1*mutation shows nuclear localization of β-catenin. About 30% of ovarian endometrioid carcinomas harbor the *ARID1A* gene mutation and show loss of BAF250a immunoreactivity [12]. Some carcinomas histologically resembling endometrioid carcinoma show aberrant p53 expression. Such tumors, especially in association with WT1 expression and high-grade atypia, should be diagnosed as HGSCs [44].

When ovarian endometrioid carcinoma is associated with uterine endometrioid carcinoma, differential diagnosis whether ovarian tumor is primary or metastatic is important. Diagnostic criteria including several factors such as tumor size, laterality, depth of invasion of uterine myometrium, background lesions (e.g., endometriosis in ovaries, atypical endometrial hyperplasia in endometrium), and molecular abnormalities have been proposed [43].

5.7 Clear Cell Tumors

Clear cell tumors present proliferation of epithelium with clear or eosinophilic cytoplasm. Some tumor cells have a hobnail appearance. These cytological features are similar to endometrial epithelium in the Arias-Stella reaction. Most clear cell tumors are malignant; benign and borderline tumors are rare.

5.7.1 Benign Clear Cell Tumor and Borderline Tumor

Benign and borderline clear cell tumors are extremely rare. Most tumors have an adenofibromatous appearance with round glands of various sizes embedded in fibrous stroma. Up to moderate nuclear atypia is observed in borderline tumors. By definition, stromal invasion of more than 5 mm is absent.

5.7.2 Clear Cell Carcinoma

CCCs comprise about 10% of ovarian cancers in the Western world [45]. In Japan, about 25% of ovarian cancers are CCCs, which is a higher proportion than in other Asian countries or among Asian women living in the USA [46, 47]. Most CCC patients are diagnosed during their fifth to seventh decades. In a Japanese multicentric study, the average patient age was 52.4 years (range, 23–73 years) [48].

Macroscopically, most CCCs are unilateral and frequently cystic with several intracystic polypoid masses of various sizes. Some can be predominantly solid. The cysts contain serous or mucinous fluid and can be hemorrhagic when the tumor is associated with an endometriotic cyst.

CCCs are characterized by a variety of histological patterns including papillary, tubulocystic, and solid patterns (Fig. 5.16) and are often admixed. The nuclear

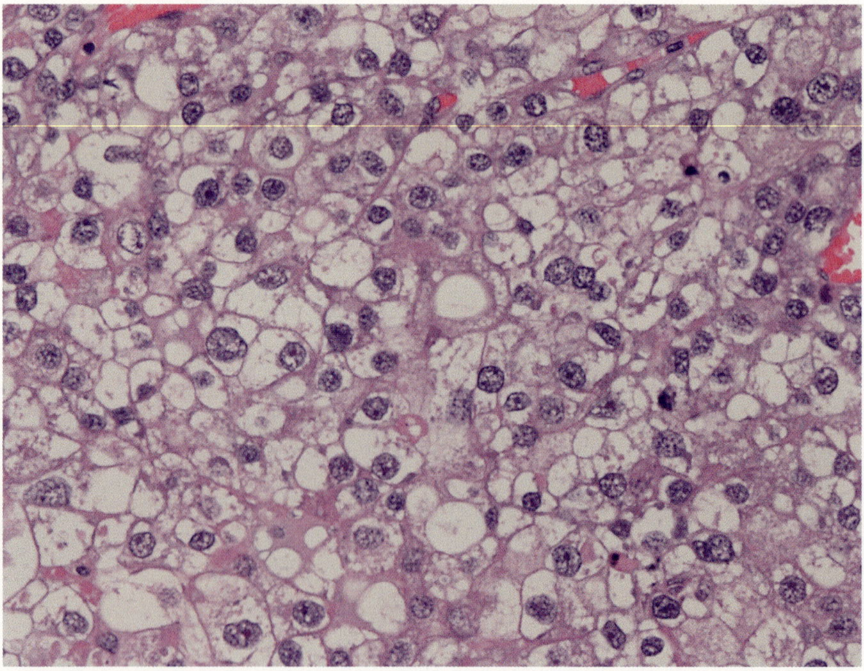

Fig. 5.16 Clear cell carcinoma. The tumor cells with clear cytoplasm and high-grade nuclear atypia growth in solid pattern

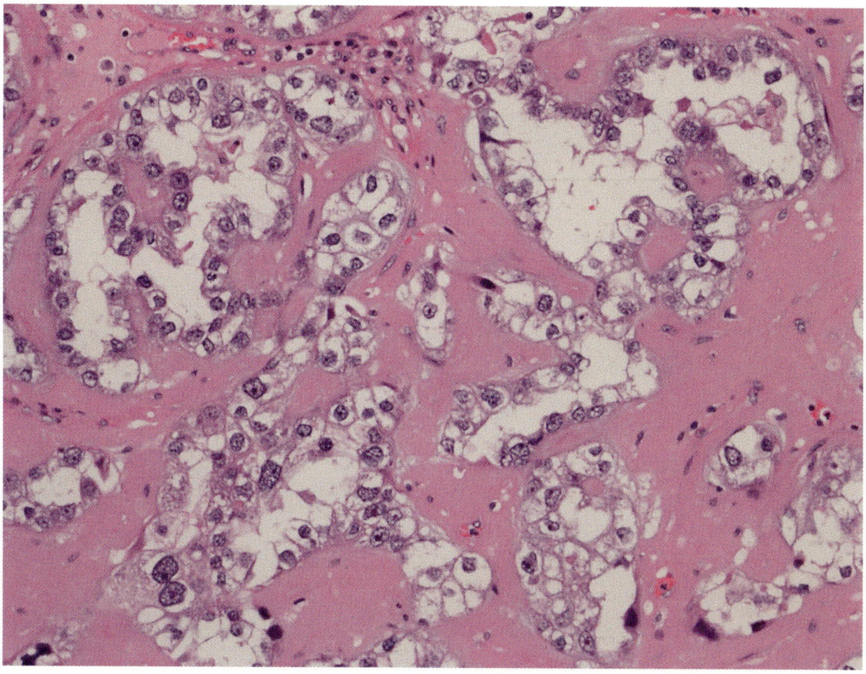

Fig. 5.17 Clear cell carcinoma. Hyalinized eosinophilic stroma is a characteristic

atypia are usually marked. Cytoplasm of tumor cells is rich in glycogen, and, hence, periodic acid-Schiff staining shows granular positivity that disappeared with diastase. The stroma often contains hyalinized eosinophilic (Fig. 5.17) or spherule-like myxoid material [49, 50]. Hyalinized eosinophilic material is derived from basement membrane materials produced by tumor cells and is immunoreactive for type IV collagen and laminin, while spherule-like myxoid material is seen at the core of papillary structures or with in solid nests of tumor cells and hyaluronan produced by tumor cells [50].

CCC tumor cells are positive for CK7 and negative for CK20. They are usually ER and PR negative. Most cases show nuclear positivity for hepatocyte nuclear factor 1β (HNF-1β) and cytoplasmic granular expression of napsin A [51, 52]. About 50% of CCC cases harbor an *ARID1A* mutation, and, hence, immunostaining for BAF250a is negative [12].

Ovarian tumors other than CCC sometimes show proliferation of tumor cells with clear cytoplasm. Some HGSCs contain clear cell component. Even though such cancers appear to be mixture of HGSC and CCC, they often present clinicopathological features of HGSCs (advanced disease, immunoreactivity for WT1, ER, and p53) and should be diagnosed as HGSCs [53]. Some endometrioid carcinomas such as secretory variant have clear cell component and mimic CCC. This type of endometrioid carcinomas lack high-grade nuclear atypia and characteristic histological pattern of CCCs [54]. Among the germ cell tumors, dysgerminoma and yolk sac tumors should be included in the differential diagnosis. Compared to CCCs, these tumors usually affect women at a younger age. Immunostaining of Oct4 and SALL4 can be used for differential diagnosis, since dysgerminomas express Oct4 and both dysgerminomas and yolk sac tumors express SALL4, while CCCs only show occasional and focal positivity for Oct4 and are negative for SALL4 [55, 56].

5.8 Brenner Tumors

Brenner tumors are characterized by the proliferation of a transitional (urothelial)-like epithelial component. Like other types of ovarian epithelial tumors, Brenner tumors are subclassified as benign, borderline/atypical proliferative, or malignant. Nonetheless, most of Brenner tumors are benign.

Formerly, a carcinoma resembling transitional cell carcinoma of the urinary tract without a benign or borderline Brenner component was designated as transitional cell carcinoma and included among transitional tumors. However, recent studies have revealed that most of such carcinomas are HGSCs or endometrioid carcinomas with a transitional-like growth pattern [57, 58]. Hence, the transitional cell carcinoma category has been abolished in the 4th edition of the WHO classification.

The immunoprofile of Brenner tumors is similar to that of the urothelium; tumor cells express CK7, p63, and urothelial markers such as uroplakin III, thrombomodulin, S-100P, and GATA3. Luminal surface cells in the epithelial nests express CK20 [59–61].

5.8.1 Benign Brenner Tumor

The mean age of the patients is 51.5 years [61]. Most pure benign Brenner tumors are small and often less than 1 cm in size. Some benign Brenner tumors are incidentally found in ovaries resected because of other diseases.

Benign Brenner tumor cells show nested growth in rich fibrous stroma with each nest containing solid growth of transitional-cell like tumor cells (Fig. 5.18). Occasionally, mucinous epithelium forms lumens within the nests. Tumor cell nuclei are ovoid and have a characteristic groove along the longitudinal axis, resulting in a coffee-bean appearance. The stroma is composed of collagen fibers and fibroblastic spindle cells without high-grade cellular atypia. Calcification is frequently present.

5.8.2 Borderline Brenner Tumor/Atypical Proliferative Brenner Tumor

Previously, these tumors were known as proliferative Brenner tumors. Most borderline Brenner tumors/atypical proliferative Brenner tumors (BBTs/APBTs) occur in women older than 50 [62]. These tumors have a large, cystic appearance with intracystic papillary excrescence. Histologically, urothelial-like cells with mild to

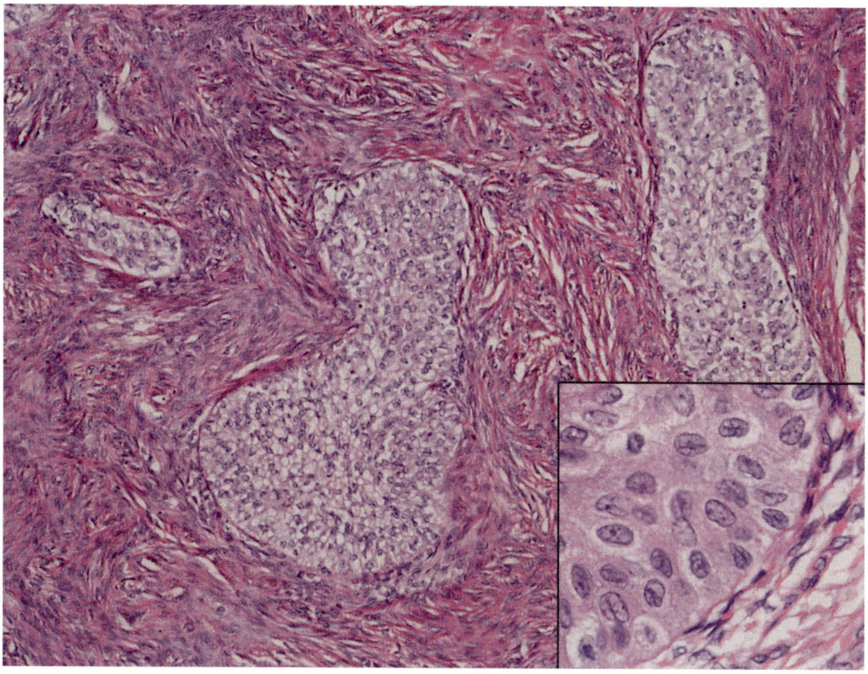

Fig. 5.18 Benign Brenner tumor. Solid tumor cell nests are embedded in fibrous stroma. The tumor cells have nuclear groove (*inset*)

moderate atypia show intracystic papillary proliferation resembling low-grade urothelial carcinoma of the urinary tract.

5.8.3 Malignant Brenner Tumor

Brenner tumors with destructive invasion are designated as malignant Brenner tumors (Fig. 5.19). Such tumors have a predilection for older women and the median age in one study was 60 years [63]. The invasive component is always associated with benign Brenner tumors or BBTs/APBTs. Rarely, these tumors may show squamous cell features.

5.9 Seromucinous Tumors

Tumors containing Müllerian mucinous epithelium were previously combined with gastrointestinal-type mucinous tumors and together classified as mucinous tumors. Rutgers et al. described borderline tumors with Müllerian-type mucinous epithelium and mixed Müllerian-type tumors containing endocervical-like mucinous cells [64, 65]. They noted an association between these tumors and endometriosis. Later, benign tumors and carcinoma of this type were described. Since these tumors are

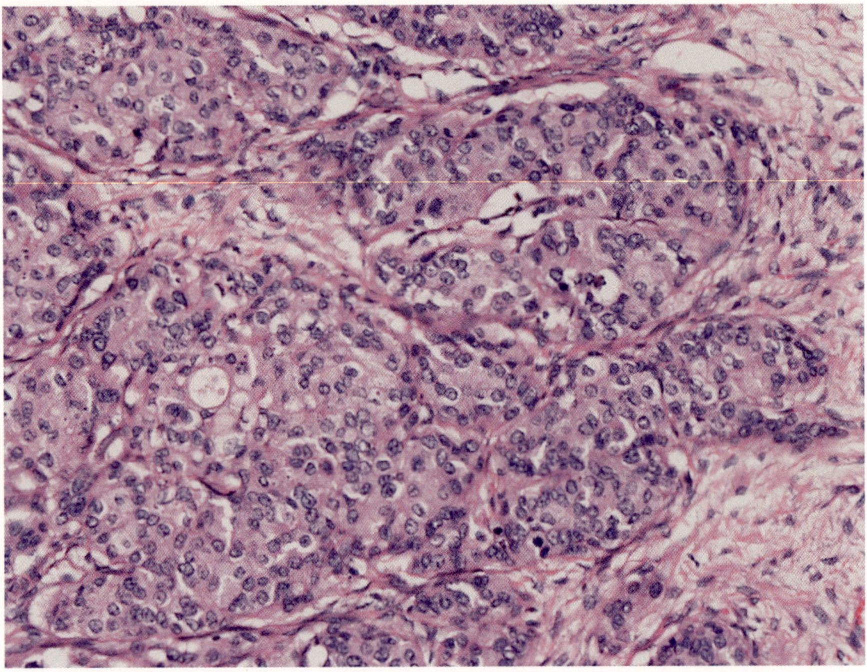

Fig. 5.19 Malignant Brenner tumor. The tumor cell nests invade into the stroma. Some tumor cell nests contain lumens. In this case, typical proliferative Brenner tumor component coexists in other fields

mainly composed of serous-type cells such as ciliated or hobnail cells and endocervical-like mucinous cells, some pathologists prefer the name of "seromucinous tumors" [66], and this term is adopted in the 4th edition of the WHO classification. However, other pathologists think that "seromucinous" is inadequate nomenclature and misleading since other types of cells besides serous and mucinous cells can also be found and these tumors are not related to serous tumors or (gastrointestinal) mucinous tumors [67].

Most cases of seromucinous tumors have borderline malignancy: benign and malignant tumors are relatively rare [66]. Both borderline and malignant seromucinous tumors show a predilection for younger women compared to other ovarian epithelial tumors.

5.9.1 Seromucinous Borderline Tumors

Some studies report that the average age of patients with seromucinous borderline tumors (SMBTs) is 34–39 years [64–66, 68]. At diagnosis, most patients have stage I disease.

Macroscopically, typical SMBTs are cystic tumors with intracystic papillary excrescences. In low-power view, SMBTs show papillary proliferation resembling

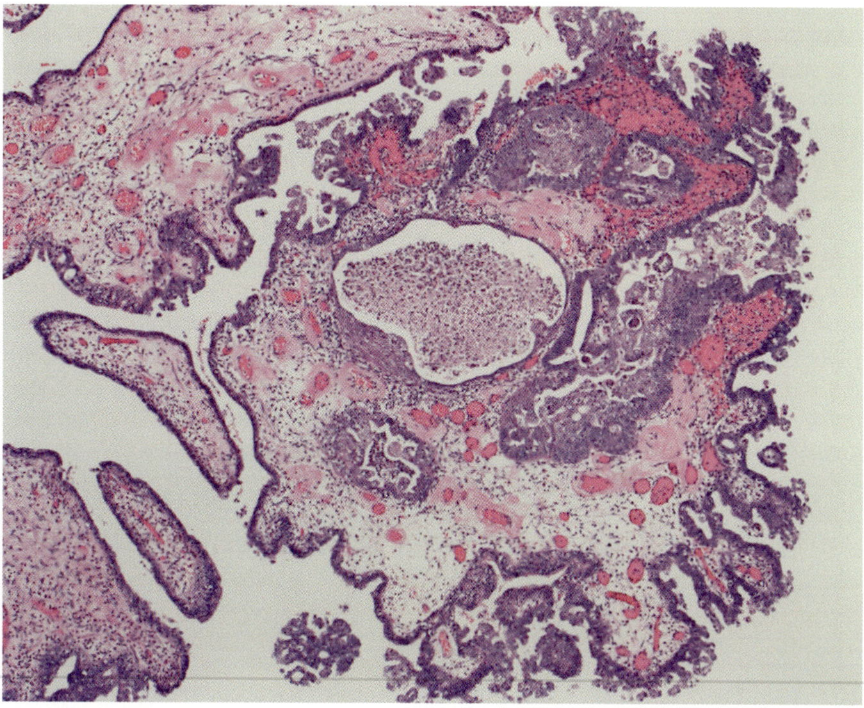

Fig. 5.20 Seromucinous borderline tumor. Intracystic branching papillary excrescence has various types of epithelium including endocervical-like mucinous cells. There are many neutrophils in the stroma

serous borderline tumors (Fig. 5.20). SMBTs are composed of a mixture of mucinous, ciliated, clear, hobnail, columnar endometrioid, indifferent, and squamous epithelium. Intracytoplasmic mucin is basophilic on staining and goblet cells are absent. Rarely, squamous cells are predominant in SMBTs [69]. Numerous neutrophils in the stroma or extracellular mucins are characteristics in SMBTs. Associated endometriosis is found in 30–50% of SMBTs. Microinvasion or intraepithelial carcinoma components are observed in some cases, but these findings do not have an impact on prognosis [66, 68].

SMBTs express CK7, vimentin, ER, and PR, but are negative for CK20, CDX2, and WT1 [70]. Squamous epithelium and cervical reserve cell-like cells express p63 [71]. About one third of SMBT cases show loss of ARID1A [13].

5.9.2 Seromucinous Carcinoma

Seromucinous carcinoma (SMC) is defined as a carcinoma composed predominantly of serous and endocervical-type mucinous epithelium. According to the largest series (19 cases) study, the age of patients ranges from 16 to 79 with a mean of 47 years [72]. The tumor is usually unilateral and solid or solid and cystic.

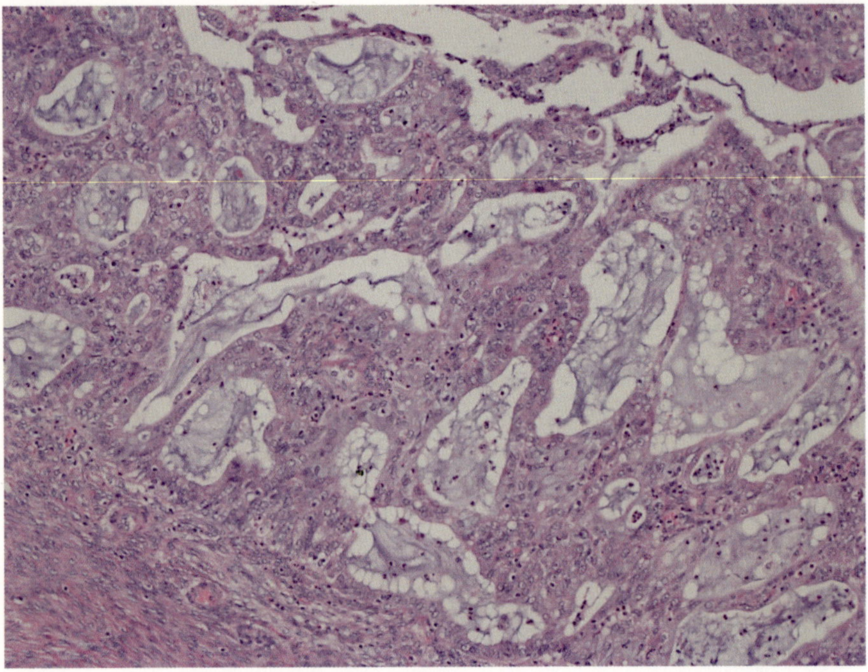

Fig. 5.21 Seromucinous carcinoma. The glands composed of endocervical-like mucinous cells show confluent proliferation without intervening stroma

The tumor is mainly composed of a mixture of endocervical-type mucinous, endometrioid, and indifferent cells with eosinophilic cytoplasm. Clear, hobnail, and squamous cells are also found in some cases. Neutrophil or eosinophil infiltration is often seen. Carcinoma is diagnosed on the basis of expansile stromal invasion showing complex papillary proliferation, confluent glandular proliferation without intervening stroma (Fig. 5.21), or infiltrative/destructive stromal invasion. Taylor et al. found endometriosis in the same ovary in 10 of the 19 cases (53%) and direct transition in 5 of those cases [72].

SMC show almost identical immunoprofile to SMBT, i.e., it is positive for CK7, ER, PR, and PAX8 and negative for CK20 and CDX2 [72].

5.10 Other Epithelial Tumors

5.10.1 Squamous Cell Carcinoma

Primary squamous cell carcinoma (SCC) of the ovary is rare. Most commonly primary ovarian SCC is malignant transformation of a mature cystic teratoma and thus should be classified as a germ cell tumor. Other background conditions of ovarian SCC are endometriosis and Brenner tumors. The prognosis of primary ovarian SCC is poor [73].

5.10.2 Undifferentiated Carcinoma

Undifferentiated carcinoma is a malignant epithelial tumor without specific differentiation. Round to polyhedral tumor cells proliferate in a sheet-like, cord, or nested manner. Brisk mitotic activity is seen.

Undifferentiated carcinoma may be seen in association with low-grade endometrioid carcinoma (dedifferentiated carcinoma). In such cases, clinical behavior is aggressive [74, 75]. The undifferentiated carcinoma component is often confused as a granulosa cell tumor or high-grade sarcoma.

Conclusion

Our understanding of ovarian epithelial tumors has been expanded, and it shows that ovarian epithelial tumors are not homogeneous, but collection of heterogeneous diseases. In the era of precision medicine, the most appropriate therapy of ovarian cancer will be different from type to type. Correct diagnosis warrants the selection of the most effective therapy.

References

1. Kurman RJ, Carcangiu ML, Herrington CS, Young RJ. Tumours of the ovary. In: Kurman RJ, Carcangiu ML, Herrington CS, Young RJ, editors. WHO classification of tumours of female reproductive organs. Lyon: International Agency for Research on Cancer; 2014. p. 11–40.
2. Medeiros F, Muto MG, Lee Y, Elvin JA, Callahan MJ, Feltmate C, Garber JE, Cramer DW, Crum CP. The tubal fimbria is a preferred site for early adenocarcinoma in women with familial ovarian cancer syndrome. Am J Surg Pathol. 2006;30:230–6.
3. Lee Y, Miron A, Drapkin R, Nucci MR, Medeiros F, Saleemuddin A, Garber J, Birch C, Mou H, Gordon RW, Cramer DW, McKeon FD, Crum CP. A candidate precursor to serous carcinoma that originates in the distal fallopian tube. J Pathol. 2007;211:26–35.
4. Kindelberger DW, Lee Y, Miron A, Hirsch MS, Feltmate C, Medeiros F, Callahan MJ, Garner EO, Gordon RW, Birch C, Berkowitz RS, Muto MG, Crum CP. Intraepithelial carcinoma of the fimbria and pelvic serous carcinoma: evidence for a causal relationship. Am J Surg Pathol. 2007;31:161–9.
5. Przybycin CG, Kurman RJ, Ronnett BM, Shih IM, Vang R. Are all pelvic (nonuterine) serous carcinomas of tubal origin? Am J Surg Pathol. 2010;34:1407–16.
6. Tang S, Onuma K, Deb P, Wang E, Lytwyn A, Sur M, Daya D. Frequency of serous tubal intraepithelial carcinoma in various gynecologic malignancies: a study of 300 consecutive cases. Int J Gynecol Pathol. 2012;31:103–10.
7. Banet N, Kurman RJ. Two types of ovarian cortical inclusion cysts: proposed origin and possible role in ovarian serous carcinogenesis. Int J Gynecol Pathol. 2015;34:3–8.
8. Körner M, Burckhardt E, Mazzucchelli L. Different proportions of aneusomic cells in ovarian inclusion cysts associated with serous borderline tumours and serous high-grade carcinomas support different pathogenetic pathways. J Pathol. 2005;207:20–6.
9. Auersperg N. Ovarian surface epithelium as a source of ovarian cancers: unwarranted speculation or evidence-based hypothesis? Gynecol Oncol. 2013;130:246–51.
10. Maeda D, Shih IM. Pathogenesis and the role of ARID1A mutation in endometriosis-related ovarian neoplasms. Adv Anat Pathol. 2013;20:45–52.
11. Jones S, Wang TL, Shih IM, Mao TL, Nakayama K, Roden R, Glas R, Slamon D, Diaz LA Jr, Vogelstein B, Kinzler KW, Velculescu VE, Papadopoulos N. Frequent mutations of chromatin remodeling gene ARID1A in ovarian clear cell carcinoma. Science. 2010;330:228–31.

12. Wiegand KC, Shah SP, Al-Agha OM, Zhao Y, Tse K, Zeng T, Senz J, McConechy MK, Anglesio MS, Kalloger SE, Yang W, Heravi-Moussavi A, Giuliany R, Chow C, Fee J, Zayed A, Prentice L, Melnyk N, Turashvili G, Delaney AD, Madore J, Yip S, McPherson AW, Ha G, Bell L, Fereday S, Tam A, Galletta L, Tonin PN, Provencher D, Miller D, Jones SJ, Moore RA, Morin GB, Oloumi A, Boyd N, Aparicio SA, Shih IM, Mes-Masson AM, Bowtell DD, Hirst M, Gilks B, Marra MA, Huntsman DG. ARID1A mutations in endometriosis-associated ovarian carcinomas. N Engl J Med. 2010;363:1532–43.
13. Wu CH, Mao TL, Vang R, Ayhan A, Wang TL, Kurman RJ, Shih IM. Endocervical-type mucinous borderline tumors are related to endometrioid tumors based on mutation and loss of expression of ARID1A. Int J Gynecol Pathol. 2012;31:297–303.
14. Fujii K, Yamashita Y, Yamamoto T, Takahashi K, Hashimoto K, Miyata T, Kawai K, Kikkawa F, Toyokuni S, Nagasaka T. Ovarian mucinous tumors arising from mature cystic teratomas-a molecular genetic approach for understanding the cellular origin. Hum Pathol. 2014;45:717–24.
15. Seidman JD, Khedmati F. Exploring the histogenesis of ovarian mucinous and transitional cell (Brenner) neoplasms and their relationship with Walthard cell nests: a study of 120 tumors. Arch Pathol Lab Med. 2008;132:1753–60.
16. Wang Y, Wu RC, Shwartz LE, Haley L, Lin MT, Shih IM, Kurman RJ. Clonality analysis of combined Brenner and mucinous tumours of the ovary reveals their monoclonal origin. J Pathol. 2015;237:146–51.
17. Tafe LJ, Muller KE, Ananda G, Mitchell T, Spotlow V, Patterson SE, Tsongalis GJ, Mockus SM. Molecular genetic analysis of ovarian brenner tumors and associated mucinous epithelial neoplasms: high variant concordance and identification of mutually exclusive RAS driver mutations and MYC amplification. Am J Pathol. 2016;186:671–7.
18. Scully RE, Young RH, Clement PB. Surface epithelial-stromal tumors and serous tumors. In: Rosai J, Sobin LH, editors. Atlas of tumor pathology. Tumors of the ovary, maldeveloped gonads, fallopian tube, and broad ligament. Washington, DC: Armed Forces Institute of Pathology; 1998. p. 51–79.
19. Nakashima N, Nagasaka T, Fukata S, Oiwa N, Nara Y, Fukatsu T, Takeuchi J. Study of ovarian tumors treated at Nagoya University Hospital, 1965-1988. Gynecol Oncol. 1990;37:103–11.
20. Cheng EJ, Kurman RJ, Wang M, Oldt R, Wang BG, Berman DM, Shih IM. Molecular genetic analysis of ovarian serous cystadenomas. Lab Invest. 2004;84:778–84.
21. Longacre TA, McKenney JK, Tazelaar HD, Kempson RL, Hendrickson MR. Ovarian serous tumors of low malignant potential (borderline tumors): outcome-based study of 276 patients with long-term (> or =5-year) follow-up. Am J Surg Pathol. 2005;29:707–23.
22. Hannibal CG, Vang R, Junge J, Frederiksen K, Kjaerbye-Thygesen A, Andersen KK, Tabor A, Kurman RJ, Kjaer SK. A nationwide study of serous "borderline" ovarian tumors in Denmark 1978-2002: centralized pathology review and overall survival compared with the general population. Gynecol Oncol. 2014;134:267–73.
23. Altman AD, Nelson GS, Ghatage P, McIntyre JB, Capper D, Chu P, Nation JG, Karnezis AN, Han G, Kalloger SE, Köbel M. The diagnostic utility of TP53 and CDKN2A to distinguish ovarian high-grade serous carcinoma from low-grade serous ovarian tumors. Mod Pathol. 2013;26:1255–63.
24. McKenney JK, Balzer BL, Longacre TA. Patterns of stromal invasion in ovarian serous tumors of low malignant potential (borderline tumors): a reevaluation of the concept of stromal microinvasion. Am J Surg Pathol. 2006;30:1209–21.
25. Maniar KP, Wang Y, Visvanathan K, Shih IM, Kurman RJ. Evaluation of microinvasion and lymph node involvement in ovarian serous borderline/atypical proliferative serous tumors: a morphologic and immunohistochemical analysis of 37 cases. Am J Surg Pathol. 2014;38:743–55.
26. Seidman JD, Soslow RA, Vang R, Berman JJ, Stoler MH, Sherman ME, Oliva E, Kajdacsy-Balla A, Berman DM, Copeland LJ. Borderline ovarian tumors: diverse contemporary viewpoints on terminology and diagnostic criteria with illustrative images. Hum Pathol. 2004;35:918–33.

27. Bell DA, Weinstock MA, Scully RE. Peritoneal implants of ovarian serous borderline tumors. Histologic features and prognosis. Cancer. 1988;62:2212–22.
28. Bell KA, Smith Sehdev AE, Kurman RJ. Refined diagnostic criteria for implants associated with ovarian atypical proliferative serous tumors (borderline) and micropapillary serous carcinomas. Am J Surg Pathol. 2001;25:419–32.
29. Boyd C, McCluggage WG. Low-grade ovarian serous neoplasms (low-grade serous carcinoma and serous borderline tumor) associated with high-grade serous carcinoma or undifferentiated carcinoma: report of a series of cases of an unusual phenomenon. Am J Surg Pathol. 2012;36:368–75.
30. Malpica A, Deavers MT, Lu K, Bodurka DC, Atkinson EN, Gershenson DM, Silva EG. Grading ovarian serous carcinoma using a two-tier system. Am J Surg Pathol. 2004;28:496–504.
31. Okoye E, Euscher ED, Malpica A. Ovarian low-grade serous carcinoma: a clinicopathologic study of 33 cases with primary surgery performed at a single institution. Am J Surg Pathol. 2016;40:627–35.
32. Ahn G, Folkins AK, McKenney JK, Longacre TA. Low-grade serous carcinoma of the ovary: clinicopathologic analysis of 52 invasive cases and identification of a possible noninvasive intermediate lesion. Am J Surg Pathol. 2016;40:1165–76.
33. Ludwick C, Gilks CB, Miller D, Yaziji H, Clement PB. Aggressive behavior of stage I ovarian mucinous tumors lacking extensive infiltrative invasion: a report of four cases and review of the literature. Int J Gynecol Pathol. 2005;24:205–17.
34. Khunamornpong S, Settakorn J, Sukpan K, Suprasert P, Siriaunkgul S. Mucinous tumor of low malignant potential ("borderline" or "atypical proliferative" tumor) of the ovary: a study of 171 cases with the assessment of intraepithelial carcinoma and microinvasion. Int J Gynecol Pathol. 2011;30:218–30.
35. Zaino RJ, Brady MF, Lele SM, Michael H, Greer B, Bookman MA. Advanced stage mucinous adenocarcinoma of the ovary is both rare and highly lethal: a Gynecologic Oncology Group study. Cancer. 2011;117:554–62.
36. Groisman GM, Meir A, Sabo E. The value of Cdx2 immunostaining in differentiating primary ovarian carcinomas from colonic carcinomas metastatic to the ovaries. Int J Gynecol Pathol. 2004;23:52–7.
37. Hu A, Li H, Zhang L, Ren C, Wang Y, Liu Y, Liu C. Differentiating primary and extragenital metastatic mucinous ovarian tumours: an algorithm combining PAX8 with tumour size and laterality. J Clin Pathol. 2015;68:522–8.
38. Moh M, Krings G, Ates D, Aysal A, Kim GE, Rabban JT. SATB2 expression distinguishes ovarian metastases of colorectal and appendiceal origin from primary ovarian tumors of mucinous or endometrioid type. Am J Surg Pathol. 2016;40:419–32.
39. Lee KR, Young RH. The distinction between primary and metastatic mucinous carcinomas of the ovary: gross and histologic findings in 50 cases. Am J Surg Pathol. 2003;27:281–92.
40. Pinto PB, Derchain SF, Andrade LA. Metastatic mucinous carcinomas in the ovary: a practical approach to diagnosis related to gross aspects and to immunohistochemical evaluation. Int J Gynecol Pathol. 2012;31:313–8.
41. Bagué S, Rodríguez IM, Prat J. Sarcoma-like mural nodules in mucinous cystic tumors of the ovary revisited: a clinicopathologic analysis of 10 additional cases. Am J Surg Pathol. 2002;26:1467–76.
42. Provenza C, Young RH, Prat J. Anaplastic carcinoma in mucinous ovarian tumors: a clinicopathologic study of 34 cases emphasizing the crucial impact of stage on prognosis, their histologic spectrum, and overlap with sarcomalike mural nodules. Am J Surg Pathol. 2008;32:383–9.
43. Scully RE, Young RH, Clement PB. Endometrioid tumors. In: Rosai J, Sobin LH, editors. Atlas of tumor pathology. Tumors of the ovary, maldeveloped gonads, fallopian tube, and broad ligament. Washington, DC: Armed Forces Institute of Pathology; 1998. p. 107–40.
44. Madore J, Ren F, Filali-Mouhim A, Sanchez L, Köbel M, Tonin PN, Huntsman D, Provencher DM, Mes-Masson AM. Characterization of the molecular differences between ovarian endometrioid carcinoma and ovarian serous carcinoma. J Pathol. 2010;220:392–400.

45. Seidman JD, Horkayne-Szakaly I, Haiba M, Boice CR, Kurman RJ, Ronnett BM. The histologic type and stage distribution of ovarian carcinomas of surface epithelial origin. Int J Gynecol Pathol. 2004;23:41–4.
46. Yahata T, Banzai C, Tanaka K, Niigata Gynecological Cancer Registry. Histology-specific long-term trends in the incidence of ovarian cancer and borderline tumor in Japanese females: a population-based study from 1983 to 2007 in Niigata. J Obstet Gynaecol Res. 2012;38:645–50.
47. Tay SK, Cheong MA. Evidence for ethnic and environmental contributions to frequency of ovarian clear cell carcinoma. Aust N Z J Obstet Gynaecol. 2014;54:225–30.
48. Takano M, Kikuchi Y, Yaegashi N, Kuzuya K, Ueki M, Tsuda H, Suzuki M, Kigawa J, Takeuchi S, Tsuda H, Moriya T, Sugiyama T. Clear cell carcinoma of the ovary: a retrospective multicentre experience of 254 patients with complete surgical staging. Br J Cancer. 2006;94:1369–74.
49. Scully RE, Young RH, Clement PB. Clear cell tumors. In: Rosai J, Sobin LH, editors. Atlas of tumor pathology. Tumors of the ovary, maldeveloped gonads, fallopian tube, and broad ligament. Washington, DC: Armed Forces Institute of Pathology; 1998. p. 141–51.
50. Kato N, Takeda J, Fukase M, Motoyama T. Alternate mucoid and hyalinized stroma in clear cell carcinoma of the ovary: manifestation of serial stromal remodeling. Mod Pathol. 2010;23:881–8.
51. Tsuchiya A, Sakamoto M, Yasuda J, Chuma M, Ohta T, Ohki M, Yasugi T, Taketani Y, Hirohashi S. Expression profiling in ovarian clear cell carcinoma: identification of hepatocyte nuclear factor-1 beta as a molecular marker and a possible molecular target for therapy of ovarian clear cell carcinoma. Am J Pathol. 2003;163:2503–12.
52. Skirnisdottir I, Bjersand K, Akerud H, Seidal T. Napsin A as a marker of clear cell ovarian carcinoma. BMC Cancer. 2013;13:524.
53. Han G, Gilks CB, Leung S, Ewanowich CA, Irving JA, Longacre TA, Soslow RA. Mixed ovarian epithelial carcinomas with clear cell and serous components are variants of high-grade serous carcinoma: an interobserver correlative and immunohistochemical study of 32 cases. Am J Surg Pathol. 2008;32:955–64.
54. Silva EG, Young RH. Endometrioid neoplasms with clear cells: a report of 21 cases in which the alteration is not of typical secretory type. Am J Surg Pathol. 2007;31:1203–8. Erratum in: Am J Surg Pathol. 2007;31:1628
55. Cheng L, Thomas A, Roth LM, Zheng W, Michael H, Karim FW. OCT4: a novel biomarker for dysgerminoma of the ovary. Am J Surg Pathol. 2004;28:1341–6.
56. Cao D, Guo S, Allan RW, Molberg KH, Peng Y. SALL4 is a novel sensitive and specific marker of ovarian primitive germ cell tumors and is particularly useful in distinguishing yolk sac tumor from clear cell carcinoma. Am J Surg Pathol. 2009;33:894–904.
57. Takeuchi T, Ohishi Y, Imamura H, Aman M, Shida K, Kobayashi H, Kato K, Oda Y. Ovarian transitional cell carcinoma represents a poorly differentiated form of high-grade serous or endometrioid adenocarcinoma. Am J Surg Pathol. 2013;37:1091–9.
58. Riedel I, Czernobilsky B, Lifschitz-Mercer B, Roth LM, XR W, Sun TT, Moll R. Brenner tumors but not transitional cell carcinomas of the ovary show urothelial differentiation: immunohistochemical staining of urothelial markers, including cytokeratins and uroplakins. Virchows Arch. 2001;438:181–91.
59. Logani S, Oliva E, Amin MB, Folpe AL, Cohen C, Young RH. Immunoprofile of ovarian tumors with putative transitional cell (urothelial) differentiation using novel urothelial markers: histogenetic and diagnostic implications. Am J Surg Pathol. 2003;27:1434–41.
60. Esheba GE, Longacre TA, Atkins KA, Higgins JP. Expression of the urothelial differentiation markers GATA3 and placental S100 (S100P) in female genital tract transitional cell proliferations. Am J Surg Pathol. 2009;33:347–53.
61. Kondi-Pafiti A, Kairi-Vassilatou E, Iavazzo C, Vouza E, Mavrigiannaki P, Kleanthis C, Vlahodimitropoulos D, Liapis A. Clinicopathological features and immunoprofile of 30 cases of Brenner ovarian tumors. Arch Gynecol Obstet. 2012;285:1699–702.

62. Roth LM, Dallenbach-Hellweg G, Czernobilsky B. Ovarian Brenner tumors. I. Metaplastic, proliferating, and of low malignant potential. Cancer. 1985;56:582–91.
63. Austin RM, Norris HJ. Malignant Brenner tumor and transitional cell carcinoma of the ovary: a comparison. Int J Gynecol Pathol. 1987;6:29–39.
64. Rutgers JI, Scully RE. Ovarian mullerian mucinous papillary cystadenomas of borderline malignancy. A clinicopathologic analysis. Cancer. 1988;61:340–8.
65. Rutgers JI, Scully RE. Ovarian mixed-epithelial papillary cystadenomas of borderline malignancy of mullerian type. A clinicopathologic analysis. Cancer. 1988;61:546–54.
66. Shappell HW, Riopel MA, Smith Sehdev AE, Ronnett BM, Kurman RJ. Diagnostic criteria and behavior of ovarian seromucinous (endocervical-type mucinous and mixed cell-type) tumors: atypical proliferative (borderline) tumors, intraepithelial, microinvasive, and invasive carcinomas. Am J Surg Pathol. 2002;26:1529–41.
67. Kurman RJ, Shih IM. Seromucinous tumors of the ovary. What's in a name? Int J Gynecol Pathol. 2016;35:78–81.
68. Rodriguez IM, Irving JA, Prat J. Endocervical-like mucinous borderline tumors of the ovary: a clinicopathologic analysis of 31 cases. Am J Surg Pathol. 2004;28:1311–8.
69. Nagai Y, Kishimoto T, Nikaido T, Nishihara K, Matsumoto T, Suzuki C, Ogishima T, Kuwahara Y, Hurukata Y, Mizunuma M, Nakata Y, Ishikura H. Squamous predominance in mixed-epithelial papillary cystadenomas of borderline malignancy of mullerian type arising in endometriotic cysts: a study of four cases. Am J Surg Pathol. 2003;27:242–7.
70. Vang R, Gown AM, Barry TS, Wheeler DT, Ronnett BM. Ovarian atypical proliferative (borderline) mucinous tumors: gastrointestinal and seromucinous (endocervical-like) types are immunophenotypically distinctive. Int J Gynecol Pathol. 2006;25:83–9.
71. Hamada T, Kiyokawa T, Nomura K, Hano H. Immunohistochemical analysis of reserve cell-like cells of ovarian müllerian mucinous/mixed epithelial borderline tumor. Int J Gynecol Pathol. 2008;27:199–206.
72. Taylor J, McCluggage WG. Ovarian seromucinous carcinoma: report of a series of a newly categorized and uncommon neoplasm. Am J Surg Pathol. 2015;39:983–92.
73. Pins MR, Young RH, Daly WJ, Scully RE. Primary squamous cell carcinoma of the ovary. Report of 37 cases. Am J Surg Pathol. 1996;20:823–33.
74. Silva EG, Deavers MT, Bodurka DC, Malpica A. Association of low-grade endometrioid carcinoma of the uterus and ovary with undifferentiated carcinoma: a new type of dedifferentiated carcinoma? Int J Gynecol Pathol. 2006;25:52–8.
75. Tafe LJ, Garg K, Chew I, Tornos C, Soslow RA. Endometrial and ovarian carcinomas with undifferentiated components: clinically aggressive and frequently underrecognized neoplasms. Mod Pathol. 2010;23:781–9.

Pathology of Non-epithelial Ovarian Tumors

6

Masaharu Fukunaga

Abstract

Non-epithelial ovarian tumors have posed pathologic diagnosis and management challenges. The World Health Organization classification of Tumors of Female Reproductive Organs was revised in 2014, and the new version addresses several new concepts and the histological classification of non-epithelial ovarian tumors and tumor-like lesions that were not previously included. In the new WHO classification, sex cord-stromal tumors is divided into three categories, pure stromal tumor, pure sex cord tumor, and mixed sex-cord tumor.

This chapter reviews recent developments regarding the pathology, differential diagnosis, immunohistochemical markers, and genetics of poorly understood non-epithelial ovarian tumors, including sex cord-stromal tumors, immature teratoma, small cell carcinoma of the ovary, hypercalcemic type, and newly described non-epithelial tumors. Many of these neoplasms and those in the differential diagnosis occur predominantly in young women, and they can be aggressive and require specific chemotherapy. Some of non-epithelial neoplasms show histologically biphasic or epithelioid features, mimicking epithelial tumors. The recent discovery of somatic mutations in FOXL2 in adult granulosa cell tumors and germline and somatic mutations in DICER1 in Sertoli-Leydig cell tumors and SMARCA4 in small cell carcinoma, hypercalcemic type, contributes immunohistochemical analyses and molecular research of these tumors. A few non-epithelial tumors are not specific to the ovary and may arise more frequently at extraovarian sites. A correct diagnosis is imperative for appropriate therapies.

M. Fukunaga, M.D.
Department of Pathology, Shin-Yurigaoka General Hospital, 255-Furusawa, Asaoku, Kawasaki, Kanagawa 215-0026, Japan
e-mail: maasafu@jikei.ac.jp

H. Katabuchi (ed.), *Frontiers in Ovarian Cancer Science*, Comprehensive Gynecology and Obstetrics, DOI 10.1007/978-981-10-4160-0_6

Keywords
Non-epithelial tumor • Sex cord-stromal tumor • Sertoli-Leydig cell tumor • Small cell carcinoma • Hypercalcemia

6.1 Introduction

The new World Health Organization (WHO) classification of Tumors of Female Reproductive Organs addresses several new concepts and histological classifications that were not previously included [1]. Non-epithelial ovarian tumors have posed pathologic diagnosis and management challenges because general diagnostic pathologists and even gynecologic pathologists rarely encounter these lesions and it is very difficult to make a correct diagnosis. Furthermore gynecologists have no or little experience of treatments of rare ovarian tumors.

This chapter reviews recent developments regarding the pathology, differential diagnosis, and genetics of poorly understood non-epithelial ovarian tumors, including pure and mixed sex cord-stromal tumors (Table 6.1), immature teratoma, small cell carcinoma of the ovary, hypercalcemic type, and newly described non-epithelial tumors. Many of these neoplasms and those in the differential diagnosis occur predominantly in young women, and some of them can be aggressive and require specific chemotherapy. Some non-epithelial neoplasm show histologically biphasic or epithelioid features, mimicking epithelial tumors. Thus, a correct diagnosis is imperative for ensuring that appropriate treatment is administered. Due to the rarity of these tumors and the lack of knowledge about them, a special review and confirmation of the diagnosis by an expert gynecological pathologist is recommended [2]. A few of these lesions are not specific to the ovary and may occur more frequently at extraovarian sites, but the mere knowledge that they occasionally occur in or involve the ovary will facilitate their recognition by pathologists [2]. In addition, the recent discovery of mutations will aid molecular diagnosis and the development of relatively specific immunohistochemical markers.

6.2 Sex Cord-Stromal Tumors: Pure Stromal Tumors

6.2.1 Fibroma, Cellular Fibroma, and Fibrosarcoma

6.2.1.1 Clinical Features

Fibroma is a benign tumor composed of fibroblasts and collagen fibers. The mean age of patients with ovarian fibroma is about 50 years. Cellular fibroma can recur, and so clinical follow-up is necessary. Fibrosarcoma is a malignant mesenchymal tumor with a poor prognosis [3]. The standard treatment involves complete resection followed by chemotherapy.

Table 6.1 WHO classification of ovarian sex cord-stromal tumors (2014) [1]

Sex cord-stromal tumors
Pure stromal tumors
Fibroma
Cellular fibroma
Thecoma
Luteinized thecoma associated with sclerosing peritonitis
Fibrosarcoma
Sclerosing stromal tumor
Signet-ring stromal tumor
Microcystic stromal tumor
Leydig cell tumor
Steroid cell tumor
Steroid cell tumor, malignant
Pure sex cord tumors
Adult granulosa cell tumor
Juvenile granuloma cell tumor
Sertoli cell tumor
Sex cord tumor with annular tubules
Mixed sex cord-stromal tumors
Sertoli-Leydig cell tumors
Well differentiated
Moderately differentiated
With heterologous elements
Poorly differentiated
With heterologous elements
Retiform
With heterologous elements
Sex cord-stromal tumors, not otherwise specified

6.2.1.2 Pathological Features

Fibroma is firm with a smooth, lobulated surface and average size is 6 cm. Cellular fibroma is mainly composed of solid components with white cut surface. Fibrosarcomas are large and soft and typically exhibit necrosis and hemorrhaging. Microscopically, fibromas are composed of fusiform and uniform cells arranged in a fascicular or whorled pattern. The stroma is fibrous with focal hyalinization or calcifications; however, approximately 10% of fibromas are hypercellular (little collagenous stroma is seen). Cellular fibroma is defined as fibroma group tumor with high cellularity, mild to moderate nuclear atypia, and 3 or few mitotic figures in 10/10HPF(high power fields). Cellular fibromas may have mitotic activity of > 4/10HPF (mitotically active cellular fibroma) [4] (Fig 6.1). Many ovarian tumors that have been reported as fibrosarcomas would now be considered to be mitotically active cellular fibromas. Fibrosarcomas are characterized by cellular spindle cell fibromatous lesions with moderate to marked nuclear atypia, 4 or more mitotic figures per 10/HPF, and atypical mitotic figures and necrosis [3] (Fig. 6.2). Fibrosarcomas are usually large and have often spread beyond the ovary at

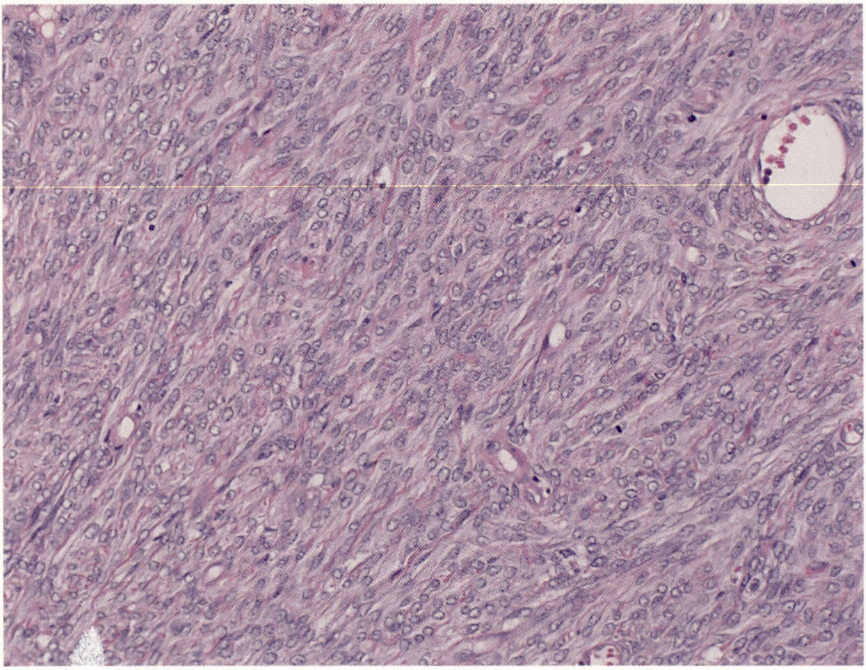

Fig. 6.1 Mitotically active cellular fibroma. Proliferating bland spindle-shaped cells and scattered mitotic figures are shown

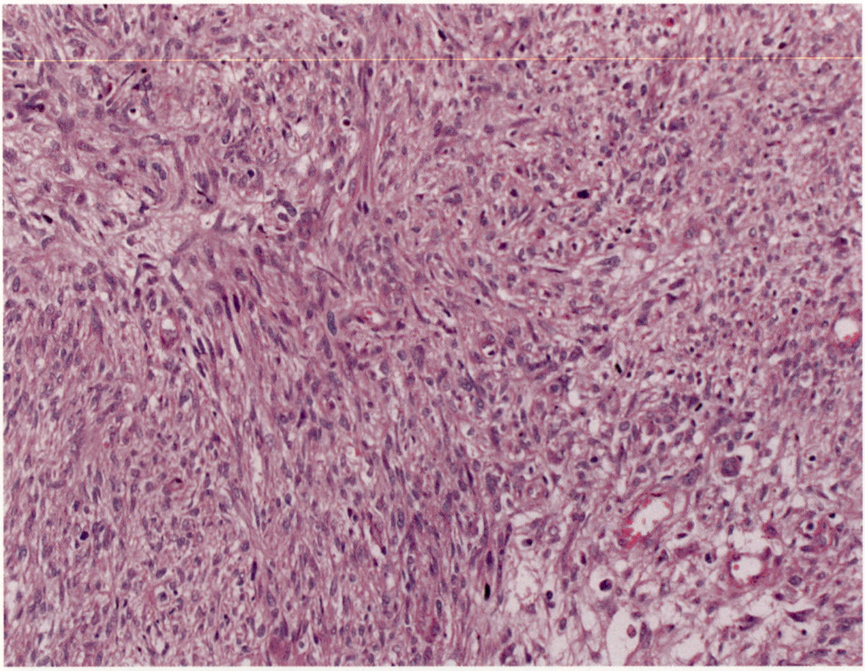

Fig. 6.2 Fibrosarcoma. The fascicular proliferation of atypical spindle cells and bizarre giant cells is shown

diagnosis. Their differential diagnoses include leiomyosarcoma, high-grade endometrial stromal sarcoma, gastrointestinal stromal sarcoma, and various types of primary or metastatic soft tissue sarcoma.

6.2.2 Thecoma

6.2.2.1 Clinical Features

Thecomas are gonadal stromal tumors that are predominantly composed of theca cell-like cells. In daily practice, thecomas are uncommon, whereas fibromas are relatively common. Thecomas usually occur in premenopausal or postmenopausal women, but can arise in children in rare cases. Luteinized thecomas occur at a younger age, usually in patients in their 20s or 30s. Premenopausal women display either endocrine-associated symptoms, such as irregular bleeding or amenorrhea, or nonspecific complaints, such as pelvic pain or abdominal distention. Luteinized thecomas can be estrogenic (50%), androgenic (11%), or nonfunctional (39%) [5]. Some patients with luteinized thecomas are virilized, whereas others show hyperestrogenic symptoms. Thecomas are benign, and excision is an appropriate treatment. The diagnosis of luteinized thecoma is restricted to luteinized thecomas associated with sclerosing peritonitis, a distinctive stromal tumor that is typically associated with sclerosing peritonitis [1].

6.2.2.2 Pathological Features

Macroscopically, thecomas are firm or hard tumors with a mean diameter of 7 cm. The cut surfaces of thecomas are solid and yellow or white. Cysts and calcifications may be present.

Histologically, thecomas are composed of fascicles or sheets of plump spindle-shaped or ovoid stromal cells that resemble the cells of the theca interna. Tumor cells have round or fusiform nuclei and amphophilic or lightly eosinophilic or clear cytoplasm (Fig. 6.3). Mitotic figures are rare. A variable number of fibroblasts are intermixed among the theca-like cells. From a practical point of view, the diagnosis of thecoma is restricted to tumors that show evidence of steroid hormone secretion, have a conspicuous tumor composed of cells with clear or vacuolated cytoplasm, or contain luteinized cells (Fig. 6.4). Immunohistochemically, most thecomas express inhibin and calretinin.

6.2.3 Sclerosing Stromal Tumor

Sclerosing stromal tumors are uncommon benign stromal tumors that mainly occur in teenagers and young women [6]. They should be treated by excision or unilateral salpingo-oophorectomy. Macroscopically, these tumors are firm and white to yellowish-white. Histologically, they are characterized by the lobular proliferation of tumor cells with staghorn or hemangiopericytomatous vascular spaces. Tumor cells include polygonal theca-like cells with vacuolated eosinophilic cytoplasm and fibroblast-like cells (Fig. 6.5). Immunohistochemically, their cells are positive for

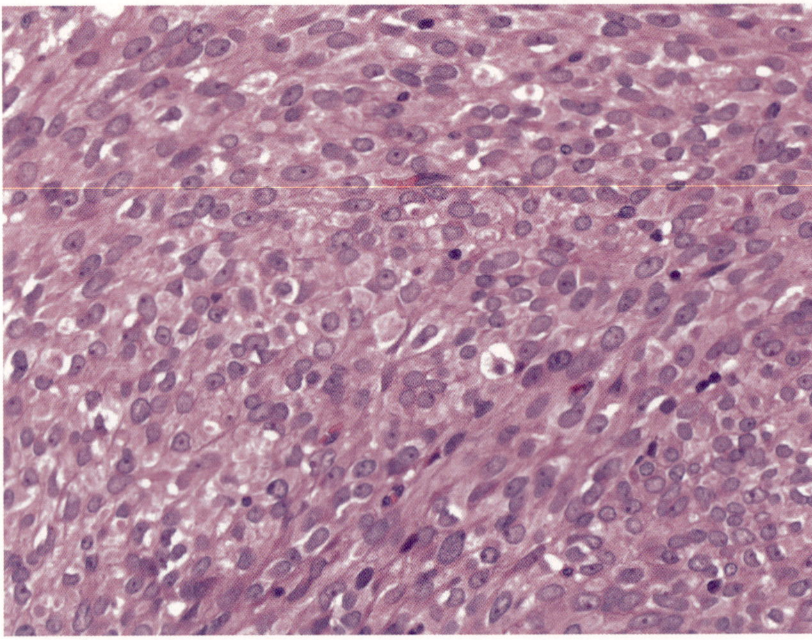

Fig. 6.3 Thecoma. Solid nests of cells with uniform round nuclei and lightly eosinophilic or clear cytoplasm are shown

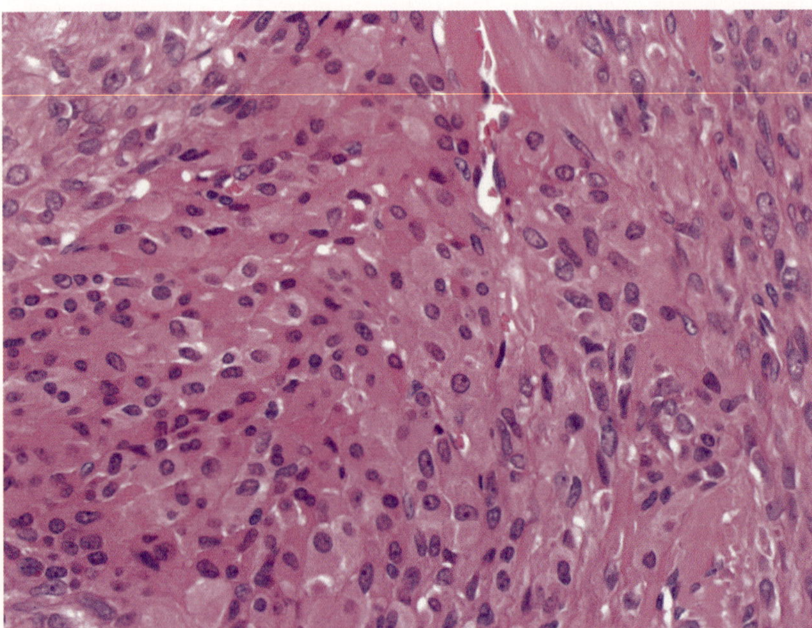

Fig. 6.4 Luteinized thecoma. Sheets of luteinized cells with abundant eosinophilic cytoplasm are shown

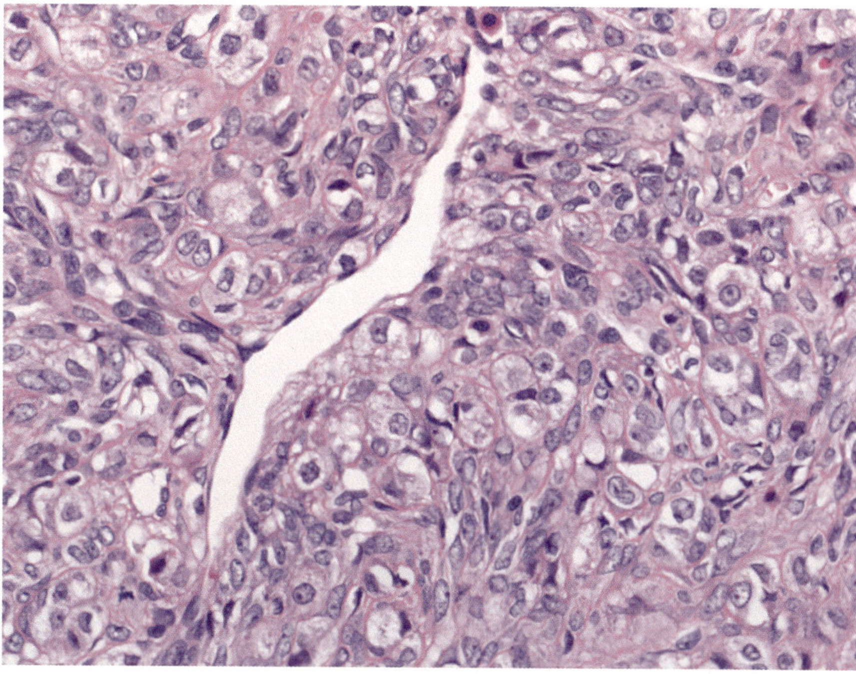

Fig. 6.5 Sclerosing stromal tumor. The tumor is composed of polygonal theca-like cells with vacuolated eosinophilic cytoplasm, fibroblast-like cells, and staghorn vascular spaces

vimentin, inhibin, calretinin, signal transducer activator of transcription 6 (STAT6), and the estrogen and progesterone receptors.

6.2.4 Microcytic Stromal Tumor

6.2.4.1 Clinical Features

This tumor has recently been described by Irving and Young [1] as a previously uncharacterized ovarian neoplasm that exhibits prominent microcystic changes and is most likely of stromal origin. The reported cases involved patients who ranged in age from 26 to 63 (mean, 45) years, and most patients presented with a pelvic mass. Hormonal manifestations are rarely seen. Microcytic stromal tumors are unilateral and do not undergo extraovarian spread.

6.2.4.2 Pathological Features

Microcystic stromal tumors are solid-cystic, solid, or predominantly cystic and display a mean diameter of 8.7 cm. Their solid components are firm and tan or white-tan. Microscopically, these ovarian tumors contain microcysts with variable amounts of solid cellular tissue and fibrous stroma. In addition, they exhibit lobular demarcation as well as sharp separation from the ovarian stroma. The microcysts are characterized by small round to oval cystic spaces. Intracytoplasmic lumens or vacuoles are also present (Fig. 6.6). The tumor cells contain moderate abundant finely granular, eosinophilic cytoplasm and bland, round to oval or spindle-shaped nuclei with fine chromatin and indistinct nucleoli [7]. Mitotic figures are very rare. This type of tumor is characterized by an absence of morphological features that would result in any other specific diagnosis in the sex cord-stroma category, an absence of epithelial elements, and an absence of teratomatous or other germ cell elements [7]. Immunohistochemically, the tumors are strongly positive for CD10 and vimentin, but do not express S-100 protein, calretinin, inhibin, epithelial membrane antigen (EMA), cytokeratin (CK), melan A, and estrogen receptors, desmin, chromogranin A, synaptophysin, WT1, or CD34 [1].

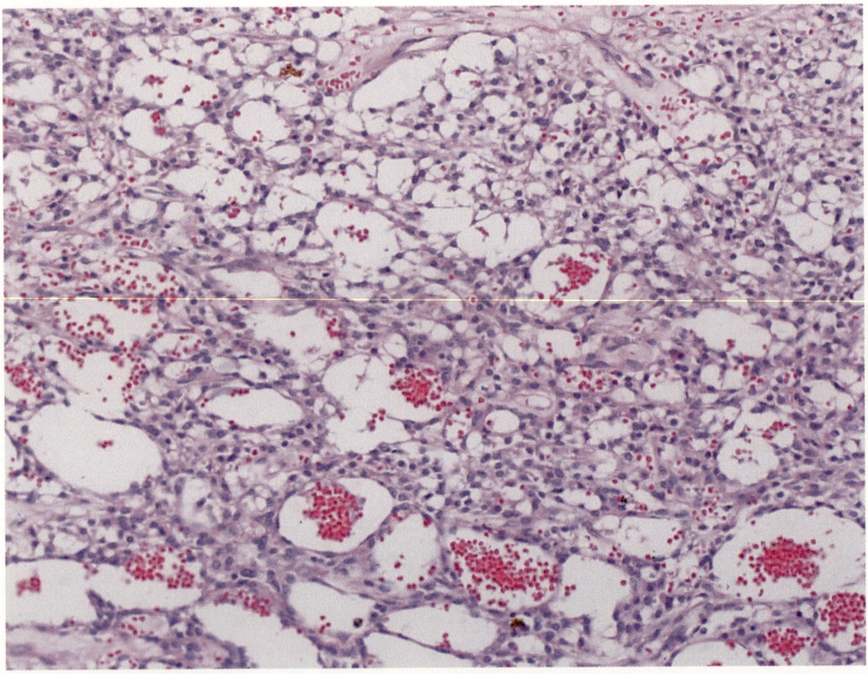

Fig. 6.6 Microcystic stromal tumor. The microcysts are characterized by small round to oval cystic spaces. Intracytoplasmic lumens or vacuoles are also present

6.3 Pure Sex Cord Tumors

6.3.1 Adult Granulosa Cell Tumor (AGCT)

6.3.1.1 Clinical Features

Granulosa cell tumor is the most common type of malignant sex cord-stromal tumor. There are two types of granulosa cell tumor, the adult type, which mainly occurs in premenopausal and postmenopausal women (mean age, 45–55 years), and juvenile granulosa cell tumors (JGCT), which mainly occur in children (mean age, 15 years) [1]. It is important that the distinction between AGCT and JGCT is made on the basis of the histology and not the patient age. The typical clinical presentation of AGCT is postmenopausal bleeding in older women and menorrhagia or amenorrhea in younger patients. Granulosa cell tumors typically secrete estrogen, and patients with these tumors exhibit endometrial hyperplasia (30–40%) or adenocarcinoma (5–10%) [8]. Granulosa cell tumors are typically unilateral and confined to the ovary at diagnosis.

The overall recurrence rate ranges from 10 to 30%. Metastases or recurrence is often detected more than 5 years after the initial treatment, particularly in the peritoneum and omentum. There is no correlation between the microscopic features of tumors, including mitotic activity, and outcomes.

6.3.1.2 Pathological Features

Macroscopically, most AGCT are solid and cystic. The solid areas are soft to firm and yellow/brown to tan. Some tumors are predominantly cystic. The average size is about 10 cm. A variety of growth patterns are observed in AGCT, including admixtures of different patterns. The cells of such tumors often grow in microfollicular or diffuse patterns. Granulosa cell tumors consist of nests and sheets of granulosa cell-like cells punctuated by small spaces, which resemble Call-Exner bodies (Fig. 6.7). Occasionally, larger follicles are sometimes observed (the macrofollicular pattern). The cells of granulosa cell tumors are often arranged in cords, trabeculae, and ribbons (Fig. 6.8). In addition, they have scant pale cytoplasm and uniform, pale, round oval nuclei. Coffee bean-like nuclear grooves were considered to be a characteristic of granulosa cell tumors, but they are not seen every case, and they also occur in many other neoplasms, including Sertoli cell tumors and Sertoli-Leydig cell tumors. Brisk mitotic figures are seen in some lesions. Some AGCT have a JGCT component, and such tumors should be classified based on their predominant histology.

Immunohistochemically, granulosa cell tumors are usually positive for inhibin, calretinin, FOXL2 (forkhead box L2), WT1, and CD56, whereas they are negative for CK7 and EMA. A missense somatic point mutation that is characteristic of AGCT has recently been identified in the FOXL2 gene [9]. This mutation is seen in approximately 95% of AGCT.

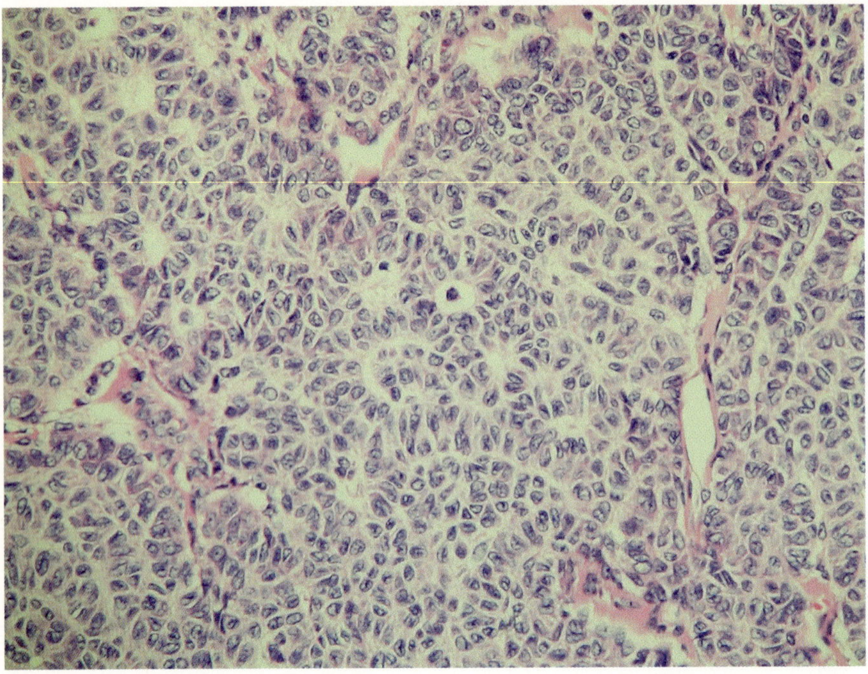

Fig. 6.7 Adult granulosa cell tumor. The tumor cells are uniform and have grooved nuclei. Note the numerous Call-Exner bodies

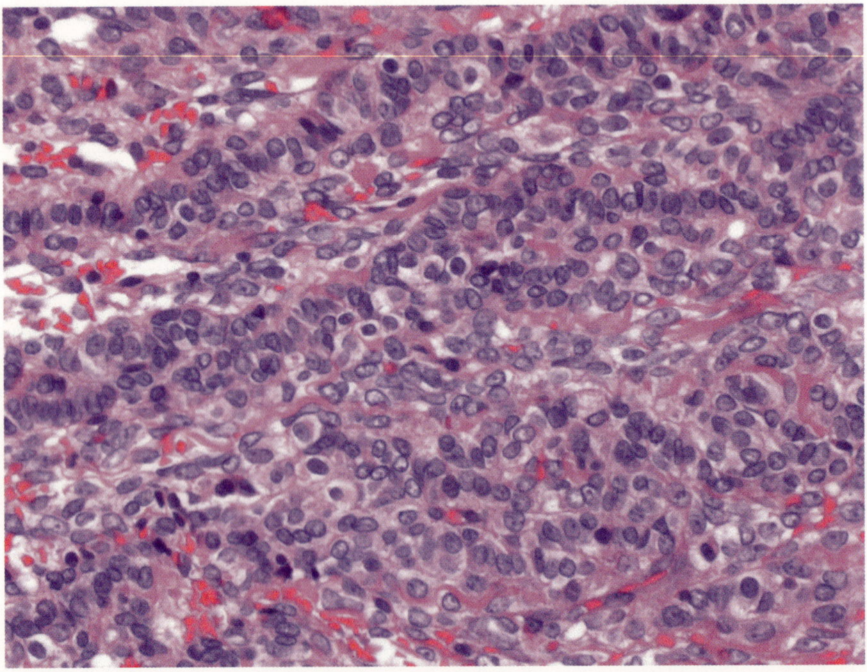

Fig. 6.8 Adult granulosa cell tumor. The tumor cells grow in cords, trabeculae, and ribbons

6.3.2 Juvenile Granulosa Cell Tumor (JGCT)

6.3.2.1 Clinical Features

Fewer than 5% of granulosa cell tumors occur in children or teenagers. Almost all JGCT are unilateral, and more than 95% of them are confined to the ovary (stage I). The symptoms of JGCT are often caused by the estrogen they secrete. Young girls frequently display isosexual pseudoprecocity, whereas older children and premenopausal women develop menstrual abnormalities or amenorrhea. Associations have been detected between JGCT and Ollier (enchondromatosis) disease and Maffucci (enchondromatosis and multiple hemangiomas) syndrome [10]. The prognosis of patients with JGCT is better than that of patients with AGCT. JGCT are less likely to recur or metastasize. The long-term survival of patients with JGCT is good, but patients whose tumors rupture or who exhibit positive peritoneal cytology or extraovarian tumor spread are at significant risk of recurrence. Inhibin and Müllerian inhibitory substance are useful tumor markers for following up patients with JGCT.

6.3.2.2 Pathological Features

The average size is about 12 cm, and most of them exhibit a mixed solid-cystic appearance, but some are completely solid or cystic. Their solid areas are yellow or tan. Hemorrhaging is sometimes seen, but necrosis is uncommon.

Microscopically, JGCT show a multinodular growth pattern, and macrofollicular, solid, and cystic growth patterns are characteristic of JGCT. Follicles often vary in size and shape and contain mucinous material (Fig. 6.9), macrofollicles are lined by one or more layers of granulosa cells and are surrounded by a rim of theca cells. Solid areas are composed of sheets of granular cells made up of an admixture of theca cells or fibroblasts. The microfollicular, insular patterns and trabeculae seen in AGCT are rarely observed in JGCT. Tumor cells have large and round nuclei and amphophilic or pink cytoplasm. In addition, they lack coffee bean-like nuclear grooves and may contain conspicuous nucleoli. Some tumor cells have enlarged pleomorphic nuclei, and multinucleated cells can also be observed (Fig. 6.10). Mitotic figures tend to be numerus with an average around 6/10HPF.

The immunohistochemical features of JGCT are similar to those of AGCT. A small minority of JGCT express FOXL2, and the FOXL2 mutation that occurs in AGCT is generally absent in JGCT [10], indicating that these two tumors, both of which are composed of granulosa cells, probably have different pathogenic mechanisms. Immunohistochemistry is of considerable value for differentiating JCGT from small cell carcinoma, hypercalcemic type (SCCHT); SCCHT does not exhibit nuclear immunoreactivity for SMARCA4 (INI1) and is focally positive for EMA, while JGCT is positive for sex cord markers, negative for EMA, and exhibits positive nuclear staining for SMARCA4.

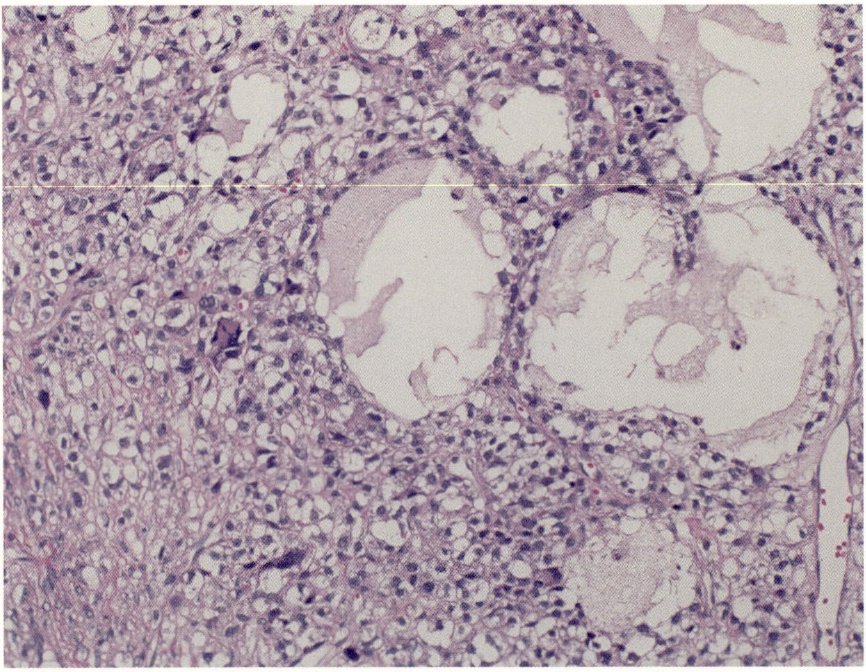

Fig. 6.9 Juvenile granulosa cell tumor. The tumor shows macrofollicular, solid, and cystic growth patterns. The follicles vary in size and shape

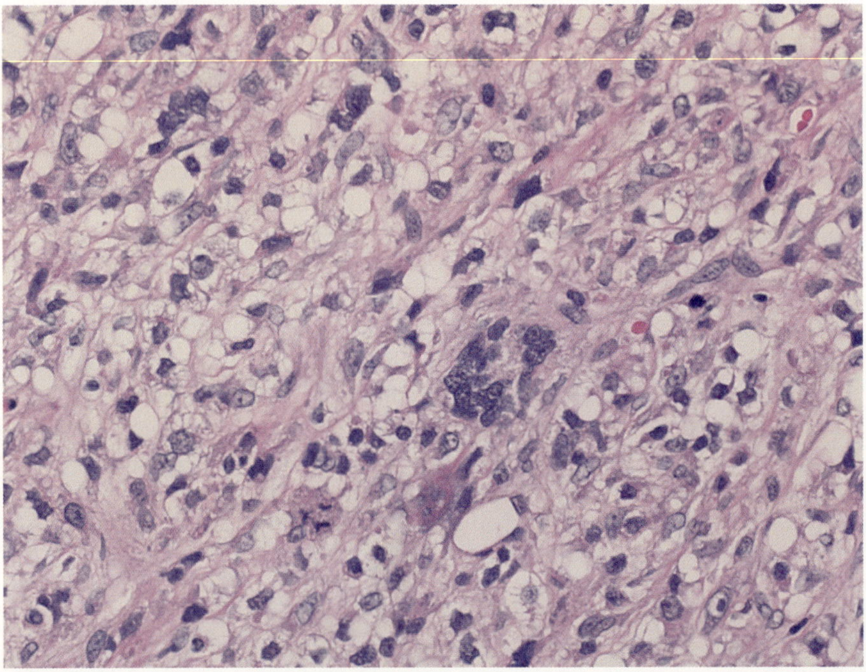

Fig. 6.10 Juvenile granulosa cell tumor. Enlarged pleomorphic nuclei and multinucleated cells are observed in solid areas

6.3.3 Sex Cord Tumor with Annular Tubules (SCTAT)

6.3.3.1 Clinical Features

About a third of patients with SCTAT have Peutz-Jeghers syndrome (PJS) [11, 12]. In these patients, the lesions are found incidentally, are often bilateral, and grossly appear to be yellow nodules of up to 3 cm in diameter. In patients without PJS (sporadic), SCTAT tumors are always unilateral, moderately large, and present as palpable masses. In patients with PJS, SCTAT presents at a mean age of 27 years, whereas it tends to appear around 34 years in patients without PJS. Subsets of both sporadic and PJS-associated SCTAT might be associated with hyperestrinism and menstrual irregularities. SCTAT is primarily treated with surgery, and PJS-associated tumors are entirely benign (albeit multifocal). About one-fifth of sporadic cases is clinically malignant and spread via the lymphatics. Recurrent lesions often occur late. Patients with PJS carry a 5–15% risk of developing sex cord-stromal tumors (SCTAT). PJS is characterized by a germline mutation of the STK 11 (serine threonine kinase 11) gene on chromosome 19p. Patients with PJS are at very high risk of gastrointestinal and non-gastrointestinal cancer (carcinoma of the gastrointestinal tract, pancreas, and breast) [13] and adenoma malignum (gastric-type mucinous adenocarcinoma) (10% risk) of the uterine cervix.

6.3.3.2 Pathological Features

SCTAT is a distinctive type of ovarian neoplasm with morphological features that are intermediate between those of granulosa cell tumors and Sertoli cell tumors. While differentiation into either of the two latter tumors can occur in some cases, Scully reported that the distinctive architecture of SCTAT, which involves simple and complex ring-shaped tubules, warrants a separate designation [11].

PJS-associated and sporadic SCATAT histologically consist of well-circumscribed round nests of cells and a mixture of simple and complex ring-shaped tubules, which contain hyalinized basement membrane-like material (Fig. 6.11). The nests or tubules are composed of uniform cells with peripherally located nuclei and a moderate amount of cytoplasm. Multiple tumorlets form single tubules or clusters of tubules, and calcifications are scattered within the ovarian stroma. Large tumors in non-PJS patients can exhibit extensive hyalinization of the tubules and stroma. Ultrastructural examinations demonstrate bundles of Charcot-Bottcher filaments in some cases of SCTAT, leading some authorities to consider this neoplasm as a subtype of Sertoli or granulosa cell tumor [14]. However, the distinctive features of SCTAT and its frequent association with PJS warrant its classification as a specific form of sex cord-stromal tumor. Immunohistochemically, SCTAT shows positive staining for inhibin, calretinin, vimentin, and CK, but is negative for EMA.

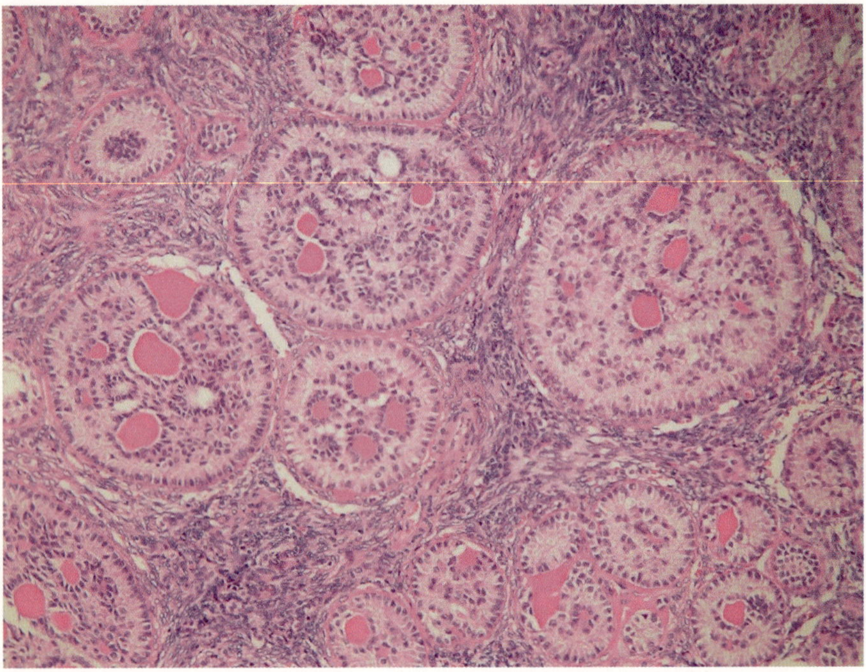

Fig. 6.11 Sex cord tumor with annular tubules. The nests and tubules are composed of uniform cells. Note the complex annular tubules surrounded by fibrous stroma

6.4 Mixed Sex Cord-Stromal Tumors

6.4.1 Sertoli-Leydig Cell Tumor (SLCT)

The WHO classification divides SLCT into retiform and well, moderately, and poorly differentiated variants. The moderately differentiated, poorly differentiated, and retiform variants sometimes contain heterologous elements.

6.4.1.1 Clinical Features

SLCT mainly arise in relatively young patients (mean age, 25 years). The retiform variant usually occurs in particularly young patients (mean age, 15 years). The symptoms of SLCT are related to the presence of an ovarian mass and virilization. Approximately 50% of SLCT secrete steroid hormones, which can also cause symptoms, and 40% of patients are virilized [15]. The serum testosterone and urine 17-ketosteroid levels of SLCT patients are increased. Most tumors are unilateral and confined to the ovary at presentation. Well-differentiated SLCT is clinically benign and does not recur after complete excision. The prognosis of patients with intermediate and poorly differentiated SLCT is generally favorable, but patients with poorly differentiated SLCT can exhibit an aggressive clinical course.

6.4.1.2 Pathological Features

Macroscopically, SLCT are usually solid and partly cystic, and the solid areas of SLCT are firm or soft and yellow or tan. Well-differentiated SLCT exhibit a mean size of 5 cm, whereas the intermediate and poorly differentiated types both display a mean size of 15 cm. Poorly differentiated tumors tend to be larger than those demonstrating intermediate differentiation [15].

Well-differentiated SLCT is histologically characterized by hollow or closed tubules lined by columnar Sertoli cells and surrounded by a fibrous stroma. Aggregates of luteinized Leydig cells are often observed (Fig. 6.12). Reinke crystalloids are rarely found in Leydig cells. Cellular atypia and mitotic figures are rare in well-differentiated SLCT.

Intermediate and poorly differentiated SLCT are composed of mature and immature Sertoli cells. Various proliferative patterns are seen in such tumors, including well-formed tubules, ill-defined tubules, trabeculae, and cord-like arrangements (Fig. 6.13). The tubules have a retiform appearance in 10–25% of intermediate and poorly differentiated tumors. The retiform tubules are branched and lined by low columnar to cuboidal cells. Bizarre cells can also be seen, but this does not appear to be an adverse prognostic finding. Cases of SLCT involving a predominant retiform growth pattern should be diagnosed as retiform variant (Fig. 6.14). In poorly

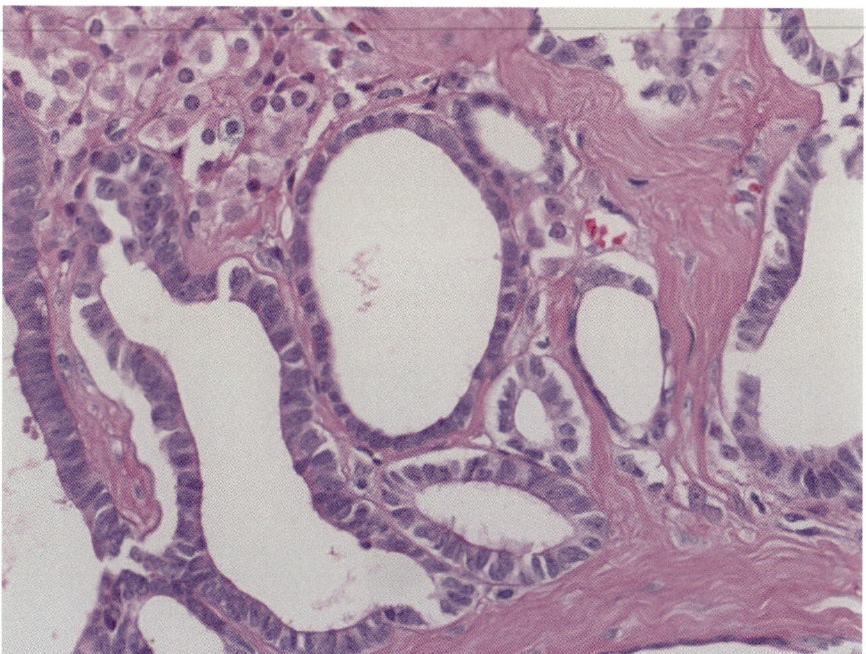

Fig. 6.12 Well-differentiated Sertoli-Leydig cell tumor. Hollow tubules lined by columnar Sertoli cells surrounded by fibrous stroma and aggregates of luteinized Leydig cells are shown

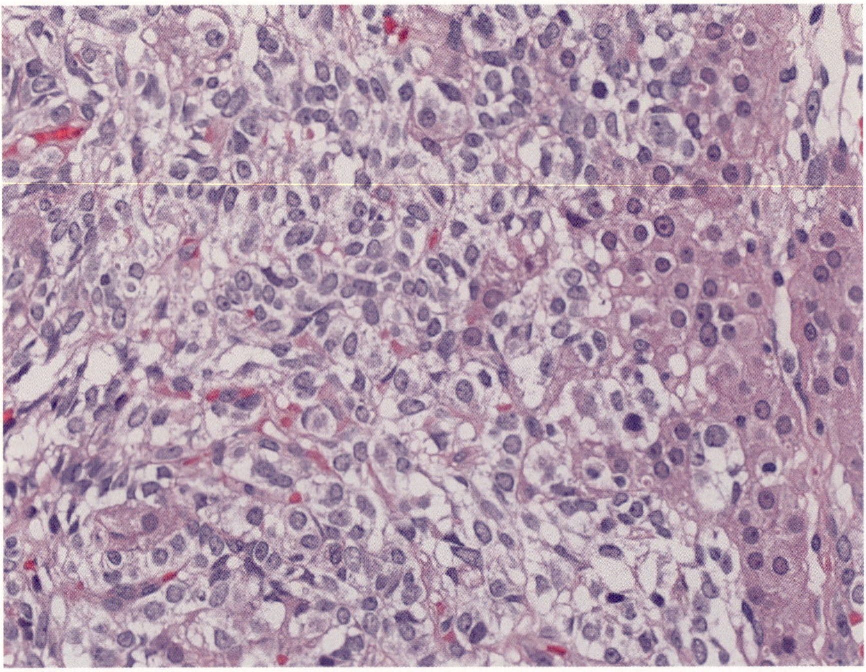

Fig. 6.13 Moderately differentiated Sertoli-Leydig cell tumor. Note the trabeculae and cord-like arrangements of Sertoli cells together with aggregates of luteinized Leydig cells

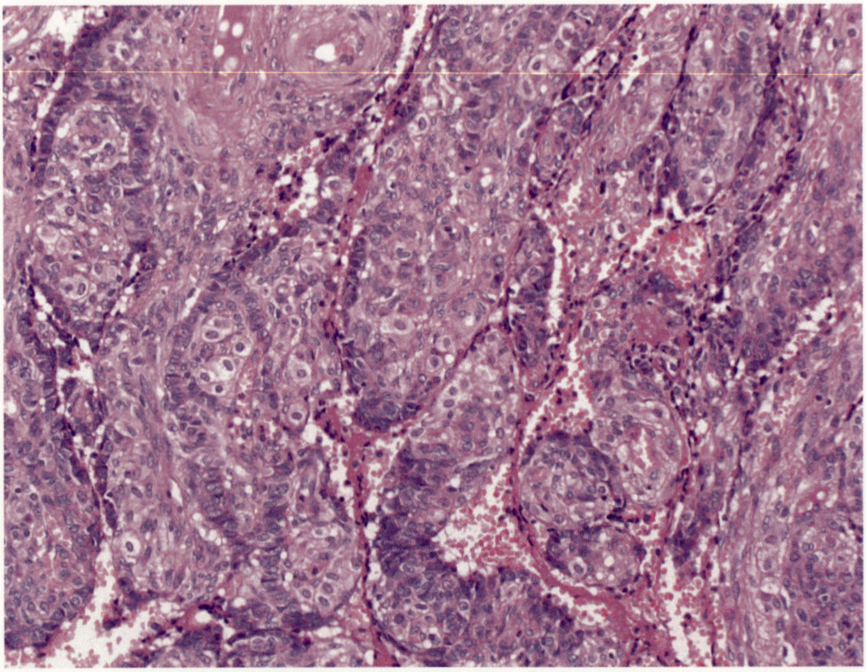

Fig. 6.14 Moderately differentiated Sertoli-Leydig cell tumor, retiform variant. Note the long and branching retiform tubules

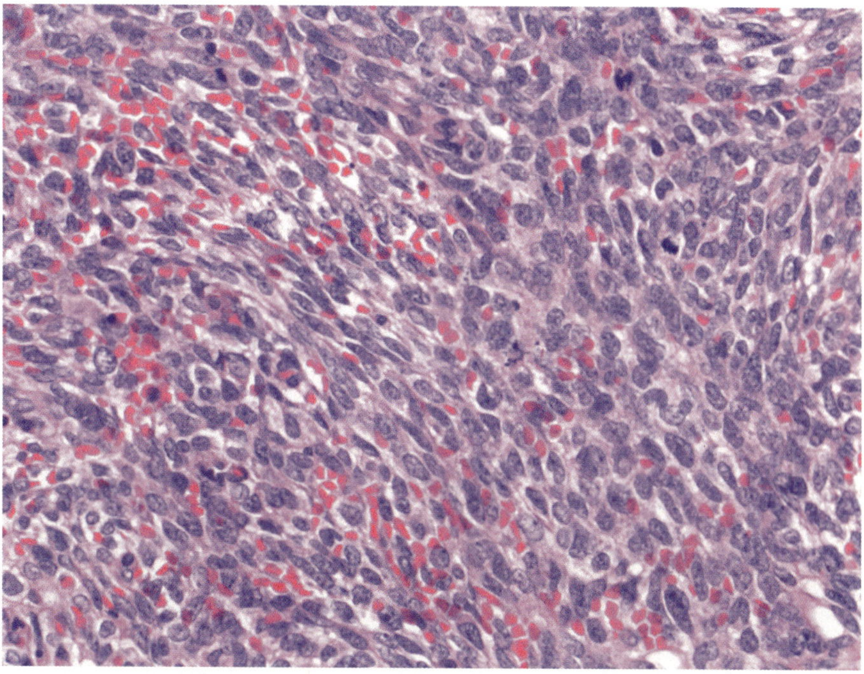

Fig. 6.15 Poorly differentiated Sertoli-Leydig cell tumor. The predominant component is derived from the sarcomatous proliferation of immature spindle-shaped cells, and brisk mitotic figures are also seen

differentiated tumors, the sarcomatous proliferation of immature stromal cells is predominant (Fig. 6.15). Brisk mitotic figures are also seen.

Heterologous elements are seen in 20–25% of intermediate and poorly differentiated SLCT. Intestinal-type mucinous epithelial tissue is the most common heterologous element (Fig. 6.16). Mucinous components can be composed of mucinous cystadenoma, a mucinous borderline tumor, or mucinous adenocarcinoma. Carcinoid cells, cartilage, neuroblasts, and rhabdomyoblasts have also been observed in such heterologous elements [16].

Immunohistochemically, most mature and immature Sertoli cells are positive for CK, but negative for EMA. Most cases of SLCT show positive membrane staining for CD99 and nuclear staining for WT1. The stromal cells of such tumors are positive for vimentin. Sertoli cells and Leydig cells are positive for inhibin (Fig. 6.17) and calretinin. Sertoli-form endometrioid adenocarcinoma of the ovary mimics SLCT, but is positive for EMA and negative for inhibin and calretinin. Histologically, Sertoli-form endometrioid adenocarcinoma displays greater cellular atypia, more irregular tubular arrangements, and necrosis.

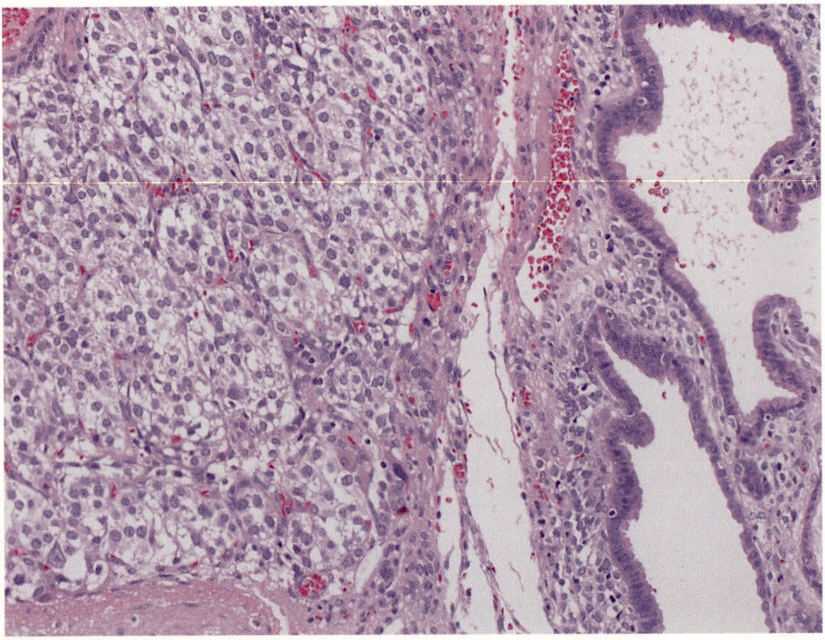

Fig. 6.16 Moderately differentiated Sertoli-Leydig cell tumor with heterologous elements. Note the intestinal-type mucinous epithelial tissue, which is the most common type of heterologous element seen in such tumors

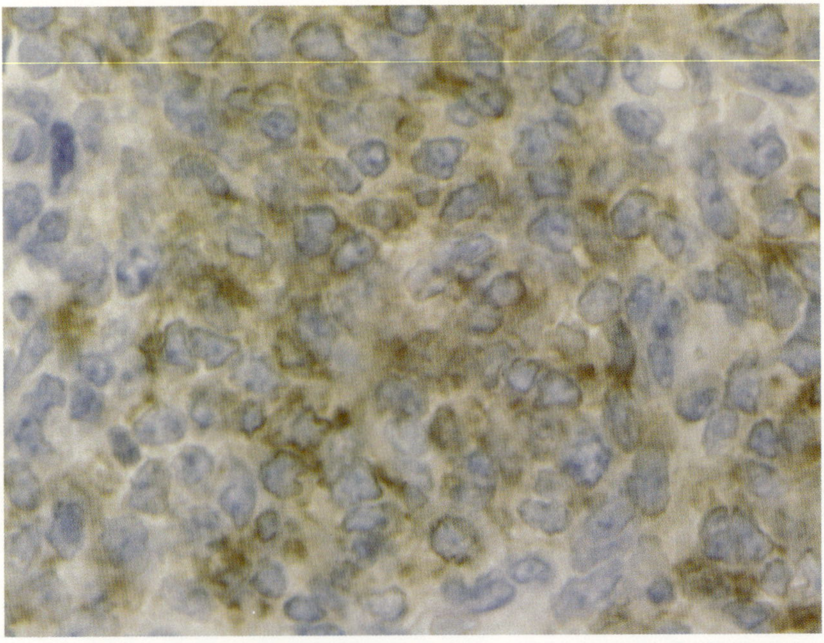

Fig. 6.17 Poorly differentiated Sertoli-Leydig cell tumor. The tumor cells are immunohistochemically positive for inhibin

6.5 Immature Teratoma

6.5.1 Clinical Features

Immature teratoma is one of most common malignant germ cell tumor of the ovary. This tumor occurs predominantly in children and young adult. The clinical presentation is nonspecific, such as abdominal discomfort, pelvic pain, abdominal swelling, or a palpable abdominal mass. They are unilateral and spread mainly to the pelvic and peritoneum by implantation.

6.5.2 Pathologic Features

Macroscopically immature teratoma is a predominantly solid tumor. The cut surface is gray or brown and soft. It may contain cysts, hemorrhage, and necrosis.

Histologically, a mixed mature and mature element is found in most tumors. Recognition of immature neuroectodermal element is most important to make a diagnosis of immature teratoma. These include sheets of mitotically active immature neuroepithelial cells, tubules lined by columnar embryonal cells with stratified hyperchromatic nuclei, nests of neuroblasts, Homer-Wright rosettes, mitotically active glia, and primitive retina with melanin pigments (Figs. 6.18 and 6.19). Immature cartilage, adipose, bone, and skeletal muscle are often present.

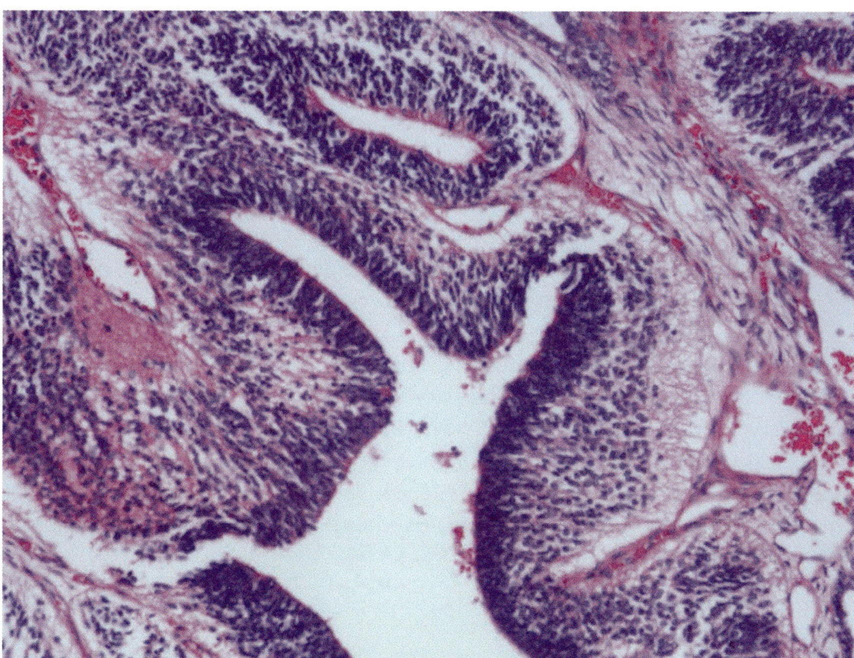

Fig. 6.18 Immature teratoma. Immature neuroectodermal tubules are prominent

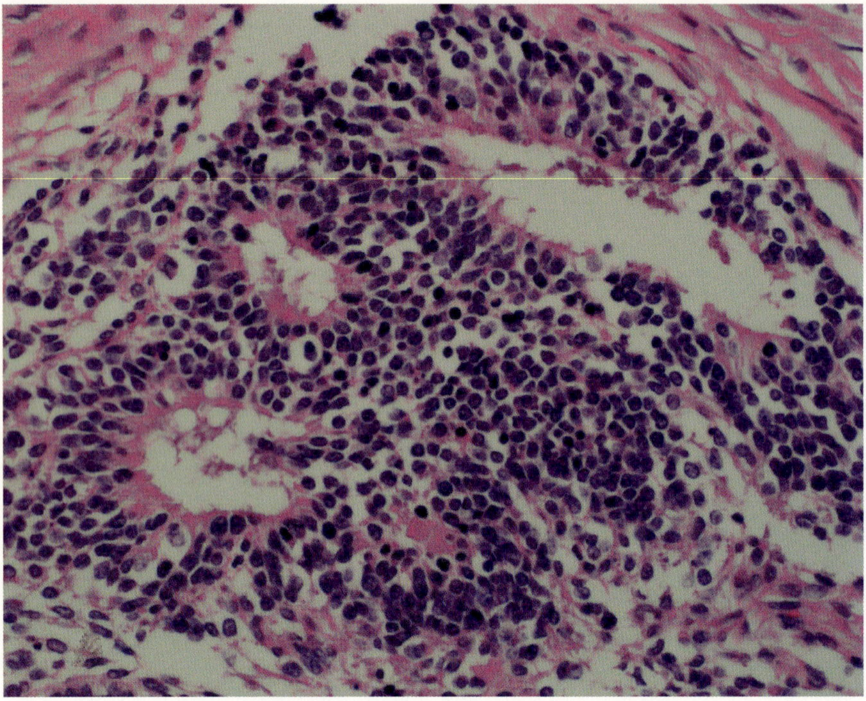

Fig. 6.19 Immature teratoma. Note neural crest-like structures and sheets of immature neural cells

Immature teratoma should be histologically graded [1]:

Grade 1: Tumors with rare foci of immature neuroepithelial tissue that occupy < low power fields (40×) in any slide (low grade).
Grade 2: Tumors with similar elements, occupying 1–3 power fields (40×) in any slide (high grade).
Grade 3: Tumors with large amount of immature neuroepithelial tissue occupying > 3 low power field (40×) in any slide (high grade).

Grade 1 cases are not treated and grade 2 and 3 are treated with same chemotherapy. Stage and grade of the primary tumor and metastases remain important predictive factor. In approximately one-third of cases, gliomatosis peritonei is observed [20]. This lesion has been considered a possible metastasis from teratoma; however, it may represent an independent lesion, probably peritoneal metaplasia [17]. The presence of gliomatosis peritonei does not indicate adverse clinical effect.

6.6 Small Cell Carcinoma of Ovary, Hypercalcemic Type

6.6.1 Clinical Features

Small cell carcinoma of the ovary, hypercalcemic type (SCCHT), is a rare neoplasm that occurs in young females. Its histogenesis is unclear, and it is categorized as a miscellaneous tumor in the revised WHO classification [1].

The reported patients with SCCHT ranged in age from 14 months to 43 (mean, 24) years [18–23]. Most patients present with signs and symptoms related to an abdominal or pelvic mass, but in rare cases, patients will present with clinical symptoms related to hypercalcemia. Approximately 66% of patients present with hypercalcemia [19]. Some studies have serologically documented the presence of parathyroid hormone-related protein. This type of ovarian carcinoma has a dismal prognosis. About 50% of such tumors have spread beyond the ovary at the time of laparotomy. The overall survival rate of SCCHT is approximately 16%.

6.6.2 Pathological Features

SCCHT typically appear as yellowish-white, soft solid tumors with marked hemorrhaging and necrosis. SCCHT exhibit a mean diameter of 15 cm. Most SCCHT are unilateral (Fig. 6.20).

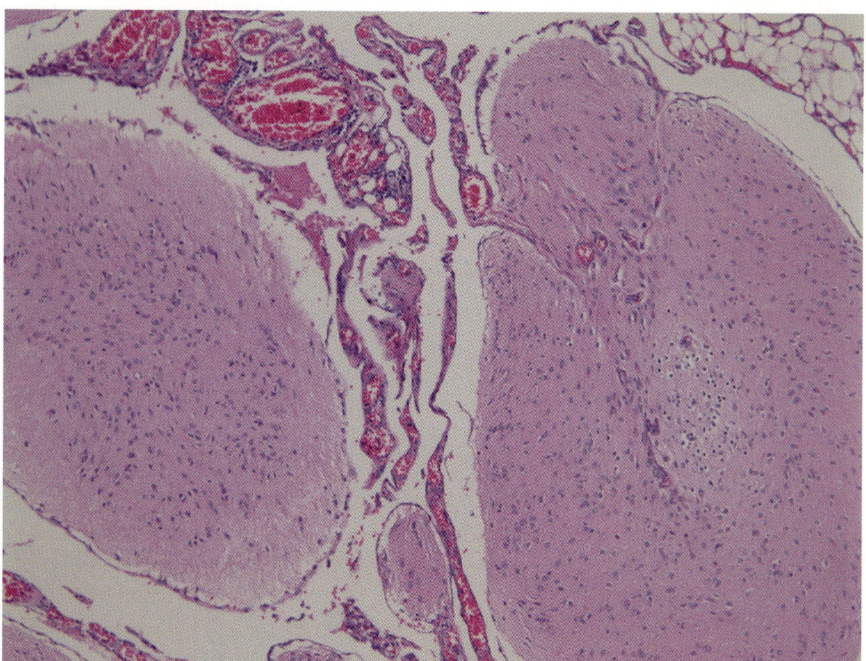

Fig. 6.20 Gliomatosis peritonei. Mature astrocytes form multiple nodes in the peritoneum

SCCHT are histologically composed of small to medium-sized round cells arranged in a solid sheet or follicular pattern (Figs. 6.21 and 6.22). Follicles that vary from small to large in size are considered to be an important feature of SCCHT, and such follicles are seen in about 80% of these tumors. The follicles contain periodic acid–Schiff-positive proteinaceous material. SCCHT usually display moderate atypia and numerous mitotic figures (typical frequency, >20/10 HPF) (Fig. 6.22). Furthermore, tumor necrosis and hemorrhaging are often prominent, whereas the stroma is fibrous but inconspicuous. In addition, a "large cell-type" variant of SCCHT, which is sometimes called "rhabdoid tumor of the ovary," is also known to exist [23] (Fig. 6.23).

Immunohistochemically, SCCHT are focally positive for EMA and low molecular weight CK. Nuclear staining for p53 is often observed, and diffuse strong nuclear staining for WT1 is seen in most cases. A minority of tumors show focal staining for neuroendocrine markers, such as CD56, chromogranin A, or synaptophysin. Staining for CD99, desmin, inhibin, calretinin, and thyroid transcription factor-1 (TTF-1) is negative.

Recently, inactivating mutations in SMARCA4, a member of the switch/sucrose non-fermenting chromatin remodeling complex, have been identified as driving events in most cases of SCCHT [24], and SCCHT exhibits complete immunohistochemical loss of SMARCA4 (INI1) (Fig. 6.24) [25]. Thus, SMARCA4 immunohistochemistry is a highly valuable tool for identifying SCCHT.

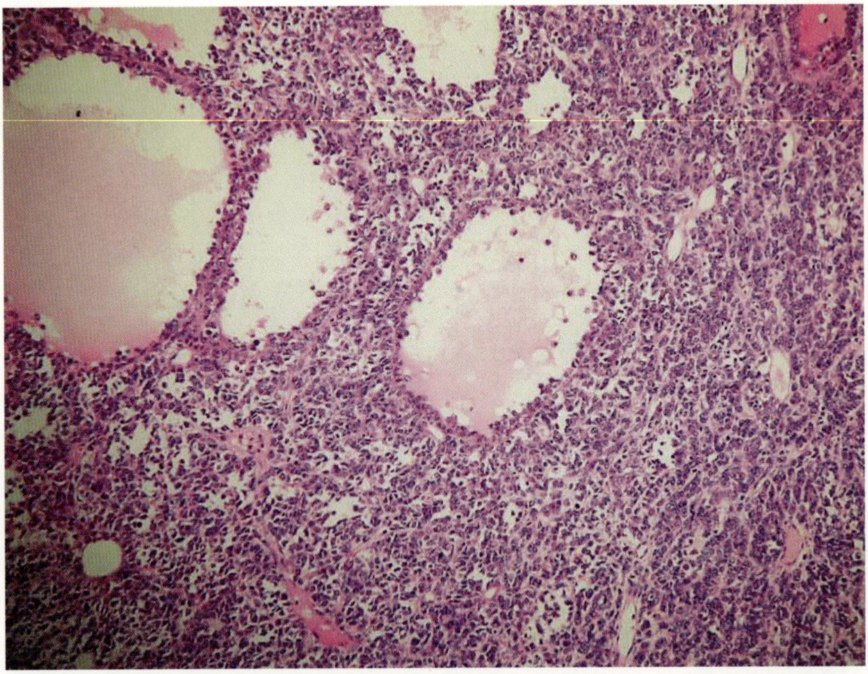

Fig. 6.21 Small cell carcinoma, hypercalcemic type. The tumor is composed of small- to medium-sized round cells arranged in solid sheets and follicular patterns

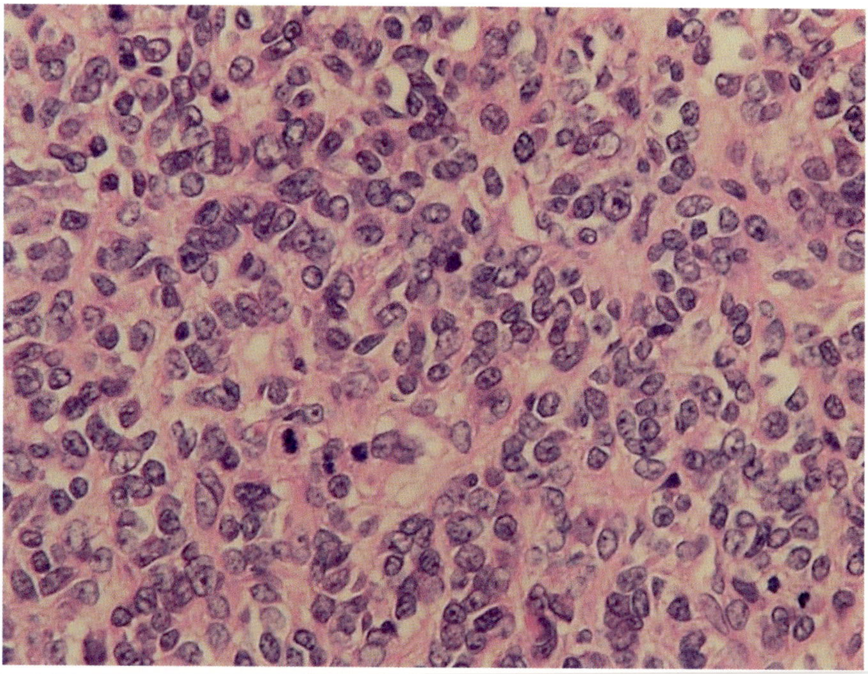

Fig. 6.22 Small cell carcinoma, hypercalcemic type. The tumor cells have hyperchromatic round or oval nuclei, a moderate amount of cytoplasm, and numerous mitotic figures

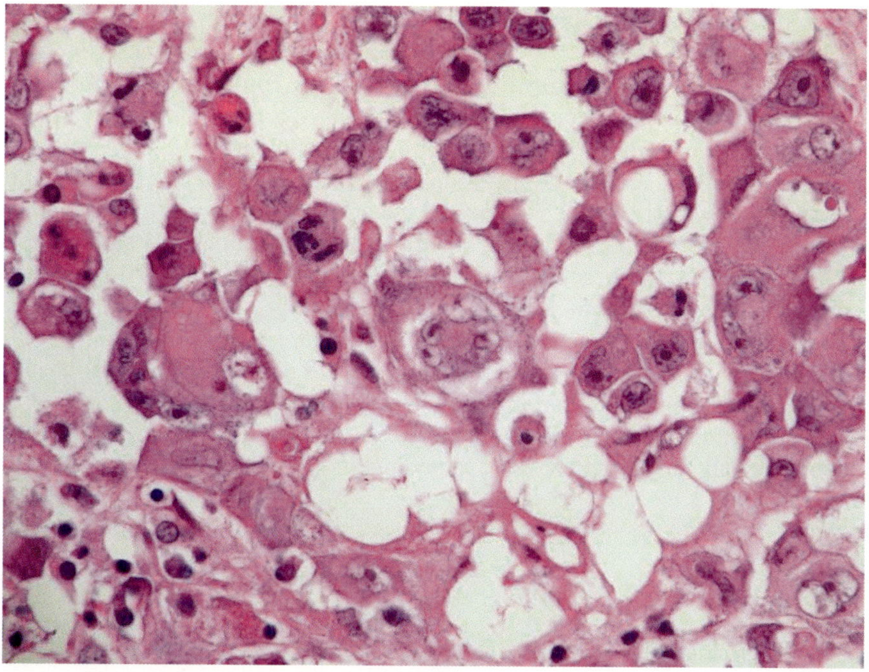

Fig. 6.23 Small cell carcinoma, hypercalcemic type, large cell variant. Note the large cells (rhabdoid cells) have eccentric nuclei and dense eosinophilic globular cytoplasm

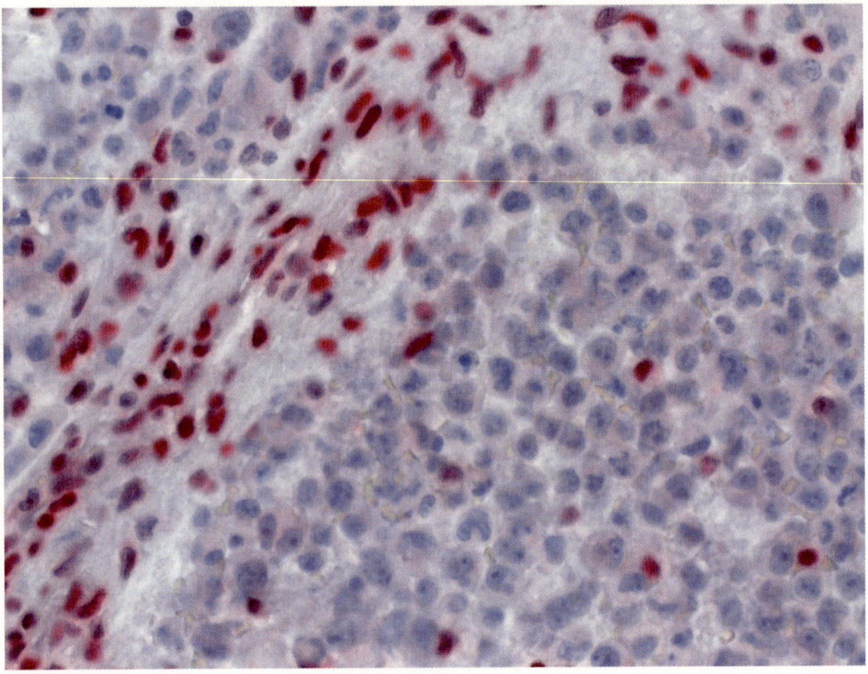

Fig. 6.24 Small cell carcinoma, hypercalcemic type. Note the complete immunohistochemical loss of SMARCA4 (INI1) (reactive cells are positive)

6.6.3 Differential Diagnosis

The differential diagnoses of SCCHT include sex cord-stromal tumors, small blue round cell tumor neoplasms, and pulmonary-type ovarian small cell carcinoma. SCCHT is often confused with granulosa cell tumors [10, 26]. Adult granulosa cell tumors are rare in the young. Most SCCHT have spread beyond the ovary at presentation, which is unusual in both variants of granulosa cell tumor. Granulosa cell tumors are usually positive for inhibin-alpha and calretinin, but negative for EMA. These features are opposite to those of SCCHT. Pulmonary-type small cell carcinoma lacks the follicular arrangement that is characteristic of SCCHT and is positive for neuroendocrine markers. SCCHT, particularly the large cell variant, can be misdiagnosed as undifferentiated carcinoma or melanoma. The large cell variant of SCCHT should always be considered in young patients with suspected undifferentiated carcinoma, and a diligent search for typical small cell carcinoma foci, including the presence of follicles, should be performed.

6.7 Solid Pseudopapillary Neoplasm of the Ovary

These tumors are histologically and immunohistochemically identical to pancreatic solid pseudopapillary neoplasms [27, 28]. The reported patients with solid pseudopapillary neoplasms of the ovary ranged in age from 17 to 57 years. Macroscopically, these tumors are solid and cystic, and histologically they exhibit diffuse, pseudopapillary, nested, and microcystic growth patterns (Fig. 6.25). In these lesions, the tumor cells have a moderate amount of pale or eosinophilic cytoplasm and uniform round nuclei. Mitoses and atypia are rare. In addition, they are positive for beta-catenin and negative for E-cadherin. The differential diagnoses of solid pseudopapillary neoplasm of the ovary include sex cord-stromal tumors, steroid cell tumors, and struma ovarii. This type of tumor rarely occurs at extrapancreatic sites [29]. Deshpande et al. [27] reported that one of three patients died of their disease and that these tumors exhibit necrosis, lymphovascular invasion, and brisk mitotic figures [27].

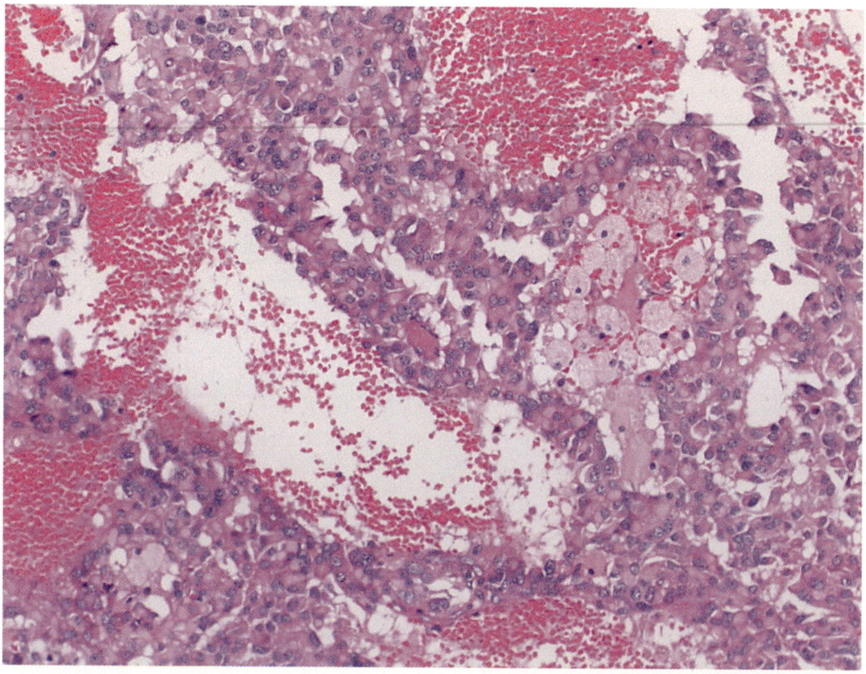

Fig. 6.25 Solid pseudopapillary neoplasm. Note the pseudopapillary, nested, and microcystic growth patterns. The tumor cells contain a moderate amount of eosinophilic cytoplasm and round nuclei

Conclusion

Non-epithelial ovarian tumors have posed pathologic diagnosis, and a correct diagnosis is imperative for appropriate therapies. Many of these neoplasms and those in the differential diagnosis occur predominantly in young women, and they can be aggressive and require specific chemotherapy. Some of non-epithelial neoplasms show histologically biphasic or epithelioid features, mimicking epithelial tumors. A few non-epithelial tumors are not specific to the ovary and may arise more frequently at extraovarian sites. The recent discovery of somatic mutations in FOXL2 in adult granulosa cell tumors and germline and somatic mutations in DICER1 in Sertoli-Leydig cell tumors and SMARCA4 in small cell carcinoma, hypercalcemic type, contributes immunohistochemical analyses and molecular research of these tumors.

References

1. Kurman RJ, Carcangiu ML, Herrington SC, et al. WHO classification of tumours of female reproductive organs. Lyon: IARC Press; 2014.
2. Foulks WD, Gore M, McCluggage WG. Rare non-epithelial ovarian neoplasms: pathology, genetics and treatment. Gynecol Oncol. 2016;142:190–8.
3. Prat J, Scully RE. Cellular fibromas and fibrosarcomas of the ovary: a comparative clinicopathologic analysis of seventeen cases. Cancer. 1981;47:2663–70.
4. Irving JA, Alkushi A, Young RH, et al. Cellular fibromas of the ovary: a study of f75 cases including 40 mitotically active tumors emphasizing their distinction from fibrosarcoma. Am J Surg Pathol. 2006;30:929–38.
5. Zhang J, Young RH, Arseneau J, et al. Ovarian stromal tumors containing lutein or Leydig cells (luteinized thecomas and stromal Leydig tumors): a clinicopathological analysis of 50 cases. Int J Gynecol Pathol. 1982;1:270–85.
6. Chalvardijan A, Scully RE. Sclerosing stromal tumors of the ovary. Cancer. 1973;31:664–70.
7. Irving JA, Young RH. Microcystic stromal tumor of the ovary. Report of 16 cases of a hitherto uncharacterized distinctive ovarian neoplasm. Am J Surg Pathol. 2009;33:367–75.
8. Pautier P, Lhomme C, Culine S, et al. Adult granulosa – cell tumor of the ovary: a retrospective study of 45 cases. Int J Gynecol Cancer. 1997;7:58–65.
9. Shah AF, Kobel M, Senz J, et al. Mutation of FOXL2 in granulosa-cell tumors of the ovary. N Engl J Med. 2009;360:2719–29.
10. Young RH, Dickersin GR, Scully RE. Juvenile granulosa cell tumor of the ovary: a clinicopathological analysis of 125 cases. Am J Surg Pathol. 1984;8:575–96.
11. Scully RE. Sex cord tumor with annular tubules. A distinctive ovarian tumor of the Peutz-Jeghers syndrome. Cancer. 1970;5:1107–21.
12. Young RH, Welch WR, Dickerson GR, Scully RE. Ovarian sex cord tumor with annular tubules. Cancer. 1982;50:1384–402.
13. Giardiello FM, et al. Very high risk of cancer in familial Peutz-Jeghers syndrome. Gastroenterology. 2000;119:1447–53.
14. Ahn GH, Chi JG, Lee SK. Ovarian sex cord tumor with annular tubules. Cancer. 1986;57:1066–73.
15. Young RH, Scully RE. Ovarian Sertoli-Leydig cell tumors: a clinicopathologic analysis of 207 cases. Am J Surg Pathol. 1985;9:543–69.
16. Young RH, Prat J, Scully RE. Ovaria Sertoli-Leydig cell tumors with heterologous elements. I. Gastrointestinal epithelium and carcinoid: a clinicopathologic analysis of 36 cases. Cancer. 1982;50:2448–58.

17. Ferguson AW, Katabuchi H, Ronnett BM, Cho KR. Glial implants in gliomatosis peritonei arise from normal tissue, not from the associated teratoma. Am J Pathol. 2001;159:51–5.
18. Dickersin GR, Kline IW, Scully RE. Small cell carcinoma of the ovary with hypercalcemia. A report of 11 cases. Cancer. 1982;49:188–97.
19. Young RH, Oliva E, Scully RE. Small cell carcinoma of the ovary, hypercalcemic type: a clinicopathologic analysis of 150 cases. Am J Surg Pathol. 1994;18:1102–16.
20. McCluggage WG, Oliva E, Connolly LE, McBride HA, Young RH. An immunohistochemical analysis of ovarian small cell carcinoma of hypercalcemic type. Int J Gynecol Pathol. 2004;23:330–6.
21. Florell SC, Bruggers CS, Matlak M, Young RH, Lowichik A. Ovarian small cell carcinoma of the hypercalcemic type in a 14-month-old: the youngest reported case. Med Pediatr Oncol. 1999;32:304–7.
22. Clement PB. Selected miscellaneous ovarian lesions: small cell carcinoma, mesothelial lesions, mesenchymal and mixed neoplasms, and non-neoplastic lesions. Mod Pathol. 2005;18:113–29.
23. Fukunaga M, Endo Y, Nomura K, Ushigome S. Small cell carcinoma of the ovary: a case report of large cell variant. Pathol Int. 1997;47:250–5.
24. Wang X, Haswell JR, Roberts CW. Molecular pathway: SW1/SNF (BAF) complexes are frequently mutated in cancer-mechanisms and potential therapeutic insights. Clin Caner Res. 2014;20:21–7.
25. Agaimy A, Thiel F, Hartmann A, Fukunaga M. SMARCA4-deficient undifferentiated carcinoma of the ovary (small cell carcinoma, hypercalcemic type): clinicopathologic and immunohistochemical studies of 3 cases. Ann Diagn Pathol. 2015;19:153–7.
26. Zaloudek C, Norris HJ. Granulosa tumors of the ovary in children. A clinical and pathologic study of 32 cases. Am J Surg Pathol. 1982;6:503–12.
27. Deshpande V, Olive E, Young RH. Solid pseudopapillary neoplasm of the ovary: a report of 3 primary ovarian tumors resembling those of the pancreas. Am J Surg Pathol. 2010;10:1514–20.
28. Abraham SC, Klimstra DS, Wilents RE, et al. Solid-pseudopapillary tumors of the pancreas are genetically distinct from pancreatic ductal adenocarcinomas and almost always harbor beta-catenin mutations. Am J Pathol. 2002;160:1361–9.
29. Fukunaga M. Pseudopapillary solid cystic tumor arising from an extrapancreatic site. Arch Pathol Lab Med. 2001;125:1368–71.

Ovarian Cancer Genome and Molecular Experimental Sciences

7

Noriomi Matsumura and Ikuo Konishi

Abstract

A large number of genomic studies have provided important insights into molecular pathogenesis of ovarian cancer. Ovarian cancer is divided into two types: type I and type II tumors. Type I ovarian tumors include clear cell, endometrioid, mucinous, and low-grade serous carcinomas, while type II tumors are mainly high-grade serous carcinomas. High-grade serous carcinomas are characterized by *TP53* gene mutations and extensive copy number alterations. Approximately half of high-grade serous ovarian carcinomas harbor homologous recombination pathway deficiency. Clear cell carcinomas are characterized by upregulation of *HNF1B* and *IL6* and mutations in *PIK3CA* and *ARID1A*. Alterations of HNF1B pathway, IL6 pathway, PI3K pathway, and SWI/SNF complex are influenced by copy number alterations and epigenetic regulation. Endometrioid carcinomas are divided into low-grade (G1–G2) and high-grade (G3) tumors, although some of high-grade serous carcinomas have been misclassified as high-grade endometrioid carcinomas. Low-grade endometrioid carcinomas harbor mutations in *CTNNB1, PTEN, KRAS, PIK3CA,* and *ARID1A*, while high-grade endometrioid carcinomas harbor *TP53* mutations. Mucinous carcinomas exhibit ERBB2/KRAS/BRAF pathway activation by *KRAS* or *BRAF* mutations or *ERBB2* amplifications. Unlike other type I tumors, half of mucinous carcinomas harbor *TP53* mutations. Low-grade serous carcinomas evolve from serous borderline tumor. *KRAS* and *BRAF* mutations are common in serous borderline tumors and low-grade serous carcinomas.

Keywords

Ovarian cancer • Genome • Genetic alterations

N. Matsumura, M.D., Ph.D. (✉)
Department of Obstetrics and Gynecology, Kindai University, Faculty of Medicine, Osaka, Japan
e-mail: noriomi@med.kindai.ac.jp

I. Konishi, M.D., Ph.D.
National Kyoto Medical Center, Kyoto, Japan

H. Katabuchi (ed.), *Frontiers in Ovarian Cancer Science*, Comprehensive Gynecology and Obstetrics, DOI 10.1007/978-981-10-4160-0_7

7.1 Introduction

There are two types of epithelial ovarian cancer: type I and type II [1]. Type I tumors grow slowly, while type II tumors behave aggressively. Type I tumors contain low-grade serous, clear cell, endometrioid, and mucinous cancers, while type II tumors are mainly high-grade serous cancers. A large number of genomic studies have provided important insights into molecular pathogenesis of ovarian cancer. This chapter summarizes genomic alterations of epithelial ovarian cancer from histology to histology.

7.2 High-Grade Serous Ovarian Carcinoma

7.2.1 Germline Mutations in Ovarian Carcinoma

Ovarian carcinoma, mainly high-grade serous, can occur via germline gene mutations in DNA repair system. In a study of 1915 ovarian carcinoma cases, 347 (18%) carried pathogenic germline mutations, 280 (15%) had mutations in BRCA1 (n = 182) or BRCA2 (n = 98), and the remaining cases had mutations in other 5 homologous recombination (HR) pathway genes (*BARD1, BRIP1, PALB2, RAD51C, RAD51D*) and four mismatch repair (MMR) genes (*MSH2, MLH1, PMS2,* and *MSH6*) [2].

7.2.2 The Genomic Landscape of High-Grade Serous Ovarian Carcinoma

The Cancer Genome Atlas (TCGA) project analyzed more than 300 high-grade serous ovarian carcinoma cases with whole-exome sequencing, SNP array (to analyze copy number alterations), mRNA expression microarray, DNA methylation microarray, and microRNA microarray [3]. The TCGA analyses identified four ovarian cancer transcriptional subtypes, three miRNA subtypes, four promoter methylation subtypes, and a transcriptional signature correlated with prognosis.

Strikingly, nearly all the high-grade serous ovarian carcinoma cases harbored somatic mutations in *TP53* (96%). Furthermore, a study by five gynecologic pathologists who reviewed the negative TP53 cases from TCGA study found that all of the negative tumors except for one were histologically misclassified. The one exception contained a homozygous deletion of the gene, indicating that all high-grade serous ovarian carcinomas have a TP53 abnormality, which is almost always a mutation [4]. Somatic gene mutations other than *TP53* occurred in less than 5% of high-grade serous ovarian carcinomas.

Additional feature of high-grade serous ovarian carcinoma is the widespread copy number alterations. The TCGA analysis identified regional copy number aberrations including 8 recurrent gains and 22 losses [3], all of which have been reported previously [5]. Focal amplifications were observed in 63 regions. The most common focal amplifications encoded *CCNE1*, *MYC*, and *MECOM* in more than 20%

of tumors. The TCGA study also identified homozygous deletions of known tumor suppressor genes, such as *PTEN*, *RB1*, and *NF1*. A focal deletion at 10q23.31 that includes only *PTEN* has been found in approximately 7% of tumors, which is associated with downregulation of *PTEN* mRNA expression [3]. Another group confirmed that *PTEN* loss is a common event in high-grade serous ovarian cancer with significantly worse prognosis [6].

Exome sequencing has a limited ability to detect gene mutation by structural rearrangement. A whole-genome sequencing analysis for 92 cases of high-grade serous ovarian carcinoma was performed focusing on the mechanism of chemoresistance [7]. Although *NF1* and *RB1* were inactivated by truncating point mutations and indels in limited number of samples (*NF1*; $n = 3$, *RB1*; $n = 2$, out of 80), inclusion of gene breakage raised the frequency of inactivating mutations to 20% for *NF1* and 17.5% for *RB1*. Gene inactivation by breakage was also seen for *PTEN* (7.5%) and *RAD51B* (5%).

Homologous recombinant (HR) pathway-deficient tumors, having extensive copy number alterations and increased single nucleotide variants, are sensitive to platinum and PARP inhibitor. HR pathway-deficient tumors tend to use error-prone nonhomologous end joining to repair DNA, leading to extensive genome DNA variations. Approximately 50% of high-grade serous ovarian carcinomas exhibit genetic or epigenetic alterations in the FA-BRCA pathway (Fig. 7.1) [3, 8]. In TCGA analysis, germline *BRCA1/2* mutations are present in 14% [3], whereas somatic *BRCA1/2* mutations have been identified in 6% [3]. Importantly, 81% of *BRCA1* and 72% of

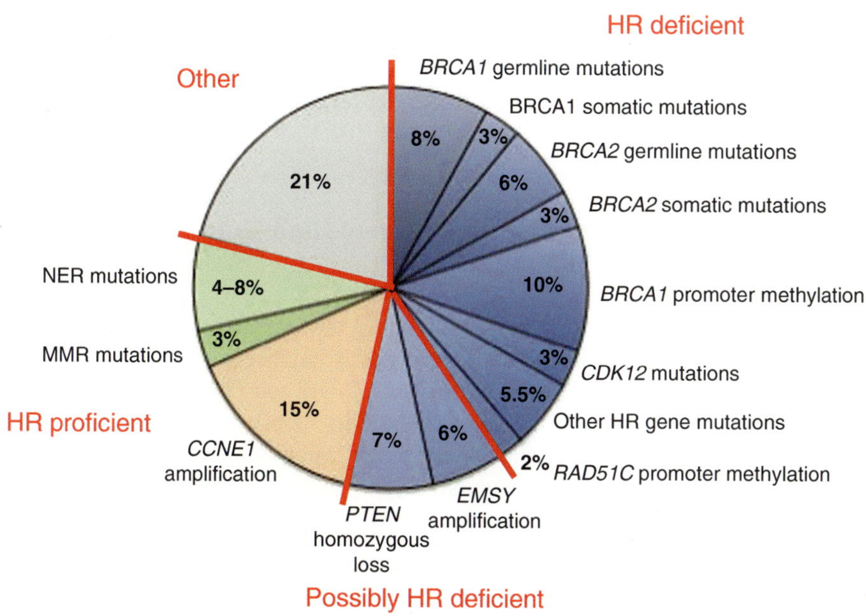

Fig. 7.1 HR-deficient and HR-proficient tumors of high-grade serous ovarian carcinoma [8]

BRCA2 mutations are accompanied by heterozygous loss [3]; thus, both alleles are inactivated. Epigenetic silencing via promoter hypermethylation occurs for *BRCA1*, but not *BRCA2*, in approximately 10% and is mutually exclusive of *BRCA1/2* mutations [3]. Other HR pathway alterations include mutations in FA genes (mainly *PALB2, FANCA, FANCI, FANCL,* and *FANCC*), in RAD genes (*RAD50, RAD51, RAD51C,* and *RAD54L*), and in DNA damage response genes (*ATM, ATR, CHEK1,* and *CHEK2*). *RAD51C* was also epigenetically silenced via promoter hypermethylation in about 2% of the cases [3]. CDK12 is known to promote the transcription of several HR pathway genes, including *BRCA1*. Inactivation mutation of *CDK12*, found in 3% of the cases [3], leads to downregulation of *BRCA1* and other HR genes [9, 10]. HR defect may also occur via indirect mechanism. PTEN inactivation has been reported to be synthetically lethal with PARP inhibition, and one of the proposed mechanisms is downregulation of *RAD51* [11, 12]. Additionally, overexpression and amplification of *EMSY*, which inhibits transcriptional activity of BRCA2 [13], is found in as high as 17% of high-grade serous ovarian carcinomas [3]. Furthermore, there may be other mechanisms of HR deficiency, such as miRNAs that target BRCA1/2 [14, 15].

HR pathway proficient tumors with *CCNE1* amplification were common in primary resistant and refractory cases [7]. Inactivation of the p53 pathway and activation of the CCNE1 pathway also contribute to chromosomal instability [16]. Alterations in nucleotide excision repair (NER) and mismatch repair (MMR) have been reported in up to 8% and 3% of high-grade serous ovarian carcinomas, which tumors are sensitive to platinum and resistant to PARP inhibitor [17].

Mechanism of acquired resistance to chemotherapy included breakage of tumor suppressor genes, reversion mutation of *BRCA1/2* mutated cases, and upregulation of *BRCA1* gene expression by demethylation of the methylated *BRCA1* promoter region in a primary tumor. Additionally, gene fusion of *ABCB1* with *SLC25A40* promoter caused upregulation of *ABCB1* expression, which can cause increased excretion of chemotherapeutic agents [7] (see also Sect. 3.4.1.1 in Chap. 3).

7.2.3 Experiments to Identify Origin of High-Grade Serous Ovarian Carcinoma

Recently, fallopian tubal epithelial cell has been thought as the origin of high-grade serous ovarian carcinoma [1]. Using a genetically engineered mouse that expresses Cre recombinase from a *Pax8* promoter, *Brca*, *Tp53*, and *Pten* genes were targeted in fallopian tubal secretory epithelial cells. This mouse model generated serous tubal intraepithelial carcinoma as the precursor lesion that gave rise to high-grade serous ovarian and peritoneal carcinomas [18]. In this model, tumor-bearing mice had higher serum CA125 levels than controls. Furthermore, the tumors had extensive copy number alterations similar to human high-grade serous ovarian carcinomas.

There is another idea regarding cell of origin of high-grade serous ovarian carcinoma. Cells of the hilum ovarian surface epithelium, the transitional area between the ovarian surface epithelium, mesothelium, and tubal epithelium, express stem cell markers and display stem cell properties. The hilum cells show increased transformation potential after inactivation of tumor suppressor genes Tp53 and Rb1. Therefore, stem cell niches in those areas are susceptible to malignant transformation and could be the origin of high-grade serous ovarian carcinoma [19].

7.3 Ovarian Clear Cell Carcinoma

7.3.1 Gene Expression of Ovarian Clear Cell Carcinoma

Ovarian clear cell carcinoma shows unique clinical features including an association with endometriosis and poor prognosis. A gene expression microarray analysis identified genes commonly expressed in both ovarian clear cell carcinoma cell lines and clinical samples, which comprise an ovarian clear cell carcinoma gene signature. The gene signature contains known markers of ovarian clear cell carcinoma, such as *HNF1B*, *VCAN*, *IL6*, and other genes that reflect oxidative stress. Expression of ovarian clear cell carcinoma signature genes was induced by treatment of immortalized ovarian surface epithelial cells with the contents of endometriotic cysts, indicating that the ovarian clear cell carcinoma signature is largely dependent on the tumor microenvironment [20].

7.3.2 DNA Methylation Analysis of Ovarian Clear Cell Carcinoma

Recently, genome-wide methylation and expression data were generated for 14 ovarian clear cell carcinoma, 32 non-ovarian clear cell carcinoma, and four normal cell lines. Consensus clustering showed that ovarian clear cell carcinoma is epigenetically distinct. Inverse relationships between expression and methylation in ovarian clear cell carcinoma were identified, suggesting functional regulation by methylation, and included 22 hypomethylated genes and 276 hypermethylated genes. The ovarian clear cell carcinoma-specific hypomethylated genes were involved in response to stress and many contain HNF1-binding sites, while the ovarian clear cell carcinoma-specific hypermethylated genes included members of the ERα network and genes involved in tumor development [21].

7.3.3 Genetic Analyses of Ovarian Clear Cell Carcinoma

ARID1A mutations were reported in 46–57% and *PIK3CA* mutations in 31–33% of ovarian clear cell carcinoma samples [22–24]. A whole-exome sequencing of 39 ovarian clear cell carcinoma samples identified recurrent somatic mutations in 426 genes [25]. In these 39 samples, *ARID1A* (62%) and *PIK3CA* (51%) were frequently mutated, and known key ovarian clear cell carcinoma-related genes such as *KRAS* (10%), *PPP2R1A* (10%), and *PTEN* (5%), as well as novel genes *MLL3* (15%),

ARID1B (10%), and *PIK3R1* (8%) were also mutated. Gene interaction analysis and functional assessment revealed that mutated genes were clustered into groups pertaining to chromatin remodeling, cell proliferation, DNA repair and cell cycle checkpointing, and cytoskeletal organization.

A copy number variation analysis based on the above exome sequencing identified frequent amplification of *MYC* (chr8q, 64%), *ZNF217* (chr20q, 54%), and *ERBB2, STAT3, HNF1B, PPM1D* (chr17q, 46%) loci as well as deletion in *SMARCA4* (chr19p, 41%), *RB1* (chr13q, 28%), *NOTCH1* (chr9q, 21%), and *SMAD4* (chr18q, 21%) loci. Other copy number alterations included amplification of *IL6, IL6R, KRAS, PIK3CA, PIK3C2B, CDK2, CDK4*, and *CCNE1*, as well as deletion of *ARID1A, SMARCC1, SMARCA2, ARID1B, CDKN1A, CDKN2A, CDKN2B*, and *TP53*. Integration of the analyses discovered that frequently mutated or amplified/deleted genes were involved in the KRAS/PI3K signaling (82%) and MYC/RB signaling (75%) pathways as well as the critical chromatin remodeling complex SWI/SNF (85%) [25] (see also Sect. 3.4.3 in Chap. 3).

7.3.4 Role of ARID1A, PIK3CA, and IL6 in the Carcinogenesis of Ovarian Clear Cell Carcinoma

Concurrent *Arid1a* inactivation and *Pik3ca* activation in mouse ovaries generated adenocarcinomas similar to human ovarian clear cell carcinomas. These tumors expressed Hnf1b, a marker of ovarian clear cell carcinoma. Furthermore, in this model, the tumor growth was promoted through sustained IL6 overproduction [26].

Ovarian clear cell carcinoma was generated in vitro by introducing *ARID1A* knockdown and mutant *PIK3CA* into a normal human ovarian epithelial cell line. Loss of *ARID1A* impairs the recruitment of the Sin3A-HDAC complex, while the *PIK3CA* mutation releases RelA from IκB, leading to NF-kB pathway activation resulting in IL6 overexpression [27].

Collectively, these findings indicate that *ARID1A* and *PIK3CA* mutations, frequently seen in ovarian clear cell carcinoma, are sufficient to generate ovarian clear cell carcinoma, associated with the specific gene expression including *HNF1B* and *IL6* (see also Sect. 3.4.3 in Chap. 3).

7.4 Ovarian Endometrioid Carcinoma

7.4.1 Genetic Analysis of Ovarian Endometrioid Carcinoma

Gene mutations in ovarian endometrioid carcinoma samples with different grades (grade 1, $n = 20$; grade 2, $n = 26$; grade 3, $n = 26$) were analyzed, and mutations in *CTNNB1* (13%, 5%, 0%), *APC* (5%, 0%, 0%), *KRAS* (10%, 12%, 0%), *PTEN* (20%, 8%, 0%), *PIK3CA* (20%, 8%, 0%), and *TP53* (15%, 46%, 65%) were found [28]. Therefore, high-grade ovarian endometrioid carcinomas are likely to harbor *TP53* mutations, while low-grade ovarian endometrioid carcinomas frequently harbor mutations of Wnt/β-catenin pathway and/or KRAS/PI3K pathway genes. In another study, *ARID1A* mutations were reported in 10 of 33 ovarian endometrioid carcinomas (30%) [23]. Another group reported mutations of *CTNNB1* (53%), *PIK3CA* (40%), *ARID1A* (30%), *PTEN* (17%), *KRAS* (33%), *PPP2R1A* (17%), and *TP53* (7%) in low-grade (grade 1 and 2) ovarian endometrioid carcinomas (n = 30) [29]. Activating mutations of the *CTNNB1* gene is associated with squamous differentiation [30].

High-grade endometrioid carcinoma tumors with TP53 mutations have expression profiles similar to those of high-grade serous carcinoma [31]. However, these tumors may have been misclassified, as suggested by more recent studies reporting a subset of high-grade serous carcinomas that display a pseudoendometrioid pattern [32] (see also Sect. 3.4.2 in Chap. 3).

7.4.2 Mouse Models of Ovarian Endometrioid Carcinoma

Like ovarian clear cell carcinomas, ovarian endometrioid carcinomas are frequently associated with endometriosis. Peritoneal endometriosis occurs in mice by the activation of an oncogenic K-ras. Additionally, expression of oncogenic K-ras and Pten deletion within the ovarian surface epithelium leads to the induction of adenocarcinomas similar to human ovarian endometrioid carcinomas [33]. In another study, inactivation of the *Pten* and *Apc* in murine ovaries resulted in the formation of endometrioid adenocarcinomas [28]. More recently, codeletion of *Arid1a* and *Pten* resulted in ovarian endometrioid carcinoma [34].

7.4.3 Microsatellite Instability (MSI) in Ovarian Endometrioid Carcinoma

Ovarian cancer, particularly endometrioid adenocarcinoma, is associated with Lynch syndrome, although the risk is much smaller than for uterine cancer. Among 71 cases with ovarian endometrioid adenocarcinoma, 7 (10%) tumors had abnormal mismatch repair (MMR) protein status, defined as complete loss of expression of MLH1, MSH2, MSH6, and/or PMS2. Each of these tumors with abnormal MMR status demonstrated MSI. Importantly, concurrent uterine tumor was present in 5/7 patients whose ovarian tumor had abnormal MMR/MSI [35].

7.4.4 Genetic Analysis of Synchronous Endometrial and Ovarian Carcinoma

Five to ten percent of women with ovarian endometrioid carcinomas present with concurrent endometrial carcinoma. Based on both targeted and exome sequencing of 18 synchronous endometrial and ovarian tumors, most (17/18) cases showed evidence of clonality. Importantly, 10 of 11 cases that fulfilled clinicopathological criteria that would lead to classification as independent endometrial and ovarian primary carcinomas showed evidence of clonality [36]. Therefore, the genome-wide analysis demonstrated that most synchronous endometrial and ovarian carcinoma tumors develop from a clonal origin.

7.5 Mucinous Ovarian Tumors

7.5.1 Origin of Mucinous Ovarian Tumors

Mucinous ovarian carcinomas typically display heterogeneity, with lesion of mucinous cystadenoma admixed with borderline tumor and carcinoma. The identical KRAS mutation in these components provides strong evidence that mucinous cystadenomas are the precursor lesions of mucinous carcinoma [37, 38].

In terms of the origin of mucinous cystadenoma, a subset develops from mucinous epithelium in mature teratomas. A microsatellite genotyping analysis of mucinous tumors associated with a teratoma revealed five of six pairs of tumors with teratoma showed a high or complete degree of allelotype matching, which differed from the somatic allelotypes of the normal control tissue [39].

It has been proposed that many of nongerm cell mucinous tumors are derived from Brenner tumors. In a study of 40 mucinous cystadenomas, 67 Brenner tumors, and 13 combined tumors, a total of 25% of tumors with a mucinous component contained a Brenner component, and 16% of tumors with a Brenner component contained a mucinous component. Mucinous tumors are typically large, whereas Brenner tumors tend to be smaller. Accordingly, the Brenner tumor is compressed by the large mucinous cystadenoma and may be overlooked [40]. This hypothesis was supported by a recent study showing that, in combined Brenner and mucinous tumors, the Brenner and mucinous components are clonally related [41] (see also Sect. 3.4.4 in Chap. 3).

7.5.2 Genetic Features of Mucinous Ovarian Tumors

KRAS-activating mutation is the most common single molecular genetic alteration in mucinous carcinomas, occurring in 65% of cases [42]. Another study identified mutations in a novel gene, *RNF43*, a zinc finger-dependent E3 ubiquitin protein ligase. *RNF43* mutations were observed with a frequency of 2/22 (9%) in mucinous ovarian borderline tumors and 6/29 (21%) in mucinous ovarian carcinomas [43]. In contrast to other type I ovarian carcinomas, *TP53* mutation is frequent in mucinous carcinomas, being present in approximately one-half of cases [42, 43]. In a genetic analysis of a total of 82 mucinous ovarian tumors, which included exome sequencing of 24 tumors and a validation cohort of benign 58 tumors for specific gene regions, benign, borderline, and carcinoma samples harbored mutations in *BRAF* (0%, 10%, 23%), *TP53* (9%, 14%, 52%), and *RNF43* (0%, 7%, 20%), respectively, which mutations were associated with progression of the disease. Other recurrent, but not associated with progression, mutations were found in *KRAS* (54%), *CDKN2A* (16%), *ARID1A* (8%), *ELF3* (6%), *GNAS* (6%), *ERBB3* (5%), and *KLF5* (5%) [44].

Overexpression and amplification of *ERRB2* was observed in 11/176 (6%) mucinous borderline tumors and 29/154 (19%) mucinous cancers. *KRAS* mutations and *ERRB2* amplification are near mutually exclusive (#41#). Thus, mutations in *KRAS*, *BRAF*, and/or *ERRB2* amplification are present in the majority of mucinous neoplasms, indicating RAS/RAF pathway activation is frequent in this tumor. (See also Sect. 3.4.4 in Chap. 3).

7.6 Serous Borderline Tumor and Low-Grade Serous Ovarian Carcinoma

It has been well established that low-grade serous ovarian carcinomas can develop from serous borderline tumor. Deletions of ch1p36 and ch9p21 are much more common in low-grade serous ovarian carcinomas than in serous borderline tumors [45]. The ch1p36 region contains several candidate tumor suppressor genes including miR-34a. Then, the ch9p21 region including the *CDKN2A/B* locus encodes three tumor suppressor proteins, p14 (Arf), p16, and p15. Thus, deletions of ch1p36 or ch9p21 may cause progression of some serous borderline tumors to low-grade serous carcinomas.

KRAS mutations occur in one-third of serous borderline tumors and log-grade serous ovarian carcinomas, and *BRAF* mutations occur in another one-third of serous borderline tumors but less commonly in low-grade serous ovarian carcinomas [46, 47]. *BRAF*-mutated advanced-stage low-grade serous ovarian carcinomas are much less common than are *BRAF*-mutated advanced-stage serous borderline tumors [48–50]. *ERBB2* and *NRAS* mutations are also detected in a small percentage of low-grade serous ovarian carcinomas [47, 51]. These mutations result in activation of the MAP kinase signal transduction pathway. Exome sequencing analyses also identified *BRAF* and *KRAS* as the most frequently mutated genes (#43#, #44#).

A better outcome has been reported for women whose tumors contain *BRAF* mutations than for women with *KRAS* mutations or wild-type *BRAF* and *KRAS* [48, 49, 52]. *BRAF* mutations correlate with the presence of cells with abundant eosinophilic cytoplasm, which may suggest cellular senescence caused by BRAF activation [53, 54] (see also Sect. 3.4.1.2 in Chap. 3).

Conclusion

Type I tumors, containing low-grade serous, clear cell, endometrioid, and mucinous cancers, are characterized by activating mutations in the ERRB2/KRAS/BRAF/MEK pathway, PI3K/AKT pathway, and Wnt pathway and inactivation mutations in the *PTEN*- and ARID1A-related chromatin remodeling. In contrast, type II tumors, mainly high-grade serous cancers, are characterized by inactivation of the TP53, deficiency of the HR pathway, and extensive copy number alterations. Representative genetic alterations are summarized in Table 7.1. These findings would lead to discovery of effective molecularly targeted drugs and their biomarkers.

Table 7.1 Representative genetic alterations in epithelial ovarian cancer

	Gene mutation	Copy number amplification	Copy number loss
High-grade serous	*TP53, BRCA1/2*	*CCNE1, MYC, MECOM*	*PTEN, RB1, NF1*
Clear cell	*ARID1A, PIK3CA*	*MYC, ZNF217, ERBB2, STAT3, HNF1B, PPM1D*	*SMARCA4, RB1, SMAD4*
Endometrioid (low-grade)	*CTNNB1, PIK3CA, KRAS, PTEN*		
Mucinous	*KRAS, TP53, BRAF, RNF43, CDKN2A*	*ERBB2*	
Low-grade serous	*KRAS, BRAF*		*CDKN2A/2B*, miR-34a

References

1. Kurman RJ, Shih IM. The dualistic model of ovarian carcinogenesis: revisited, revised, and expanded. Am J Pathol. 2016;186:733–47.
2. Norquist BM, Harrell MI, Brady MF, et al. Inherited mutations in women with ovarian carcinoma. JAMA Oncol. 2016;2:482–90.
3. Cancer Genome Atlas Research Network. Integrated genomic analyses of ovarian carcinoma. Nature. 2011;474:609–15.
4. Vang R, Levine DA, Soslow RA, et al. Molecular alterations of TP53 are a defining feature of ovarian high-grade serous carcinoma: a rereview of cases lacking TP53 mutations in the cancer genome atlas ovarian study. Int J Gynecol Pathol. 2016;35:48–55.
5. Etemadmoghadam D, deFazio A, Beroukhim R, et al. Integrated genome-wide DNA copy number and expression analysis identifies distinct mechanisms of primary chemoresistance in ovarian carcinomas. Clin Cancer Res. 2009;15:1417–27.
6. Martins FC, Santiago ID, Trinh A, et al. Combined image and genomic analysis of high-grade serous ovarian cancer reveals PTEN loss as a common driver event and prognostic classifier. Genome Biol. 2014;15:526.
7. Patch AM, Christie EL, Etemadmoghadam D, et al. Whole-genome characterization of chemoresistant ovarian cancer. Nature. 2015;521:489–94.
8. Konstantinopoulos PA, Ceccaldi R, Shapiro GI, et al. Homologous recombination deficiency: exploiting the fundamental vulnerability of ovarian cancer. Cancer Discov. 2015;5:1137–54.
9. Bajrami I, Frankum JR, Konde A, et al. Genome-wide profiling of genetic synthetic lethality identifies CDK12 as a novel determinant of PARP1/2 inhibitor sensitivity. Cancer Res. 2014;74:287–97.
10. Joshi PM, Sutor SL, Huntoon CJ, et al. Ovarian cancer-associated mutations disable catalytic activity of CDK12, a kinase that promotes homologous recombination repair and resistance to cisplatin and poly(ADP-ribose) polymerase inhibitors. J Biol Chem. 2014;289:9247–53.
11. Mendes-Pereira AM, Martin SA, Brough R, et al. Synthetic lethal targeting of PTEN mutant cells with PARP inhibitors. EMBO Mol Med. 2009;1:315–22.
12. Shen WH, Balajee AS, Wang J, et al. Essential role for nuclear PTEN in maintaining chromosomal integrity. Cell. 2007;128:157–70.
13. Hughes-Davies L, Huntsman D, Ruas M, et al. EMSY links the BRCA2 pathway to sporadic breast and ovarian cancer. Cell. 2003;115:523–35.
14. Moskwa P, Buffa FM, Pan Y, et al. miR-182-mediated downregulation of BRCA1 impacts DNA repair and sensitivity to PARP inhibitors. Mol Cell. 2011;41:210–20.
15. Choi YE, Pan Y, Park E, et al. MicroRNAs down-regulate homologous recombination in the G1 phase of cycling cells to maintain genomic stability. Elife. 2014;3:e02445.

16. Bagheri-Yarmand R, Biernacka A, Hunt KK, et al. Low molecular weight cyclin E overexpression shortens mitosis, leading to chromosome missegregation and centrosome amplification. Cancer Res. 2010;70:5074–84.
17. Ceccaldi R, O'Connor KW, Mouw KW, et al. A unique subset of epithelial ovarian cancers with platinum sensitivity and PARP inhibitor resistance. Cancer Res. 2015;75:628–34.
18. Perets R, Wyant GA, Muto KW, et al. Transformation of the fallopian tube secretory epithelium leads to high-grade serous ovarian cancer in Brca;Tp53;Pten models. Cancer Cell. 2013;24:751–65.
19. Flesken-Nikitin A, Hwang CI, Cheng CY, et al. Ovarian surface epithelium at the junction area contains a cancer-prone stem cell niche. Nature. 2013;495:241–5.
20. Yamaguchi K, Mandai M, Oura T, et al. Identification of an ovarian clear cell carcinoma gene signature that reflects inherent disease biology and the carcinogenic processes. Oncogene. 2010;29:1741–52.
21. Yamaguchi K, Huang Z, Matsumura N, et al. Epigenetic determinants of ovarian clear cell carcinoma biology. Int J Cancer. 2014;135:585–97.
22. Jones S, Wang TL, Shih IM, et al. Frequent mutations of chromatin remodeling gene ARID1A in ovarian clear cell carcinoma. Science. 2010;330:228–31.
23. Wiegand KC, Shah SP, Al-Agha OM, et al. ARID1A mutations in endometriosis-associated ovarian carcinomas. N Engl J Med. 2010;363:1532–43.
24. Matsumoto T, Yamazaki M, Takahashi H, et al. Distinct β-catenin and PIK3CA mutation profiles in endometriosis-associated ovarian endometrioid and clear cell carcinomas. Am J Clin Pathol. 2015;144:452–63.
25. Murakami R, Matsumura N, Higasa K, et al. Exome sequencing landscape analyses in ovarian clear cell carcinoma shed light on key chromosomal regions and mutation gene networks. Am J Pathol. (in press)
26. Chandler RL, Damrauer JS, Raab JR, et al. Coexistent ARID1A-PIK3CA mutations promote ovarian clear-cell tumorigenesis through pro-tumorigenic inflammatory cytokine signalling. Nat Commun. 2015;6:6118.
27. Kim M, Lu F, Zhang Y. Loss of HDAC-mediated repression and gain of NF-κB activation underlie cytokine induction in ARID1A- and PIK3CA-mutation-driven ovarian cancer. Cell Rep. 2016;17:275–88.
28. Wu R, Hendrix-Lucas N, Kuick R, et al. Mouse model of human ovarian endometrioid adenocarcinoma based on somatic defects in the Wnt/beta-catenin and PI3K/Pten signaling pathways. Cancer Cell. 2007;11:321–33.
29. McConechy MK, Ding J, Senz J, et al. Ovarian and endometrial endometrioid carcinomas have distinct CTNNB1 and PTEN mutation profiles. Mod Pathol. 2014;27:128–34.
30. Saegusa M, Hashimura M, Yoshida T, et al. Beta- Catenin mutations and aberrant nuclear expression during endometrial tumorigenesis. Br J Cancer. 2001;84:209–17.
31. Tothill RW, Tinker AV, George J, et al. Novel molecular subtypes of serous and endometrioid ovarian cancer linked to clinical outcome. Clin Cancer Res. 2008;14:5198–208.
32. Soslow RA, Han G, Park KJ, et al. Morphologic patterns associated with BRCA1 and BRCA2 genotype in ovarian carcinoma. Mod Pathol. 2012;25:625–36.
33. Dinulescu DM, Ince TA, Quade BJ, et al. Role of K-ras and Pten in the development of mouse models of endometriosis and endometrioid ovarian cancer. Nat Med. 2005;11:63–70.
34. Guan B, Rahmanto YS, RC W, et al. Roles of deletion of Arid1a, a tumor suppressor, in mouse ovarian tumorigenesis. J Natl Cancer Inst. 2014;106:dju146.
35. Aysal A, Karnezis A, Medhi I, et al. Ovarian endometrioid adenocarcinoma: incidence and clinical significance of the morphologic and immunohistochemical markers of mismatch repair protein defects and tumor microsatellite instability. Am J Surg Pathol. 2012;36:163–72.
36. Anglesio MS, Wang YK, Maassen M, et al. Synchronous endometrial and ovarian carcinomas: evidence of clonality. J Natl Cancer Inst. 2016;108:djv428.
37. Mok SC, Bell DA, Knapp RC, et al. Mutation of K-ras protooncogene in human ovarian epithelial tumors of borderline malignancy. Cancer Res. 1993;53:1489–92.

38. Cuatrecasas M, Villanueva A, Matias-Guiu X, et al. K-ras mutations in mucinous ovarian tumors: a clinicopathologic and molecular study of 95 cases. Cancer. 1997;79:1581–6.
39. Wang Y, Shwartz LE, Anderson D, et al. Molecular analysis of ovarian mucinous carcinoma reveals different cell of origins. Oncotarget. 2015;6:22949–58.
40. Seidman JD, Khedmati F. Exploring the histogenesis of ovarian mucinous and transitional cell (Brenner) neoplasms and their relationship with Walthard cell nests: a study of 120 tumors. Arch Pathol Lab Med. 2008;132:1753–60.
41. Wang Y, RC W, Shwartz LE, et al. Clonality analysis of combined Brenner and mucinous tumours of the ovary reveals their monoclonal origin. J Pathol. 2015;237:146–51.
42. Mackenzie R, Kommoss S, Winterhoff BJ, et al. Targeted deep sequencing of mucinous ovarian tumors reveals multiple overlapping RAS-pathway activating mutations in borderline and cancerous neoplasms. BMC Cancer. 2015;15:415.
43. Ryland GL, Hunter SM, Doyle MA, et al. RNF43 is a tumour suppressor gene mutated in mucinous tumours of the ovary. J Pathol. 2013;229:469–76.
44. Ryland GL, Hunter SM, Doyle MA, et al. Mutational landscape of mucinous ovarian carcinoma and its neoplastic precursors. Genome Med. 2015;7:87.
45. Kuo KT, Guan B, Feng Y, et al. Analysis of DNA copy number alterations in ovarian serous tumors identifies new molecular genetic changes in low-grade and high-grade carcinomas. Cancer Res. 2009;69:4036–42.
46. Singer G, Oldt R 3rd, Cohen Y, et al. Mutations in BRAF and KRAS characterize the development of low-grade ovarian serous carcinoma. J Natl Cancer Inst. 2003;95:484–6.
47. Jones S, Wang TL, Kurman RJ, et al. Low-grade serous carcinomas of the ovary contain very few point mutations. J Pathol. 2012;226:413–20.
48. Grisham RN, Iyer G, Garg K, et al. BRAF mutation is associated with early stage disease and improved outcome in patients with low-grade serous ovarian cancer. Cancer. 2013;119:548–54.
49. Wong KK, Tsang YT, Deavers MT, et al. BRAF mutation is rare in advanced-stage low-grade ovarian serous carcinomas. Am J Pathol. 2010;177:1611–7.
50. Ardighieri L, Zeppernick F, Hannibal CG, et al. Mutational analysis of BRAF and KRAS in ovarian serous borderline (atypical proliferative) tumours and associated peritoneal implants. J Pathol. 2014;232:16–22.
51. Emmanuel C, Chiew YE, George J, et al. Genomic classification of serous ovarian cancer with adjacent borderline differentiates RAS pathway and TP53-mutant tumors and identifies NRAS as an oncogenic driver. Clin Cancer Res. 2014;20:6618–30.
52. Tsang YT, Deavers MT, Sun CC, et al. KRAS (but not BRAF) mutations in ovarian serous borderline tumour are associated with recurrent low-grade serous carcinoma. J Pathol. 2013;231:449–56.
53. Zeppernick F, Ardighieri L, Hannibal CG, et al. BRAF mutation is associated with a specific cell type with features suggestive of senescence in ovarian serous borderline (atypical proliferative) tumors. Am J Surg Pathol. 2014;38:1603–11.
54. Maniar KP, Wang Y, Visvanathan K, et al. Evaluation of microinvasion and lymph node involvement in ovarian serous borderline/atypical proliferative serous tumors: a morphologic and immunohistochemical analysis of 37 cases. Am J Surg Pathol. 2014;38:743–55.

Strategies for the Management of Epithelial Ovarian Cancer

8

Nozomu Yanaihara and Aikou Okamoto

Abstract

Ovarian cancer is the most lethal gynecological malignancy worldwide. Ovarian cancer mostly responds to primary treatment; however, patients with advanced stage disease have a high recurrence rate, and the 5-year survival rate is estimated to be below 45%. The basic primary treatment of epithelial ovarian cancer comprises surgical intervention, which aims to completely eradicate the tumor, and platinum–taxane-based combination chemotherapy, followed by optimal follow-up. In this context, fundamental strategies for the management of epithelial ovarian cancer are discussed based on the current clinical practice guidelines.

Keywords

Chemotherapy • Molecular targeted therapy • Surgical management

8.1 Introduction

Optimal treatment strategies for epithelial ovarian cancer are well documented in the current clinical practice guidelines; these guidelines are based on the evidence obtained from clinical studies performed worldwide [1–3]. In Japan, the fourth edition of the Japan Society of Gynecologic Oncology guidelines for the treatment of ovarian cancer was published in 2015 with the overall task to improve the prognosis of ovarian cancer [3]. Basic primary treatment for epithelial ovarian cancer includes surgical intervention (staging laparotomy and debulking surgery)

N. Yanaihara, M.D., Ph.D. (✉) • A. Okamoto, M.D., Ph.D.
Department of Obstetrics and Gynecology, The Jikei University School of Medicine, 3-25-8 Nishi-Shinbashi, Minato-ku, Tokyo 105-8461, Japan
e-mail: yanazou@jikei.ac.jp

H. Katabuchi (ed.), *Frontiers in Ovarian Cancer Science*, Comprehensive Gynecology and Obstetrics, DOI 10.1007/978-981-10-4160-0_8

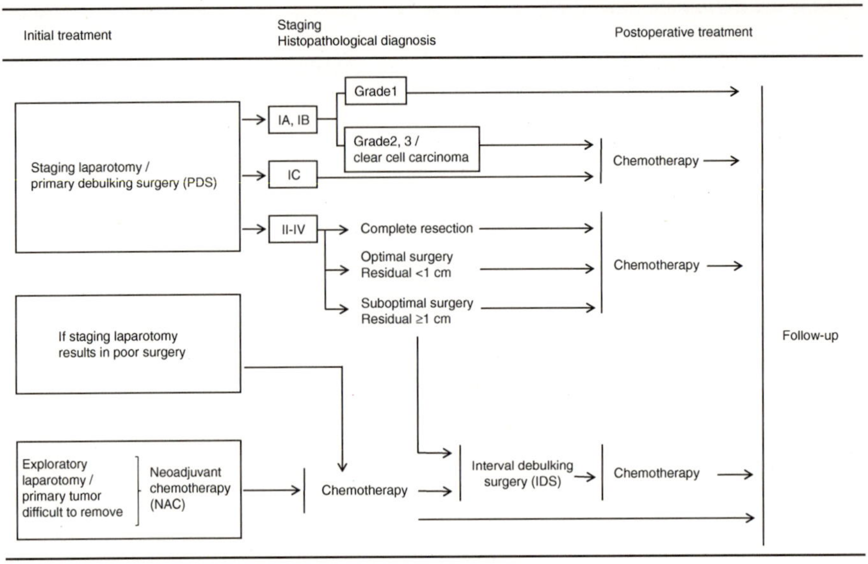

Fig. 8.1 Flowchart of fundamental strategies for the management of epithelial ovarian cancer. Cited from Komiyama et al. [3] with slight modifications

and chemotherapy (postoperative and neoadjuvant) followed by optimal follow-up. Fundamental strategies for the management of epithelial ovarian cancer are shown in the flowchart (Fig. 8.1) [3].

8.2 Surgical Management

8.2.1 Early (Localized to the Ovary)-Staged Ovarian Cancer

The primary aim of surgery for early ovarian cancer is to resect the tumor and define a precise pathological diagnosis to obtain definitive staging according to the International Federation of Gynecology and Obstetrics guidelines. Optimal staging laparotomy, which can reveal important information for subsequent treatment, includes bilateral salpingo-oophorectomy, total hysterectomy, omentectomy, peritoneal cytology, pelvic/para-aortic lymph node dissection (biopsy), and biopsies from sites in the abdominal cavity. Both retroperitoneal lymph node dissection up to the renal veins and intraperitoneal (IP) biopsy of the Douglas pouch, parietal peritoneum, surface of the diaphragm, intestinal tract, mesentery, and suspected lesions are informative factors for accurate staging. It is well known that the comprehensive surgical staging is important to disclose occult advanced disease [4, 5]. Therefore, if the final diagnosis of ovarian cancer is confirmed after initial surgery (incomplete surgery and/or staging), staging laparotomy by re-laparotomy should be performed [3]. Although retroperitoneal lymph node metastases have been observed in 5%–21% of patients with pT1 diseases, there is no strong evidence based on randomized clinical trials to indicate that lymph node dissections have any impact on the prognosis of early ovarian cancer [6].

The clinical requirement of preserving fertility in young patients with ovarian cancer may be present. The basic fertility-sparing surgical procedure for early ovarian cancer includes disease-side salpingo-oophorectomy, omentectomy, and peritoneal cytology with informed consent after providing detailed information about fertility preservation and the potential risk of disease recurrence [3]. In addition, staging laparotomy, including the biopsy of the contralateral ovary, pelvic/para-aortic lymph nodes, and sites in the abdominal cavity, should be considered to exclude the possibility of advanced disease. The basic indication for fertility-sparing surgery is stage IA disease with grade 1 or 2 of the serous, mucinous, or endometrioid histotype. In addition, stage IC (localized to one ovary with negative ascites cytology) with grade 1 or 2 of non-clear histotype or stage IA of clear cell histotype can also be considered for fertility-sparing surgery.

8.2.2 Advanced Stage (Stage II or More) Ovarian Cancer

Maximal debulking surgery to achieve complete visible disease resection is recommended for advanced ovarian cancer because no residual tumor at the end of surgery has been shown to be associated with prolonged patient survival [3, 7]. In general, complete surgery is defined if there is no residual tumor detectable by macroscopic evaluation, optimal surgery is defined as residual tumors of <1 cm in diameter, and suboptimal surgery is defined if the residual tumors are ≥ 1 cm in diameter. Surgical procedures that may lead to achieve complete resection include bowel resection, peritoneal stripping, diaphragm resection, bulky lymph node removal, splenectomy, and other procedures. Therefore, multidisciplinary expert surgical and medical management may be required. Conversely, indications for pelvic/para-aortic lymph node dissection in advanced ovarian cancer remain to be elucidated. A retrospective review of three randomized trials for advanced ovarian cancer indicated that lymphadenectomy might offer benefit mainly to patients with advanced ovarian cancer but without gross residual disease [8]. A multicenter randomized clinical trial, however, demonstrated that there was no difference in overall survival (OS) between patients with systemic lymphadenectomy and those with removed bulky nodes [9]. Altogether, systemic retroperitoneal lymphadenectomy could be considered if optimal surgery has been achieved in patients with advanced ovarian cancer.

If primary surgery for advanced ovarian cancer results in a suboptimal outcome, interval debulking surgery (IDS) should be considered as a treatment option during chemotherapy [3]. There have been two controversial randomized clinical trials about the value of this treatment strategy: the Gynecological Cancer Cooperative Group of the European Organization for Research and Treatment of Cancer (EORTC) trial, which showed IDS to have improved survival [10], and the Gynecologic Oncology Group phase III treatment trial, which reported negative effects of IDS for these patients [11].

Although the fundamental treatment strategy for advanced ovarian cancer has generally been primary debulking surgery (PDS) followed by chemotherapy, therapeutic benefit of neoadjuvant chemotherapy (NAC) followed by IDS is still debated. Till date, two large randomized clinical trials (the EORTC 55971/NCIC OV13 and CHORUS trials) have demonstrated that the prognosis of advanced ovarian cancer with NAC + IDS was not inferior to that of PDS followed by chemotherapy [12, 13]. In addition, a recent phase III noninferiority trial (the JCOG 0602 trial) comparing PDS with NAC + IDS conducted by the Japan Clinical Oncology Group supports the idea that NAC + IDS is becoming more widely accepted [14]. Based on these results, NAC + IDS could be considered as a treatment option for patients with advanced ovarian cancer in whom an optimal outcome by primary surgery cannot be expected because of its extensive dissemination and metastasis, poor patient condition, and serious complications [1–3]. The performance status and the American Society of Anesthesiologists (ASA) physical status classification are generally used for evaluating the patient's general condition. Patient's age (particularly of the elderly), general condition, nutrition status, and clinical stage should be taken into consideration for choosing appropriate surgery. It should be noted that the incidences of intraoperative and perioperative complications are frequent in elderly patients. Because it is thought that maximal debulking surgery should also be performed in elderly patients, NAC with the improvement of the general condition followed by IDS (hopefully complete surgery) should be considered in these patients [15].

8.2.3 Risk-Reducing Salpingo-Oophorectomy (RRSO)

Recent accumulating evidence has revealed that prophylactic bilateral salpingo-oophorectomy is associated with a reduced risk of breast, ovarian, fallopian tube, and primary peritoneal cancers in women with *BRCA1* or *BRCA2* mutations [16, 17]. Therefore, RRSO, under the institutional ethics committee approval, is recommended for the patients carrying *BRCA1/2* mutations, along with genetic counseling by clinical geneticists and careful pathological review [3].

8.2.4 Laparoscope-Assisted Surgery

There is no difference in terms of the survival benefit for selected patients with early ovarian cancer between open laparotomy and minimally invasive procedures, such as laparoscope-assisted surgery, performed by experienced gynecologic oncologists [18]. In addition, it is noted that laparoscopic inspection for observing intraperitoneal cavity and for staging in patients with advanced ovarian cancer can be a useful method [19]. However, quite a few randomized trials of laparoscope-assisted surgery for ovarian cancer have been conducted till date, but laparoscope-assisted surgery is not currently recognized as a standard procedure that can replace open laparotomy [3]. In patients with advanced cancer, however, the minimally invasive procedure may be substituted for open laparotomy to observe the abdominal cavity and collect tissue samples [3]. Furthermore, in general, laparoscope-assisted approach can be used for prophylactic bilateral salpingo-oophorectomy.

8.2.5 Intraoperative Pathological Evaluation

Although the diagnosis of ovarian cancer may be made by preoperative evaluation and intraoperative findings, the judgment between benign and borderline malignancies is occasionally difficult. Intraoperative rapid pathological examination using frozen sections may help to select the optimal surgical procedure and avoid an unnecessary second surgical procedure in such cases [1–3].

8.3 Frontline Chemotherapy

8.3.1 Standard Chemotherapy

Standard frontline chemotherapies include (1) conventional TC therapy with paclitaxel (3-h intravenous infusion at 175 or 180 mg/m^2) followed by carboplatin (1-h intravenous infusion of area under the curve [AUC] of 5 or 6) on day 1, given every 3 weeks for 6 cycles, and (2) dose-dense TC therapy with paclitaxel (1-h intravenous infusion at 80 mg/m^2 on days 1, 8, and 15) plus carboplatin (1-h intravenous infusion at an AUC of 6 on day 1), given every 3 weeks for 6 cycles. Significant improvement in both progression-free survival (PFS) and overall survival (OS) with a dose-dense schedule when compared with conventional therapy in stage II–IV ovarian cancer was documented by the JGOG3016 trial [20, 21]. However, higher toxicity, which is a potential reason to discontinue treatment, was observed in dose-dense regimens.

As frontline chemotherapy, other than conventional TC therapy, DC therapy with docetaxel (1-h intravenous infusion at 70 or 75 mg/m^2) followed by carboplatin (1-h intravenous infusion at an AUC of 5) on day 1, given every 3 weeks for 6 cycles, and also PLD-C therapy with pegylated liposomal doxorubicin (1-h intravenous infusion at 30 mg/m^2) followed by carboplatin (1-h intravenous infusion at an AUC of 5) on day 1, given every 4 weeks for 6 cycles, can be considered as alternatives [3]. In addition, for frail and elderly patients who may not be able to tolerate these combination therapies, cisplatin or carboplatin monotherapy is recommended [3].

It has been suggested that response rates to standard first-line chemotherapy, which is conventionally used for high-grade serous carcinoma (HGSC), are less in rare ovarian cancer subtypes, such as low-grade serous carcinoma, clear cell carcinoma (CCC), and mucinous carcinoma [22]. However, at present, there is insufficient evidence to support the modification of standard chemotherapy according to tumor histopathology [3]. A randomized phase III trial (the JGOG3017/GCIG trial) of paclitaxel/carboplatin versus irinotecan/cisplatin as a first-line chemotherapy for stage IC-IV CCC showed no significant difference in 2-year PFS and OS rates [23].

Postoperative chemotherapy can be avoided for patients with stage IA or IB, grade 1 disease, as confirmed by optimal staging laparotomy [3], based on evidence from a Cochrane meta-analysis of five randomized clinical trials, including the ACTION and ICON1 trials. This meta-analysis aimed to evaluate the benefit of postoperative chemotherapy for early ovarian cancer and found that adjuvant platinum-based chemotherapy was effective in the majority of early ovarian cancer patients, except in the subpopulations involving patients with stage IA or IB, grade 1 disease [24].

8.3.2 Intraperitoneal Chemotherapy

IP chemotherapy after optimal surgery can be considered for advanced ovarian cancer [3], although this delivery method may have greater toxicity associated with catheter complications, such as infection, abdominal pain, and abdominal discomfort. The GOG172 trial demonstrated that IP chemotherapy conveyed a survival advantage to stage III ovarian cancer patients with no more than 1 cm of residual disease [25]. The IP chemotherapy regimen used in this trial was 24-h intravenous infusion of paclitaxel at 135 mg/m^2 on day 1, followed by IP cisplatin at 100 mg/m^2 on day 2, and IP paclitaxel at 60 mg/m^2 on day 8, given every 3 weeks for 6 cycles. A recent Cochrane meta-analysis of nine randomized clinical trials reported reliable estimates of survival benefits for IP chemotherapy for advanced ovarian cancer [26].

8.3.3 After Primary Treatment

In general, observation rather than maintenance chemotherapy is recommended for patients who exhibit no evidence of disease progression (complete remission) after initial treatment because the usefulness of maintenance chemotherapy has not yet been demonstrated through several randomized clinical trials [27–30]. However, maintenance with molecular targeted drugs, which is described in a later section, has been shown to increase PFS when the agents were concurrently used with TC therapy followed by maintenance therapy. If complete remission is not achieved by initial treatment (partial remission or progression), additional treatment (second-line chemotherapy and radiotherapy), participation in a clinical trial, or best supportive care should be considered [1, 3].

8.4 Molecular Targeted Therapy

The use of bevacizumab (a monoclonal antibody targeting vascular endothelial growth factor) should be considered in combination with chemotherapy and as subsequent maintenance therapy with careful patient selection and appropriate monitoring for adverse events [3]. Two large randomized trials (the GOG218 and ICON7 trials) have evaluated the benefit of bevacizumab with conventional TC therapy as a frontline treatment for ovarian cancer [31, 32]. There were several differences between the two trials regarding patient characteristics and the dose and duration of bevacizumab. Both trials showed that PFS, but not OS, was significantly improved if bevacizumab was concurrently used with TC therapy and followed by maintenance therapy compared to the control arm (conventional TC therapy). Subgroup analysis of the ICON7 trial showed that both the PFS and OS of patients at high risk of disease progression (stage IV, inoperable stage III, or stage III with a residual tumor >1 cm) were significantly prolonged by the addition of bevacizumab [33]. Since neither of these trials documented a significant impact on OS, the consensus and license situations differ among counties in terms of the incorporation of bevacizumab into frontline therapies.

Molecular targeted agents with a potential for use in the treatment of ovarian cancer as a frontline therapy include poly ADP-ribose polymerase (PARP) inhibitors (including olaparib, niraparib, veliparib, and rucaparib) and immune checkpoint inhibitors (including anti-CTLA-4 antibody, anti-PD-1 antibody, and anti-PD-L1 antibody). We should not overlook the ongoing clinical trials regarding the use of these molecular targeted agents in a variety of clinical settings, including frontline, maintenance, and recurrent disease with or without cytotoxic agents in ovarian cancer treatment [34, 35].

8.5 Optimal Follow-Up After Primary Treatment

Because there is a lack of strong evidences in terms of the optimal follow-up interval and methods after initial treatment, clinical practice based on current guidelines varies [1–3]. In general, routine visit could be every 1–3 months for 2 years, followed by every 3–6 months for 3 years, and every 1 year for year 6 onward. History taking and pelvic examination should be considered at every visit, whereas CA125 measurement and imaging studies, including transvaginal ultrasonography and computed tomography scanning, may be ordered as clinically required. Early intervention for patients with a complete clinical remission after initial treatment who have elevated CA125 levels without any symptoms of recurrent disease remains to be elucidated. A phase III trial (the MRC OV05-EORTC 55955 trial) evaluating the utility of CA125 monitoring for ovarian cancer recurrence demonstrated that early intervention based on elevated CA125 levels alone had no clinical benefit compared with the treatment after the clinical evidence of relapse [36]. Therefore, early intervention in response to elevated CA125 levels alone is not necessarily recommended at present [3]. Although one may argue the usefulness of CA125 measurement as a part of follow-up, it may be useful as a clue to identify patients with surgically resectable recurrence [1, 3].

Conclusion

Ovarian cancer is one of the most challenging cancers affecting women, with 5-year survival rates below 45% [37]. Multidisciplinary therapy of surgery with chemotherapy remains the fundamental strategies for first-line therapy of ovarian cancer. In the past decades, only a few clinical trials have been able to achieve an improved overall survival. Many current practice guidelines are based on evidence generated by clinical trials that have been conducted through international collaboration. Further ongoing clinical trials addressing IP chemotherapy, NAC + IDS, and the integration of molecular targeted agents may result in greater impact on the outcome for patients with ovarian cancer.

References

1. NCCN Clinical Practice Guidelines in Oncology™. Ovarian cancer including fallopian tube cancer and primary peritoneal cancer. V.2.2015. Available at: http://www.nccn.org/professionals/physician_gls/pdf/ovarian.pdf.
2. Ledermann JA, Raja FA, Fotopoulou C, Gonzalez-Martin A, Colombo N, Sessa C, ESMO Guidelines Working Group. Newly diagnosed and relapsed epithelial ovarian carcinoma: ESMO Clinical Practice Guidelines for diagnosis, treatment and follow-up. Ann Oncol. 2013;24:vi24–32.
3. Komiyama S, Katabuchi H, Mikami M, Nagase S, Okamoto A, Ito K, et al. Japan Society of Gynecologic Oncology guidelines 2015 for the treatment of ovarian cancer including primary peritoneal cancer and fallopian tube cancer. Int J Clin Oncol. 2016;21:435–46.
4. Garcia-Soto AE, Boren T, Wingo SN, Heffernen T, Miller DS. Is comprehensive surgical staging needed for thorough evaluation of early-stage ovarian carcinoma? Am J Obstet Gynecol. 2012;206:242.e241–5.
5. Timmers PJ, Zwinderman AH, Coens C, Vergote I, Trimbos JB. Understanding the problem of inadequately staging early ovarian cancer. Eur J Cancer. 2010;46:880–4.
6. Maggioni A, Benedetti Panici P, Dell'Anna T, Landoni F, Lissoni A, Pellegrino A, et al. Randomised study of systematic lymphadenectomy in patients with epithelial ovarian cancer macroscopically confined to the pelvis. Br J Cancer. 2006;95:699–704.
7. du Bois A, Reuss A, Pujade-Lauraine E, Harter P, Ray-Coquard I, Pfisterer J. Role of surgical outcome as prognostic factor in advanced epithelial ovarian cancer: a combined exploratory analysis of 3 prospectively randomized phase 3 multicenter trials: by the Arbeitsgemeinschaft Gynaekologische Onkologie Studiengruppe Ovarialkarzinom (AGO-OVAR) and the Groupe d'Investigateurs Nationaux Pour les Etudes des Cancers de l'Ovaire (GINECO). Cancer. 2009;115:1234–44.
8. du Bois A, Reuss A, Harter P, Pujade-Lauraine E, Ray-Coquard I, Pfisterer J, Arbeitsgemeinschaft Gynaekologische Onkologie Studiengruppe Ovarialkarzinom; Groupe d'Investigateurs Nationaux pour l'Etude des Cancers Ovariens. Potential role of lymphadenectomy in advanced ovarian cancer: a combined exploratory analysis of three prospectively randomized phase III multicenter trials. J Clin Oncol. 2010;28:1733–9.
9. Panici PB, Maggioni A, Hacker N, Landoni F, Ackermann S, Campagnutta E, et al. Systematic aortic and pelvic lymphadenectomy versus resection of bulky nodes only in optimally debulked advanced ovarian cancer: a randomized clinical trial. J Natl Cancer Inst. 2005;97:560–6.
10. van der Burg ME, van Lent M, Buyse M, Kobierska A, Colombo N, Favalli G, et al. The effect of debulking surgery after induction chemotherapy on the prognosis in advanced epithelial ovarian cancer. Gynecological Cancer Cooperative Group of the European Organization for Research and Treatment of Cancer. N Engl J Med. 1995;332:629–34.

11. Rose PG, Nerenstone S, Brady MF, Clarke-Pearson D, Olt G, Rubin SC, Gynecologic Oncology Group, et al. Secondary surgical cytoreduction for advanced ovarian carcinoma. N Engl J Med. 2004;351:2489–97.
12. Vergote I, Tropé CG, Amant F, Kristensen GB, Ehlen T, Johnson N, European Organization for Research and Treatment of Cancer-Gynaecological Cancer Group; NCIC Clinical Trials Group, et al. Neoadjuvant chemotherapy or primary surgery in stage IIIC or IV ovarian cancer. N Engl J Med. 2010;363:943–53.
13. Kehoe S, Hook J, Nankivell M, Jayson GC, Kitchener H, Lopes T, et al. Primary chemotherapy versus primary surgery for newly diagnosed advanced ovarian cancer (CHORUS): an open-label, randomised, controlled, non-inferiority trial. Lancet. 2015;386:249–57.
14. Onda T, Satoh T, Saito T, Kasamatsu T, Nakanishi T, Nakamura K, et al. Comparison of treatment invasiveness between upfront debulking surgery versus interval debulking surgery following neoadjuvant chemotherapy for stage III/IV ovarian, tubal, and peritoneal cancers in a phase III randomised trial: Japan Clinical Oncology Group Study JCOG0602. Eur J Cancer. 2016;64:22–31.
15. Glasgow MA, Yu H, Rutherford TJ, Azodi M, Silasi DA, Santin AD, Schwartz PE. Neoadjuvant chemotherapy (NACT) is an effective way of managing elderly women with advanced stage ovarian cancer (FIGO stage IIIC and IV). J Surg Oncol. 2013;107:195–200.
16. Rebbeck TR, Kauff ND, Domchek SM. Meta-analysis of risk reduction estimates associated with risk-reducing salpingo-oophorectomy in BRCA1 or BRCA2 mutation carriers. J Natl Cancer Inst. 2009;101:80–7.
17. Domchek SM, Friebel TM, Singer CF, Evans DG, Lynch HT, Isaacs C, et al. Association of risk-reducing surgery in BRCA1 or BRCA2 mutation carriers with cancer risk and mortality. JAMA. 2010;304:967–75.
18. Ghezzi F, Malzoni M, Vizza E, Cromi A, Perone C, Corrado G, et al. Laparoscopic staging of early ovarian cancer: results of a multi-institutional cohort study. Ann Surg Oncol. 2012;19:1589–94.
19. Fagotti A, Ferrandina G, Fanfani F, Garganese G, Vizzielli G, Carone V, et al. Prospective validation of a laparoscopic predictive model for optimal cytoreduction in advanced ovarian carcinoma. Am J Obstet Gynecol. 2008;199:642.e1.
20. Katsumata N, Yasuda M, Takahashi F, Isonishi S, Jobo T, Aoki D, Japanese Gynecologic Oncology Group, et al. Dose-dense paclitaxel once a week in combination with carboplatin every 3 weeks for advanced ovarian cancer: a phase 3, open-label, randomised controlled trial. Lancet. 2009;374:1331–8.
21. Katsumata N, Yasuda M, Isonishi S, Takahashi F, Michimae H, Kimura E, Japanese Gynecologic Oncology Group, et al. Long-term results of dose-dense paclitaxel and carboplatin versus conventional paclitaxel and carboplatin for treatment of advanced epithelial ovarian, fallopian tube, or primary peritoneal cancer (JGOG 3016): a randomised, controlled, open-label trial. Lancet Oncol. 2013;14:1020–6.
22. Mackay HJ, Brady MF, Oza AM, Reuss A, Pujade-Lauraine E, Swart AM, Gynecologic Cancer InterGroup, et al. Prognostic relevance of uncommon ovarian histology in women with stage III/IV epithelial ovarian cancer. Int J Gynecol Cancer. 2010;20:945–52.
23. Sugiyama T, Okamoto A, Enomoto T, Hamano T, Aotani E, Terao Y, et al. Randomized phase III trial of Irinotecan plus cisplatin compared with paclitaxel plus carboplatin as first-line chemotherapy for ovarian clear cell carcinoma: JGOG3017/GCIG trial. J Clin Oncol. 2016;34:2881–7.
24. Winter-Roach BA, Kitchener HC, Dickinson HO. Adjuvant (post-surgery) chemotherapy for early stage epithelial ovarian cancer. Cochrane Database Syst Rev. 2009:CD004706.
25. Armstrong DK, Bundy B, Wenzel L, Huang HQ, Baergen R, Lele S, Gynecologic Oncology Group, et al. Intraperitoneal cisplatin and paclitaxel in ovarian cancer. N Engl J Med. 2006;354:34–43.
26. Jaaback K, Johnson N, Lawrie TA. Intraperitoneal chemotherapy for the initial management of primary epithelial ovarian cancer. Cochrane Database Syst Rev. 2016:CD005340.

27. Markman M, Liu PY, Wilczynski S, Monk B, Copeland LJ, Alvarez RD, et al. Phase III randomized trial of 12 versus 3 months of maintenance paclitaxel in patients with advanced ovarian cancer after complete response to platinum and paclitaxel-based chemotherapy: a Southwest Oncology Group and Gynecologic Oncology Group Trial. J Clin Oncol. 2003;21:2460–5.
28. Pfisterer J, Weber B, Reuss A, Kimmig R, du Bois A, Wagner U, et al. Randomized phase III trial of topotecan following carboplatin and paclitaxel in first-line treatment of advanced ovarian cancer: a gynecologic cancer intergroup trial of the AGO-OVAR and GINECO. J Natl Cancer Inst. 2006;98:1036–45.
29. De Placido S, Scambia G, Di Vagno G, Naglieri E, Lombardi AV, Biamonte R, et al. Topotecan compared with no therapy after response to surgery and carboplatin/paclitaxel in patients with ovarian cancer: multicenter Italian trials in ovarian cancer (MITO-1) randomized study. J Clin Oncol. 2004;22:2635–42.
30. Pecorelli S, Favalli G, Gadducci A, Katsaros D, Panici PB, Carpi A, et al. Phase III trial of observation versus six courses of paclitaxel in patients with advanced epithelial ovarian cancer in complete response after six courses of paclitaxel/platinum-based chemotherapy: final results of the after-6 protocol 1. J Clin Oncol. 2009;27:4642–8.
31. Burger RA, Brady MF, Bookman MA, Fleming GF, Monk BJ, Huang H, Gynecologic Oncology Group, et al. Incorporation of bevacizumab in the primary treatment of ovarian cancer. N Engl J Med. 2011;365:2473–83.
32. Perren TJ, Swart AM, Pfisterer J, Ledermann JA, Pujade-Lauraine E, Kristensen G, ICON7 Investigators, et al. A phase 3 trial of bevacizumab in ovarian cancer. N Engl J Med. 2011;365:2484–96.
33. Oza AM, Cook AD, Pfisterer J, Embleton A, Ledermann JA, Pujade-Lauraine E, ICON7 trial investigators, et al. Standard chemotherapy with or without bevacizumab for women with newly diagnosed ovarian cancer (ICON7): overall survival results of a phase 3 randomised trial. Lancet Oncol. 2015;16:928–36.
34. Crafton SM, Bixel K, Hays JL. PARP inhibition and gynecologic malignancies: a review of current literature and on-going trials. Gynecol Oncol. 2016;142:588–96.
35. Hamanishi J, Mandai M, Konishi I. Immune checkpoint inhibition in ovarian cancer. Int Immunol. 2016;28:339–48.
36. Rustin GJ, van der Burg ME, Griffin CL, Guthrie D, Lamont A, Jayson GC, et al. Early versus delayed treatment of relapsed ovarian cancer (MRC OV05/EORTC 55955): a randomised trial. Lancet. 2010;376:1155–63.
37. Webb PM, Jordan SJ. Epidemiology of epithelial ovarian cancer. Best Pract Res Clin Obstet Gynaecol. 2017;41:3–14.

9 Strategies for the Management of Epithelial Ovarian Borderline Tumors

Kimio Ushijima

Abstract

Borderline ovarian tumor (BOT) has distinct characteristics from benign or carcinoma of the ovary. BOT occurs more often in young women, so usually fertility preservation should be considered. BOT has some histologic subtypes and different clinical behavior. So the clinical management for BOT should be decided individually. Serous borderline tumor (SBT) shows relatively higher incidence of extra ovarian peritoneal implant lesion than other subtypes, and micropapillary pattern (MP) has worse prognosis. As other subtypes, mucinous boderline tumor (intestinal type) and seromucinous boderline tumor are existed. Intestinal type has tendency to be large tumor and having histologic heterogeneity. Seromucinous BOT has similar character with SBT. Prognosis of BOT is much better than carcinoma, but advanced cases with invasive implant have high incidence of recurrence.

Standard surgical procedure for BOT is staging laparotomy for ovarian cancer excepting systemic lymphadenectomy by open surgery. In young women fertility-sparing surgery is accepted. Laparoscopy itself has no relation with worse prognosis. Restaging surgery is necessary after cystectomy. Accurate pathological diagnosis and appropriate surgical treatment are most important for the management of BOT. Adjuvant chemotherapy has no evidence of clinical benefit even for advanced-stage BOT.

Keywords

Borderline ovarian tumor • Serous borderline tumor • Mucinous borderline tumor • Seromucinous borderline tumor • Restaging surgery • Laparoscopic surgery

K. Ushijima, M.D., Ph.D.
Department of Obstetrics and Gynecology, Kurume University School of Medicine, 67 Asahi Machi, Kurume 830 0011, Japan
e-mail: kimi@med.kurume-u.ac.jp

H. Katabuchi (ed.), *Frontiers in Ovarian Cancer Science*, Comprehensive Gynecology and Obstetrics, DOI 10.1007/978-981-10-4160-0_9

9.1 Introduction

Borderline ovarian tumor (BOT) was defined by the World Health Organization (WHO) histologically as exhibiting atypical epithelial proliferation, greater than seen in benign counterparts without destructive stromal invasion. BOT also was recognized as having intermediate clinical behavior between benign and malignant ovarian tumor [1]. The incidence of BOT is increasing [2]. From the data of the Japan Society of Obstetrics and Gynecology, Gynecologic Oncology Committee, in 1998, 300 cases from 89 institutions, in 2007, 968 cases from 269 institutions, and, in 2013, 1903 cases from 423 institutions were reported [3]. The increasing tendency is more remarkable than the increase of number of institutions. Furthermore, comparing with carcinoma, BOT occurs 10 years younger than carcinoma does, so fertility-sparing treatment strategy should be usually considered.

BOT has various histologic types having different clinical behavior. Also, diagnostic accuracy of BOT is relatively low preoperatively and at surgery. Due to these unique characteristics, different treatment strategy from invasive carcinoma should be planned, but it is still controversial. In this chapter, it is explained how we should make the treatment strategy for typical histologic types of BOT.

9.2 Characteristics of Serous Borderline Tumor

Serous borderline tumor (SBT) is diagnosed by the stratified serous epithelial cells resembling the fallopian tube with a hierarchical pattern of branching and a varying degree of nuclear atypia with an absence of frank invasion. About 30% of SBT occur in bilateral ovaries, and 20–40% of cases have extra ovarian peritoneal implants [4]. Some SBT has worse prognostic pathologic features, such as micropapillary pattern (SBT-MP), microinvasion, extraovarian implant, and bilateral tumors. Each characteristic often coexists in same patient. Especially in SBT-MP, surface involvement, bilateral appearance, and peritoneal implants are found more frequently and show remarkably worse prognosis than usual SBT (Fig. 9.1) [5]. Among peritoneal

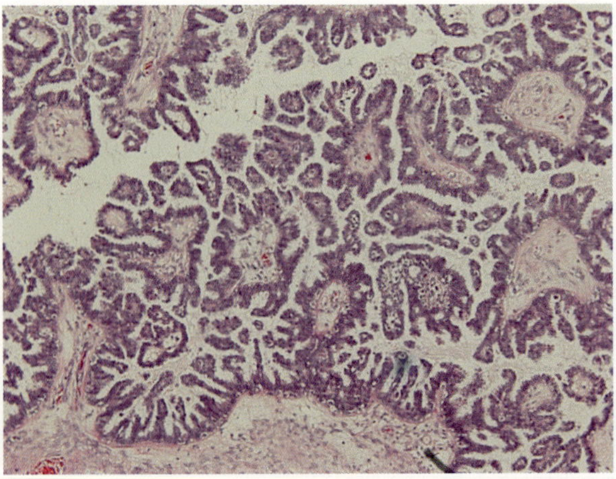

Fig. 9.1 Serous borderline tumor, micropapillary pattern. Non-hierarchial pattern is shown with micropapillary projection five times longer than width at least 5 mm in dimension with fibrous stalks

implants, invasive implant has more aggressive behavior but less frequently (12% of all implants) than noninvasive implant [5]. Retroperitoneal lymph node involvement was found in 20%–30% of SBT, but most of them were not significantly prognostic, suggesting lymph nodes via peritoneal route and not through lymphatic channels [6].

The prognosis of SBT is excellent in stage I tumor, and advanced-stage SBT with noninvasive implant still has 90% in 5-year survival rate. Nevertheless, longtime follow-up should be required, because recurrence may occur in longer period as about 20 years [7].

9.3 Characteristics of Mucinous Borderline Tumor and Seromucinous Borderline Tumor

Mucinous borderline tumor (MBT) is diagnosed by the proliferation of mucinous epithelial tumor cells with intermediate (variable) nuclear atypia and an absence of frank stromal invasion. In 2014 WHO tumor classification about mucinous tumors was revised. Only intestinal-type mucinous ovarian tumor was classified as mucinous tumor. And tumor with two or more epithelial types, such as endocervical-type mucinous, serous epithelium, and rarely endometrioid or squamous epithelium, was newly classified as seromucinous type [8]. These two tumors should be discriminated, because their clinical characteristics are apparently different [9]. MBT intestinal type is more frequently (85% of MBT), and usually large and multicystic tumor, and mostly confined to the ovary. Seromucinous BOT includes tumors which were used to be called as endocervical-like mucinous, mixed Müllerian mucinous, and mixed serous, endometrial, or squamous borderline epithelium. Prognosis of MBT was excellent in stage I tumor. Seromucinous BOT has 40% of bilateral tumors, and more than 20% are stage II–III tumors like SBT [4]. Also clinical behavior of seromucinous BOT resembles with SBT [10].

MBT has often heterogeneous histology, containing areas of cystadenoma or mucinous carcinoma. The discordant diagnosis of frozen section and permanent diagnosis occurs in 34% of MBT [11]. The prognosis of MBT is also excellent, but around 10% of MBT has recurred during 5–10 years period as mucinous carcinoma. Most recurrent cases have the possibility of sampling error at the primary tumor resection because of more heterogeneity (benign, borderline, intraepithelial carcinoma, microinvasion, invasive carcinoma) in huge mucinous tumor [12]. If borderline is suspicious, adequate pathologic sampling is needed. National Cancer Institute-sponsored ovarian tumor workshop proposed that one section per cm (<10 cm) and two sections per cm (>10 cm) should be obtained for the accurate diagnosis [13].

9.4 Surgical Management of BOT

9.4.1 Standard Surgical Procedure

Standard surgical procedure for BOT is staging laparotomy for ovarian cancer excepting systemic lymphadenectomy by open surgery. Lymphadenectomy can be omitted even for stage II and III disease, as there is no difference in the recurrence or survival rate between with and without lymphadenectomy [14]. No residuals at surgery would be very important as a favorite prognostic factor. If suspected peritoneal lesions are found by intra-abdominal examination, removing such lesions should be considered, or taking peritoneal biopsies from several sites should be considered if there are no suspected peritoneal lesions [15]. Appendectomy is to be added for MBT.

For patients who wish to preserve fertility, in addition to salpingo-oophorectomy on the affected side + omentectomy + peritoneal cytology, detailed intra-abdominal examination should be considered [15].

9.4.2 Laparoscopic Surgery and Restaging Surgery

BOT which was diagnosed accurately has excellent prognosis. Some surgical factors are related to recurrence of BOT, such as cystectomy, incomplete resection, and intraoperative spillage. Recently, laparoscopic surgery (LS) has become a standard procedure for benign ovarian tumor resection. LS was often employed for BOT with preoperative diagnosis as a benign tumor. LS has the potential risk of recurrence such as rupture of cyst, tumor cell dissemination, and trocar site metastasis. Most recurrent cases after LS had received conservative therapy. Nevertheless, LS itself had no relation with worse prognosis [16].

Restaging surgery is planned when unexpected final pathological result of BOT is obtained after primary surgery. The upstaging rate varies 7–40% among the studies, and it was always remarkably higher in SBT, especially SBT-MP histology has high risk of upstage [17]. Most positive findings of upstaged cases are peritoneal implant or positive washing cytology (Fig. 9.2). The standard procedure of restaging surgery for BOT is as follows. Disease-side unilateral salpingo-oophorectomy (USO), careful inspection of peritoneum, random biopsy at peritoneum, infracolic omentectomy, appendectomy (in case of MBT), and washing cytology should be

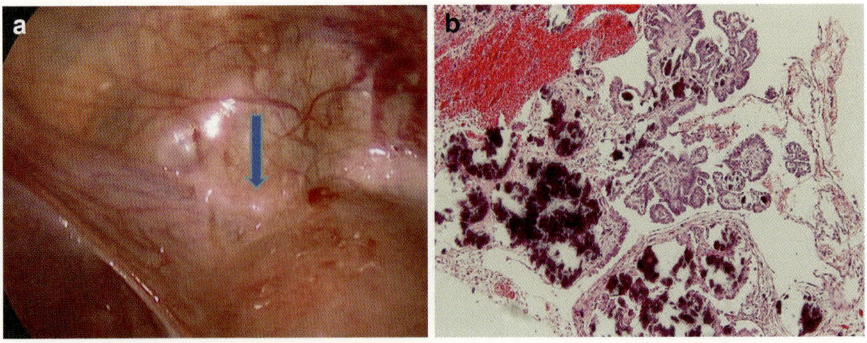

Fig. 9.2 Peritoneal implant in serous borderline tumor. (**a**) Small nodule on Douglas pouch peritoneum showed peritoneal (non invasive) implant (**b**)

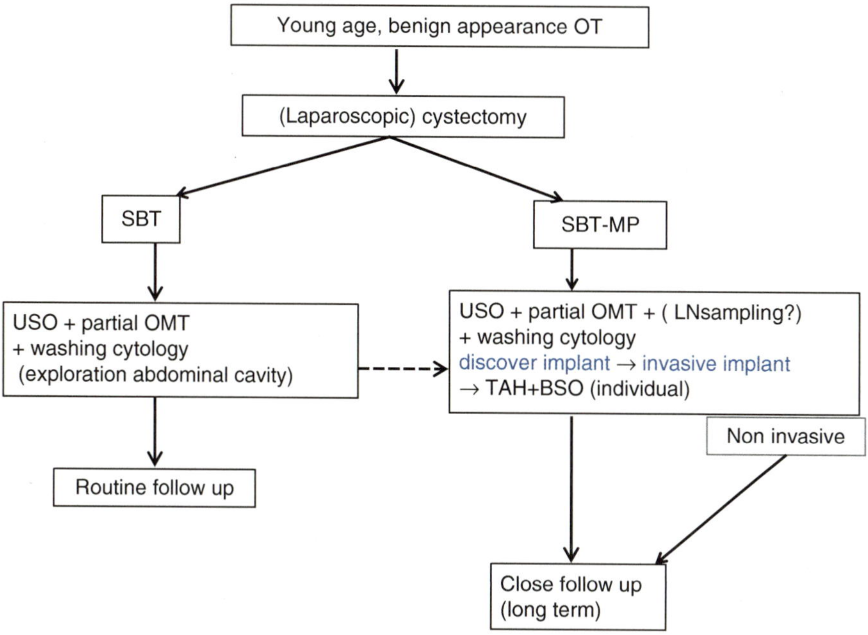

Fig. 9.3 Management strategy for serous BOT. *OT* ovarian tumor, *SBT* serous borderline tumor, *SBT-MP* serous borderline tumor with micropapillary pattern, *USO* unilateral salpingo-oophorectomy, *OMT* omentectomy, *TAH* total abdominal hysterectomy, *BSO* bilateral salpingo-oophorectomy

performed. If peritoneal implant is found, fertility preservation may be abandoned in some cases (Fig. 9.3). On the other hand, MBT has low incidence of upstaged cases as 4% [17]. Therefore, in case of MBT intestinal type, restaging surgery may be not required, if at least USO was already performed. Nevertheless, recheck the pathology by full-sectioned specimen which should be done to avoid missing the worse prognostic findings, such as intraepithelial carcinoma, microinvasive carcinoma, or mucinous carcinoma. In seromucinous BOT, therapeutic strategies are almost same as SBT (Fig. 9.4).

In cases with bilateral tumors, surgical approach may be individualized. Conservative procedure, such as USO plus cystectomy or bilateral cystectomy, has risk of recurrence. Both procedures retrospectively have shown no significant difference of recurrence rate as 26%, so less invasive strategy may be chosen for fertility outcomes [18].

About the adjuvant therapy, BOT was often described to be chemoresistant because of its low proliferation rate. There is no prospective study about the adjuvant chemotherapy for BOT. In a retrospective study for 80 patients with stages II to IV SBT, 3-year progression-free survival (PFS) was 89.9% without adjuvant chemotherapy group. On the other hand, PFS was 70.6% with adjuvant chemotherapy group [19]. A recent meta-analysis showed no survival difference between patients with adjuvant chemotherapy and surgery only [20].

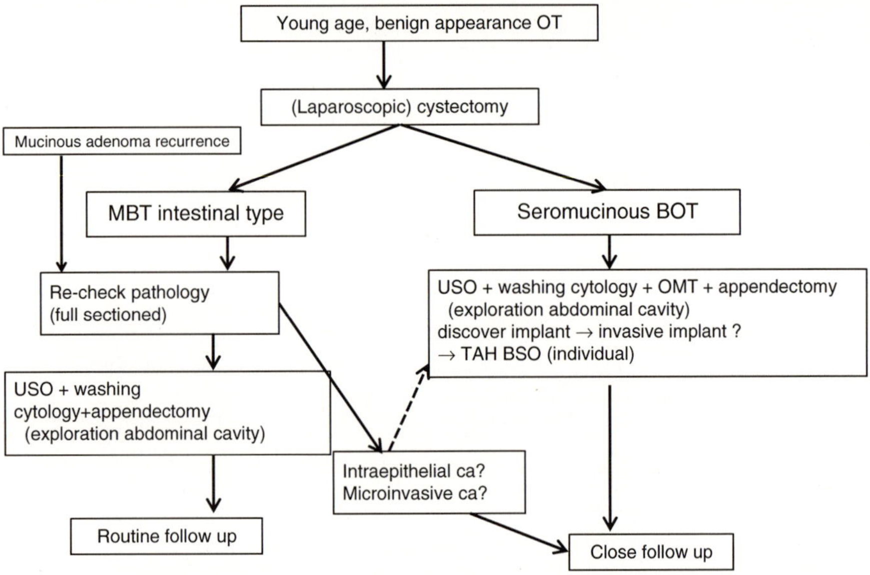

Fig. 9.4 Management strategy for mucinous and seromucinous BOT. *MBT* mucinous borderline tumor

Conclusion

In conclusion, BOT mainly consists of three different types, SBT, intestinal MBT, and seromucinous MBT. Each type shows different characteristics, and each has unique clinical features which influence prognosis. Accordingly, we should not treat them uniformly under the simple diagnosis of "borderline tumor." Inadequate or overtreatment should be avoided. To propose the optimal treatment strategy for patient, close communication with the pathologist and discussion with individual patient are essential.

References

1. McCluggage WG. Ovarian borderline tumours: a review with emphasis on controversial areas. Diag Histopathol. 2011;17:178–91.
2. Skı'rnisdo´ ttir I, Garmo H, Wilander E, Holmberg L. Borderline ovarian tumors in Sweden 1960–2005: trends in incidence and age at diagnosis compared to ovarian cancer. Int J Cancer. 2008;123:1897–901.
3. Saito T, Katabuchi H. Annual Report of the Committee on Gynecologic Oncology, Japan Society of Obstetrics and Gynecology: Patient annual report for 2013 and treatment annual report for 2008. J Obstet Gynaecol Res. 2016;42:1069–79.
4. Plat J. Chapter 6: Surface epithelial-stromal tumors:Serous tumors. In: Pathology of the ovary. Philadelphia: Saunders; 2004. p. 83–102.

5. Bell DA, Longacre TA, Plat J, Kohn EC, Soslow RA, Ellenmson LH, Malpica A, Stoler M, Kurman RJ. Serous borderline (low malignant potential atypical proliferative) ovarian tumors: workshop perspective. Hum Pathol. 2004;35:934–48.
6. Seidman JD, Kurman RJ. Ovarian serous borderline tumors: a critical review of the literature with emphasis on prognostic factor. Hum Pathol. 2000;31:539–57.
7. Silva E, Gershenson DM, .Malpica A, Deavers M. The recurrence and the overall survival rates of ovarian serous borderline neoplasms with noninvasive implants is time dependent. Am J Surg Pathol 2006;30:1367–1371.
8. Kurman RJ, Carcngiu ML, Herrington CS, Young RH. Chapter 1: Tumors of Ovary, Seromucionus tumors. In: WHO classification of tumours of female reproductive organs. Lyon: International Agency for Research on Cancer; 2014. p. 38–40.
9. Hart WR. Mucinous tumors of the ovary: a review. Int J Gynecol Pathol. 2005;24:4–25.
10. Shappell HW, Riopel MA, Smith Sehdev AE, Ronnett BM, Kurman RJ. Diagnostic criteria and behavior of ovarian seromucinous (endocervical-type mucinous and mixed cell-type) tumors: atypical proliferative (borderline) tumors, intraepithelial, microinvasive, and invasive carcinomas. Am J Surg Pathol. 2002;26:1529–41.
11. Pongsuvareeyakul T, Khunamornpong S, Settakorn J, Sukpan K, Suprasert P, Siriaunkgul S. Accuracy of frozen-section diagnosis of ovarian mucinous tumors. Int J Gynecol Cancer. 2012;22:400–6.
12. Koskas M, Uzan C, Gouy S, Pautier P, Lhomme C, Haie-Meder C, et al. Prognositic factors of a large retrospective series of mucinous borderline tumors of the ovary (excluding peritoneal pseudomyxoma). Am J Surg Oncol. 2011;18:40–8.
13. Chiesa AG, Deavers MT, Veras E, Silva EG, Gershenson D, Malpica A. Ovarian intestinal type mucinous borderline tumors: are we ready for a nomenclature change? Int J Gynecol Pathol. 2010;29:108–12.
14. Cardon I, Leunen K, Van Gorp T, Amant F, Neven P, Vergote I. Management of borderline ovarian neoplasms. J Clin Oncol. 2007;25:2928–37.
15. Komiyama S, Katabuchi H, Mikami M, Nagase S, Okamoto A, Ito K, et al. Japan Society of Gynecologic Oncology guidelines 2015 for the treatment of ovarian cancer including primary peritoneal cancer and fallopian tube cancer. Int J Clin Oncol. 2016;21:435–46.
16. Morice P, Uzan C, Fauvet R, Gouy S, Duvillard P, Darai E. Borderline ovarian tumour: pathological diagnostic dilemma and risk factors for invasive or lethal recurrence. Lancet Oncol. 2012;13:e103–15.
17. Zapardiel I, Rosenberg P, Peiretti M, Zanagnolo V, Sanguineti F, Aletti G, Landoni F, Bocciolone L, Colombo N, Maggioni A. The role of restaging borderline ovarian tumors: single institution experience and review of the literature. Gynecol Oncol. 2010;119:274–7.
18. Vasconcelos I, de Sousa Mendes M. Conservative surgery in ovarian borderline tumours; a meta-analysis with emphasis on recurrence risk. Eur J Cancer. 2015;51:620–31.
19. Shih K, Zhou Q, Aghajanian C, Huh J, Soslow R, Morgan J, Iasonos A, Chi D, Barakat R, Abu-Rustum N. Patterns of recurrence and role of adjuvant chemotherapy in stage II–IV serous ovarian borderline tumors. Gynecol Oncol. 2010;119:270–3.
20. Vasconcelos I, Olschewski J, Braicu I, Sehouli J. Limited efficacy of platinum-based adjuvant treatment on the outcome of borderline ovarian tumors. Eur J Gynecol Reprod Biol. 2015;186:26–33.

Strategies for the Management of Non-epithelial Ovarian Tumors

10

Satoru Kyo

Abstract

The rarity of non-epithelial ovarian tumors provides many challenging aspects for the clinician, with most general gynecologists only seeing a patient every several years. The first barrier to the management of these tumors is the difficulty of pathological diagnosis, and specialists in pathology must therefore be involved in the diagnostic process. The second barrier is a lack of clinical practice guidelines, due to the paucity of reliable clinical studies resulting from the rarity of such patients. A more advanced information base can be found in the field of testicular cancer, and some treatment strategies have thus been based on clinical studies of testicular tumors. Fortunately, the prognosis of patients with non-epithelial ovarian tumors is not poor in the early clinical stages, and fertility-sparing operations can be selected although there are some unresolved issues concerning the indication of this type of surgery. Furthermore, established chemotherapies have been associated with a favorable prognosis. Recent advances in molecular biology have identified a variety of genetic alterations in these tumors, some of which can be useful as biomarkers. Further basic research to dissect the molecular mechanisms of carcinogenesis of these tumors is now necessary to develop novel molecular-targeting approaches that can be combined with existing chemotherapeutic regimens, such as BEP (bleomycin, etoposide, and cisplatin), that have been shown to be effective in this type of tumors.

Keywords

Granulosa cell tumor • Germ cell tumor • Fertility-sparing surgery • BEP

S. Kyo, M.D., Ph.D.
Department of Obstetrics and Gynecology, Shimane University Faculty of Medicine, 89-1, Enya-Cho, Izumo, Shimane 693-8501, Japan
e-mail: satoruky@med.shimane-u.ac.jp

H. Katabuchi (ed.), *Frontiers in Ovarian Cancer Science*, Comprehensive Gynecology and Obstetrics, DOI 10.1007/978-981-10-4160-0_10

10.1 Introduction

Malignant non-epithelial ovarian tumors are relatively rare, but account for approximately 10% of ovarian malignancies. Although there are few reliable clinical trials on the treatment of these tumors, surgical procedures and appropriate chemotherapy regimens have now been established. Each of these tumors has characteristic clinical features that are helpful for proper preoperative diagnosis. In the latest World Health Organization (WHO) classification guidelines for ovarian cancer [1], non-epithelial tumors encompass a large variety of types, including mesenchymal tumors (low- and high-grade endometrioid stromal tumors), mixed epithelial and stromal tumors (adenosarcomas and carcinosarcomas), pure stromal tumors (e.g., fibromas and thecomas), pure sex cord-stromal tumors (SCSTs, e.g., adult granulosa cell tumors or AGCTs and juvenile granulosa cell tumors or JGCTs), mixed SCSTs (e.g., Sertoli-Leydig cell tumors), and germ cell tumors (see Table 6.1 in Chap. 6). Considering relatively high prevalence of SCSTs and malignant ovarian germ cell tumors (MOGCTs) in malignant ovarian tumors, this chapter focuses on the management strategies for these tumors, with a discussion on the molecular aspects of each.

10.2 Ovarian Sex Cord-Stromal Tumors (SCSTs)

10.2.1 Clinical Features of Ovarian SCSTs

In Japanese population, the SCSTs account for 0.3–0.5% of malignant ovarian neoplasia [2–4]. Among the various SCSTs, two types of pure sex cord tumor, namely, AGCTs and JGCTs, are representative. They are usually characterized by age at diagnosis, with the former commonly arising in perimenopausal and early postmenopausal women and the latter in younger patients (most often 10–30 years of age). Although patient age is informative, clinical symptoms are variable in SCSTs, and a definitive diagnosis can only be made by pathological examination of the dissected tumors. Approximately 50% of patients with granulosa cell tumor (GCT) exhibit estrogen-related symptoms, such as atypical bleeding and menstrual disorders, and may have abdominal symptoms, including distension and pain. Elevation of serum estradiol (E2) levels is representative of this disease, but is only observed in 70% of patients [5], meaning that it has limitations as a diagnostic marker and that a diagnosis of GCT cannot therefore be ruled out simply by the absence of elevated serum E2.

Some differences in clinical behavior are observed between AGCTs and JGCTs, with JGCTs appearing to have more favorable clinical outcome with less likelihood of recurrence and metastasis. However, when recurrence occurs in JGCT, it is typically early (within a few years), while AGCTs are likely to have late onset of recurrence [6]. About 80–90% of SCSTs are diagnosed as Stage I, and 95% are unilateral. The SEER (Surveillance, Epidemiology, and End Results) Program of the National Cancer Institute (NCI) has demonstrated that 5-year survival of Stage I and II patients is excellent (95%), but is poorer in Stage III and IV patients (59%), suggesting that surgical staging may be as important in GCTs as it is in epithelial ovarian cancer [7]. Of additional clinical relevance is the accompaniment of endometrial disorders alongside GCTs caused by tumor-produced estrogen, with 50% of patients having endometrial hyperplasia and up to 10% having endometrial cancer. This is an important issue because the presence of such disorders, particularly endometrial cancer, may affect operative procedures such as the addition of pelvic and para-aortic lymphadenectomy. Preoperative and postoperative evaluation of the endometrium is therefore required to detect endometrial neoplasms.

Although Sertoli-Leydig cell tumors are representative of the mixed type of SCSTs, they are rare and account for <0.5% of ovarian neoplasms, in which moderately and poorly differentiated forms are more common [1]. Sertoli-Leydig cell tumors have been reported in patients with a wide range of ages, but with a mean age of 25 years [8]. Between 40% and 60% of patients are virilized, while occasional patients have estrogenic manifestations [9]. Androgenic manifestations include amenorrhea, hirsutism, breast atrophy, clitoral hypertrophy, and hoarseness [1]. Patients typically present with abdominal pain, ascites, or tumor rupture. About 2–3% of tumors are found to have spread beyond the ovary at presentation, but lymph node metastases are rare [1]. The prognosis of Sertoli-Leydig cell tumors is favorable overall, but this depends significantly on the particular grade. Well-differentiated tumors are associated with close to 100% survival, while tumors with moderate differentiation are clinically malignant in about 10% of cases. Poorly differentiated tumors behave in a malignant fashion, with recurrence usually within 2 years and occurring in the peritoneal cavity [1].

10.2.2 Molecular Aspects of Ovarian SCSTs

No reports exist regarding genetic susceptibility to AGCT and in families with multiple AGCTs. There are few somatic molecular abnormalities in AGCTs, but recent molecular analyses have identified a frequent somatic mutation in approximately 95% of AGCTs in the *FOXL2* (forkhead box protein L2) gene, which encodes a nuclear transcription factor expressed mainly in the adult ovary and which is critically important for the development of granulosa cells [9]. The reported somatic mutation in *FOXL2* is a recurrent missense mutation in codon C134W (402C>G). Of particular interest is that this mutation is rare in other types of SCST, suggesting that it is specific to AGCTs. It may therefore be useful as a molecular marker for the differential diagnosis of SCSTs, especially in cases with equivocal clinical features.

In contrast to *FOXL2* mutations, FOXL2 expression itself is specific to most SCSTs, and immunostaining for this protein can therefore be used as a marker for these tumors. FOXL2 immunostaining has shown higher sensitivity for the diagnosis of SCSTs compared to α-inhibin and calretinin, the two traditional immunomarkers for SCSTs, and FOXL2 staining is typically more intense in positive cases than either [10]. In SCSTs that are negative for FOXL2 expression, α-inhibin and/or calretinin immunostaining has been shown to yield positive results [9]. Thus, FOXL2 is a sensitive and specific marker for SCSTs. Although most AGCTs carry a somatic mutation in the *FOXL2* gene, the mutation does not affect expression of the protein, and positive immunostaining has thus also been confirmed in AGCTs. In summary, FOXL2 staining is detectable in nearly all SCST cases, even those with a FOXL2 mutation, and that together with α-inhibin and calretinin, forms part of an immunomarker panel that results in positive staining with at least one marker in essentially all cases of SCST.

In contrast to AGCTs, JGCTs arise in the context of a variety of genetic syndromes, including Ollier's disease (a rare bone disease characterized by multiple enchondromatosis) and Maffucci's syndrome (enchondromatosis with hemangiomas) [6, 11, 12]. In Ollier's disease and Maffucci's syndrome, somatic mutations in *IDH1* (isocitrate dehydrogenase 1) and *IDH2* (isocitrate dehydrogenase 2) have been frequently reported, suggesting that mutation of these genes plays a key role in the pathogenesis of these diseases [13]. Somatic *DICER1* (a gene encoding an RNase III endonuclease involved with the processing of microRNA) mutations have occasionally been reported in JGCTs, with one study describing low-frequency (1 out of 14 patients) "hotspot" mutations in the gene [14]. In contrast, mutations in *DICER1* are found in 60% of Sertoli-Leydig cell tumors [14]. Germline mutations are also seen in familiar multinodular goiter with Sertoli-Leydig cell tumors, and tumor susceptibility includes pleuropulmonary blastoma in childhood [1]. Sertoli-Leydig cell tumors have been associated with cervical embryonal rhabdomyosarcoma in four cases [1].

In conclusion, the characteristic genetic difference between AGCTs and JGCTs is the status of *FOXL2* gene. The former tumors have very frequent mutations in *FOXL2,* while the latter tumors rarely have them, suggesting that AGCTs and JGCTs arise in different molecular pathways. Sertoli-Leydig cell tumors frequently have mutations in *DICER1*.

10.2.3 Treatment Strategy of Ovarian SCSTs

The key to success in the treatment is surgery. Considering the relatively worse 5-year survival of advanced cases (59% in Stages III and IV) [7], primary surgery should have the basic aim of tumor debulking, including the complete dissection of peritoneal disseminations, as well as strict surgical staging [15]. Retrospective studies have reported that retroperitoneal lymph node metastasis is very rare in SCSTs [16] and that lymphadenectomy can therefore be omitted [15]. One important issue is that preoperative and intraoperative differential diagnoses of GCTs from epithelial ovarian cancers are occasionally difficult. It is essential, therefore, not to delay radical surgeries, including lymphadenectomy and staging laparotomy, in such situations [15].

Fertility-sparing surgery for SCSTs has been accepted due to the rarity of bilateral occurrence (especially in Stage I disease) and because of the excellent prognosis for these patients, with the 5-year survival of Stage I–II patients being reported as 95% [4]. In particular, most patients with JGCTs are candidates for fertility-sparing surgery, considering the age of the patients. However, while radical surgery and adjuvant chemotherapy are recommended by some clinicians for better prognosis, quality of life and long-term morbidity should be considered for such young patients. Although Stage IA disease appears to be an appropriate indication for fertility-sparing surgery, it remains unclear whether this approach should be recommended for patients with Stage IC or more advanced disease, with the indication for Stage IC disease being particularly controversial.

Adjuvant chemotherapy is not recommended for GCTs with Stage I disease, because most cases can be cured by surgery alone, without recurrence. This concept is based on the biology of such indolent tumors, in that they usually have slow growth rates and are less effective to chemotherapy compared with faster-growing tumors. Furthermore, slow growth generates longer disease-free intervals, even without chemotherapy. Nevertheless, some researchers recommend chemotherapy for Stage IC disease in the presence of poor prognostic factors, such as nuclear atypia, high mitotic index, aneuploidy, or age >40 years [17]. Adjuvant therapy may be considered for patients with more advanced stages, residual tumor burden, or risk factors for recurrence, although there is no strong evidence to support prognostic improvement, and considerable caution is required given that adjuvant chemotherapy for young patients is likely to significantly affect long-term morbidity and quality of life. The risk factors for Stage I disease have been found to be a rupture of the membranes, a tumor diameter more than 10–15 cm, poorly differentiated Sertoli-Leydig tumors, and moderately differentiated Sertoli-Leydig tumors with heterologous elements [15].

In adjuvant therapy, combination chemotherapies with cisplatin, vinblastine, and bleomycin (PVB) or with bleomycin, etoposide, and cisplatin (BEP) have been used, with an EORTC (European Organization for Research and Treatment of Cancer) study using PVB in 38 AGCT patients (7 primary and 31 recurrent cases) exhibiting a 61% response rate [18], while a Gynecologic Oncology Group (GOG) study using BEP in 57 SCST patients (16 primary and 41 recurrent cases) had a 37% response rate [19]. Taxanes in conjunction with cisplatin have also been used for GCTs, with relatively high response rates (54%) observed [20]. However, there have been no randomized control trials (RCTs) comparing BEP and taxane-based chemotherapies, and for the time being, BEP appears to be the standard regimen for the treatment of GCTs.

The Japan Society of Gynecologic Oncology published the guidelines for the treatment of ovarian tumors [21], and the flow chart for the treatment of SCSTs is shown in Fig. 10.1.

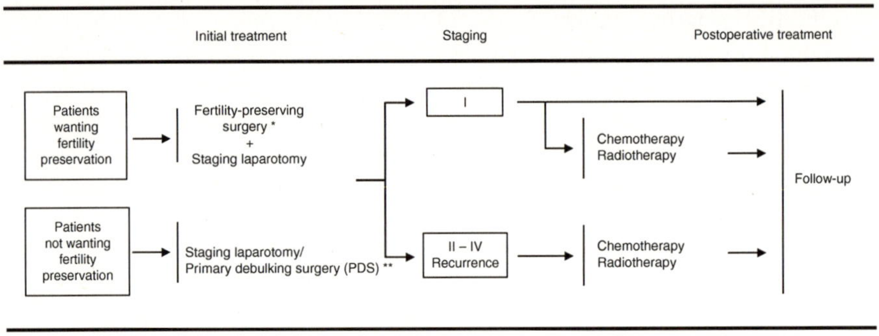

Fig. 10.1 Treatment of malignant sex cord-stromal tumors. *Fertility-preserving surgery—affected-side salpingo-oophorectomy + omentectomy + peritoneal cytology + detailed intra-abdominal examination. **Lymph node dissection (biopsy) can be omitted. Reprint with permission from ref. 21

10.3 Malignant Ovarian Germ Cell Tumors (MOGCTs)

10.3.1 Clinical Features of MOGCTs

In Japanese population, the MOGCTs account for 3–4% of malignant ovarian neoplasia [2–4] and have very characteristic clinical features. Firstly, they represent 80% of preadolescent ovarian malignancies. Secondly, they have excellent sensitivity to chemotherapy. Thirdly, most cases show unilateral occurrence. These features permit the possibility of fertility-sparing treatment in such patients.

Malignant transformation in ovarian mature cystic teratoma is the most frequent type of MOGCT, accounting for 38% of MOGCT patients in Japan, while yolk sac tumors, dysgerminomas, and immature teratomas account for 23%, 17%, and 11%, respectively. Grading of immature teratoma is a recent important issue, with these tumors having been graded from 1 to 3, depending on the amount of immature neuroectodermal component in tissue specimens [22]. Recently, however, a two-tiered (low- and high-grade) system has been more commonly used [23]. In this new system, Grade 1 is categorized as low grade, while Grades 2 and 3 are classified as high grade. The latter is considered as an indication for chemotherapy irrespective of clinical staging, but chemotherapy can be omitted in low-grade (Grade 1) tumors. The recurrence rates of immature teratoma are 18%, 37%, and 70%, in Grade 1, 2, and 3 tumors, respectively [22], with 3-year disease-free survivals after fertility-sparing surgery being 100%, 70%, and 66% [24], respectively. While most MOGCTs have extremely high sensitivity to chemotherapy, dysgerminomas have high sensitivity to irradiation as well, and this can therefore be a potent tool for local control of such tumors. Yolk sac tumors, embryonal carcinomas, and non-gestational choriocarcinomas are rare and sometimes have mixed components of each histology type. Since tumor diameter and histological type are considered as important prognostic factors in these mixed germ cell tumors, careful pathological examination is required, with a sufficient number of histological sections [20, 24]. Large tumors of high-grade immature teratoma, or those composed of yolk sac or choriocarcinoma components in over one third of histological specimens, have a worse prognosis, while tumors with <10 cm diameter have good overall prognosis irrespective of the histological composition [25].

The initial symptoms and signs of MOGCTs include subacute pain or palpation of the pelvic mass, which are observed in 80–90% of patients [26]. Some present as acute abdominal cases due to rupture of the membranes, bleeding from tumors, or torsion. It should be noted that it is not uncommon to find that patients being treated for appendicitis or other abdominal conditions, especially those that are young or preadolescent, are occasionally diagnosed during surgery as having these tumors.

Elevation of specific tumor markers is one of the characteristics of MOGCTs, in particular AFP (alpha-fetoprotein) for yolk sac tumors, hCG (human chorionic gonadotropin) for choriocarcinomas, LDH (lactate dehydrogenase) for dysgerminomas, and SCC (squamous cell carcinoma antigen) for malignant transformation of mature cystic teratomas. However, there are a considerable number of patients without significant elevation of these markers, meaning that their diagnostic value is limited. Nevertheless, their expression can be useful to monitor residual postoperative tumor burden, as well as treatment efficacy and recurrence during follow-up.

The clinical stage of MOGCTs is determined according to the guidelines established for epithelial ovarian cancers. Extraovarian lesions of MOGCTs mainly consist of retroperitoneal lymph node metastases and peritoneal dissemination. A SEER study of 760 cases of MOGCT reported that 76% of cases were Stages I and II, while 24% were Stages III and IV [27]. The prognostic factors for MOGCT have been studied by multivariate analysis, with clinical stage and preoperative levels of tumor marker (AFP and hCG) found to be independent prognostic factors for survival in one report [28], while SEER has reported that patient age at diagnosis, clinical stage, and histological type (i.e., yolk sac tumor) were independent prognostic factors [27]. SEER also reported that patients with retroperitoneal metastasis have significantly worse 5-year survival compared to those without retroperitoneal metastasis (83% vs. 96%) and that retroperitoneal metastasis is another independent prognostic factor [29].

10.3.2 Molecular Aspects of Ovarian Germ Cell Tumors

A wide variety of molecular studies, including genome sequencing and transcriptome profiling, have characterized the biological features of MOGCTs and their potential biomarkers. The characteristic features reported for the main histological subtypes of MOGCTs are summarized in Fig. 10.2, with pure dysgerminoma and yolk sac tumors having been found to be mainly non-diploid (i.e., tetraploid, polyploid, or aneuploid), while only 8% of immature teratomas are thought to be non-diploid [30]. DNA copy number analyses have revealed that part or whole gains of chromosomal arm 12p are frequent among both MOGCTs and testicular germ cell tumors [31]. A transcriptome profiling study comparing dysgerminoma and yolk

	Ploidy	CGH	miRNA	mRNA	Protein
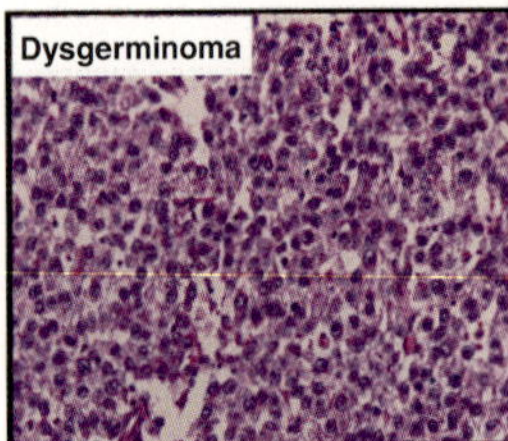 Dysgerminoma	Non-diploid (91%)	Gain 1q 7q 8 12 19 21 Loss 13	miR-146b-5p miR-155 miR-182	CASP8 CDH3 CXCL10 IL6R NANOG PDPN PLBD1 POU5F1	GATA4 KIT KRT8 LIN28A NANOG PAD14 PDPN POU5F1 SMAD3 TFAP2C
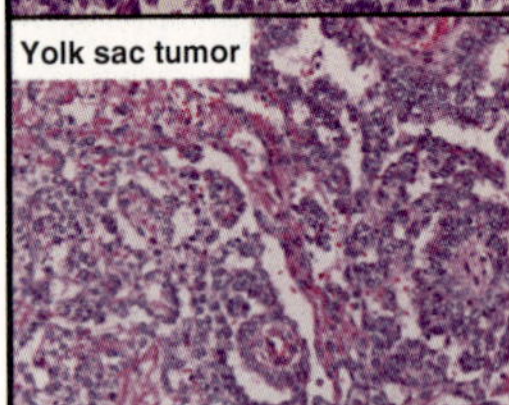 Yolk sac tumor	Non-diploid (86%)	Gain 1q 12p 20q Loss 1p	miR-122 miR-200b miR-200c miR-302a miR-302c miR-375 miR-638	BMP1 TGFB2	AE1/AE3 AFP FUT4 GATA4 GATA6 GGT1 GPC3 LIN28A PAD14
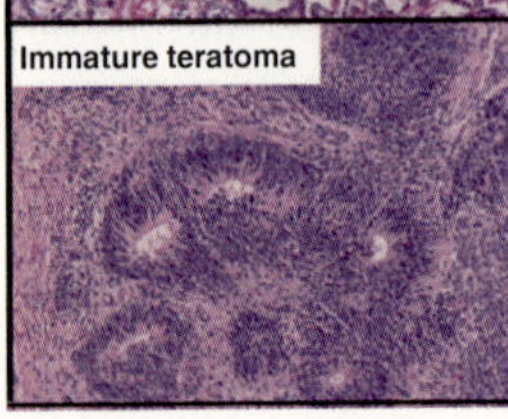 Immature teratoma	Diploid (92%)	No Characteristic alterations	No specific miRNAs	Non-studied	LIN28A PAD14 SOX2

Fig. 10.2 Representative molecular characteristics of the main histological subtypes of MOGCTs. Hematoxylin- and eosin-stained sections of the subtypes are illustrated to the left; dysgerminoma (growing with sheets or nests of polygonal cells with round vesicular nuclei, abundant clear cytoplasm with glycogen, and well-defined cell membranes), yolk sac tumor (commonly with reticular (*left side*) and endodermal sinus (*right side*) growth patterns) and immature teratoma (with variable amounts of immature embryonal-type tissues, mostly in the form of neuroectodermal tubules and rosettes (as shown)). The typical diploid or non-diploid, copy number alterations reported in ≥30% of the subtypes and aberrantly expressed miRNAs, mRNAs, and proteins are also listed. Adapted with alterations from Endocr Rev. 2013; 34: 339–376

sac tumors revealed that a subset of eight WNT/β-catenin signaling components is sufficient to distinguish between the two histological subtypes [32]. Immunohistochemical analysis from the same study indicated that cytoplasmic β-catenin is expressed in all histological subtypes, but with only weak focal staining in dysgerminoma, and that β-catenin nuclear accumulation is observed only in yolk sac tumors and teratomas [32]. Other work has indicated that the IL6R (interleukin 6 receptor) and C-X-C motif chemokine 10 (CXCL10), known to be involved in cytokine signaling and immune responses, are overexpressed in dysgerminomas [30]. Upregulation of IL6R expression prevents premature entry into meiosis and maintains an immature germ cell population in the human fetal ovary [33]. On the other hand, the expression of CXCL10 and its receptor CXCR3 can lead to tumor recruitment of T-lymphocytes [34], which is in keeping with the observation of infiltration of T-lymphocytes in dysgerminoma, although the biological function and significance of this phenomenon remains unclear.

The pluripotency genes, NANOG (nanog homeobox), POU5F1 (POU domain, class 5, transcription factor 1), POU5F1B (POU domain, class 5, transcription factor 1B), and PDPN (podoplanin), have also been found to be overexpressed in dysgerminoma [35] and seminoma [36]. The fact that the expression pattern for these genes is similar between dysgerminoma and seminoma indicates that common tumorigenic pathways exist for a subgroup of ovarian and testicular germ cell tumors and/or that such expression patterns represent the remnant traits of their mutual precursor, i.e., the primordial germ cell. Other groups have reported that the cell signaling genes *BMP1* (bone morphogenetic protein 1) and *TGFB2* (transforming growth factor-beta 2) are overexpressed in yolk sac tumors [32, 37]. The TGF-β/BMP signaling pathway regulates embryonic development, and its biological relevance is underlined by the fact that mutations in the BMP receptor Alk6b (activin receptor-like kinase 6b) impairs germ cell differentiation and initiates germ cell tumors in zebra fish [38].

Several microRNA (miRNA) expression profiling studies have identified that two miRNA clusters, namely, miR-302-367 and miR-371-373, are overexpressed in MOGCTs when compared with nonmalignant control tissues [35, 37, 39, 40]. The coordinate overexpression of these miRNAs appears to be specific for MOGCTs, with no similar findings having been reported for other malignancies or diseases to date. Gene ontology analysis has shown that the downregulated mRNA targets for miR-302-367 and miR-371-373 mediate cellular processes important in oncogenesis and malignant progression, supporting the functional significance of these miRNA clusters in the biology of MOGCTs [35]. On the other hand, the most significantly overexpressed miRNA in yolk sac tumors has been reported to be miR-375 [37, 40]. Dysregulation of miR-375 has been observed for various tumor types, including head and neck, esophageal, lung, and gastric cancers [30]. Signaling pathway analyses of miR-375-regulated genes have indicated the involvement of cell cycle regulation, focal adhesion, MAPK (mitogen-activated protein kinase), TGF-β, WNT, and VEGF (vascular endothelial growth factor) pathways [41]. In dysgerminoma, three other miRNAs have been identified as being highly expressed, namely, miR-0146b-5p, miR-155, and miR-182 [37, 40]. Although the specific functions of these miRNAs remain unclear, they are known to be overexpressed in other tumor types, including breast, lung, cervix, and colon cancers, and interactions with *BRCA1* (breast cancer associated gene 1) have been reported [30].

In regard to potential biomarkers for MOGCTs, protein expression analyses have indicated that pluripotency/developmental factors and histology-specific markers may be the two most important functional categories. POU5F1 and NANOG are significantly expressed more often in dysgerminoma, for example, supporting their application as biomarkers for this subtype [42, 43]. The pluripotency factor SOX2 (sex-determining region Y-box 2), on the other hand, has been shown to be more significantly expressed in immature teratoma and to be very specific to this subtype [30, 43]. Primordial germ cells do not express SOX2 and remain capable of proliferation, and thus the absence of SOX2 expression in dysgerminoma underlines their strong resemblance to this progenitor cell type.

In addition to POU5F1, PDNP has also been proposed as a diagnostic marker of dysgerminoma [30]. In contrast, the differential diagnosis of yolk sac tumor is difficult due to its complex and varied histological appearance, especially between yolk sac tumor and clear cell carcinoma of the ovary, and good markers for this tumor type are limited. Mixed tumors exhibit further complexity, with small components of yolk sac tumor growing in close proximity to other subtypes such as immature teratoma. In the past, AFP has been a famous tumor marker for yolk sac tumors [44], but the diagnostic use of AFP immunohistochemistry has low sensitivity and specificity [45]. Alternatively, the transcription factor GATA6 (GATA-binding factor 6) has been shown to be more frequently expressed in yolk sac tumors than dysgerminomas, with GATA4 (GATA-binding factor 4) being expressed in dysgerminoma, yolk sac tumors, and immature teratomas [46]. The differential expression pattern of GATA4 and GATA6 may thus be used as a marker to distinguish between yolk sac tumors and dysgerminomas.

10.3.3 Treatment Strategy of Ovarian Germ Cell Tumor

Surgery is the primary treatment of MOGCTs. Since most patients with MOGCTs are of preadolescent or reproductive ages and have unilateral tumors, fertility-sparing surgery should be considered, especially considering the fact that patients with MOGCTs are extremely sensitive to chemotherapy. Unilateral salpingo-oophorectomy of the affected side with omentectomy and peritoneal cytology are the basic procedures in operation for MOGCTs. A routine biopsy of the contralateral ovary should be avoided to preserve ovarian function, unless macroscopic findings are detected [47]. However, since dysgerminoma occasionally (in 10–15% of cases) occurs bilaterally, careful examination of the contralateral ovary is necessary [48]. Stage III and IV patients who desire fertility-sparing surgery can be permitted this option, with a focus on tumor debulking [47, 49], based on the evidence that fertility-sparing surgery does not adversely affect prognosis [26, 27, 50–52].

Intraoperative frozen section analysis is necessary irrespective of the type of surgery undertaken (fertility-sparing or otherwise). However, the diagnostic accuracy of such an analysis is of limited value, and it is recommended to avoid overtreatment during the operation. In the event that a differential diagnosis is required to distinguish the tumor from types that do not permit fertility-sparing surgery, it may be appropriate to initially perform fertility-sparing surgery without overtreatment and then reoperate if necessary after postoperative pathological examination.

When patients do not require fertility-sparing surgery, standard operative procedures for epithelial ovarian malignancies should be performed, with the addition of pelvic and para-aortic lymphadenectomy, although the prognostic impact of retroperitoneal lymphadenectomy is not proven. A recent retrospective study of 1083 patients with MOGCTs that were deemed to be at clinical Stage I at the time of surgery reported no significant difference in the 5-year survival between patients with and without retroperitoneal lymphadenectomy, including patients who were upstaged to FIGO (International Federation of Gynecology and Obstetrics) Stage IIIC after lymphadenectomy [53]. On multivariate analysis, lymphadenectomy was not an independent predictor of survival when controlling for age, histology, and race. Moreover, the presence of lymph node metastasis had no significant effect on survival [54]. Thus, neither lymphadenectomy nor lymph node metastasis was an independent predictor of survival in patients with MOGCTs confined to the ovary. This probably reflects the highly chemosensitive nature of these tumors, and retroperitoneal lymphadenectomy can thus be omitted [54].

There are issues about the selection of surgical procedures and postoperative treatments in each tumor type. It remains unresolved whether patients with Stage I (Grade III) immature teratoma, pathologically diagnosed after ovarian cystectomy for mature cystic teratoma, require the addition of adnexectomy [55]. It has been accepted, however, that there is no need for chemotherapy in patients with Stage IA dysgerminoma or Stage IA (Grade I) immature teratoma [47]. Furthermore, in patients with Stage IA dysgerminoma that undergo operation with incomplete surgical staging, chemotherapy can be delayed until there is evidence of relapse, since these tumors have been shown to respond well to chemotherapy upon recurrence [56].

The current standard chemotherapy regimen for MOGCTs is BEP (bleomycin, etoposide, and cisplatin), based on the clinical trial results for testicular germ cell tumors, as well as the excellent cure rates achieved in early-stage patients (almost 100%) and even in advanced patients (at least 75%) [57]. Despite the lack of Phase III trials, BEP is strongly recommended as standard chemotherapy regimen for MOGCTs, although special attention should be paid to guarantee the best outcomes with this approach. Firstly, drug doses should be maintained, without reckless reduction. Only in the case of pyrogenic neutropenia, or thrombocytopenia with bleeding, can a 20% decrease in etoposide be permitted [58]. Secondly, the drugs should not be substituted for alternatives. In testicular tumors, the attempt to omit bleomycin in favor of decreasing pulmonary toxicity has been shown to fail, worsening the prognosis of the patient [59]. Furthermore, a change from cisplatin to carboplatin has also been reported to adversely affect prognosis [60]. Thirdly, treatment schedule compliance is strictly important. Even with the presence of neutropenia, the next cycle of chemotherapy must commence at day 22 [61], and although the presence of severe bone marrow suppression, such as neutropenia <500 per mm^3 or thrombocytopenia $<10^5$ per mm^3, may permit delay of the next cycle of chemotherapy, it should only do so for a maximum of 3 days [62]. This compliance requirement is thus quite different from more common epithelial tumors of the ovary. Finally, and as mentioned above, postoperative adjuvant chemotherapy with BEP can be omitted in patients with Stage IA dysgerminoma and Stage I (Grade 1) immature teratoma [44] and is in fact recommended to be omitted in young patients (<15 years old) with immature teratoma [63, 64].

One of the critical issues in chemotherapy for MOGCTs is how many cycles should be performed, since there have been no RCTs to assess the optimal number. Based on GOG78 (in which one arm of the trial performed three cycles of BEP for early-stage MOGCTs), the NCCN (National Comprehensive Cancer Network) guidelines now recommend three cycles of BEP [55, 57]. In the BEP protocol, however, accumulative pulmonary toxicity caused by bleomycin and secondary neoplasms induced by etoposide should be a concern. The rate of occurrence of pulmonary toxicity from bleomycin is 0–2% over three cycles of BEP and is 6–18% over four or more cycles. A pulmonary function test performed during bleomycin therapy is unfortunately not a good predictor of toxicity, since it has been shown to have a relatively low sensitivity and specificity [65, 66]. Secondary neoplasms triggered by etoposide are also accumulative, and the rate of occurrence is very low (0.4%) with a total dose of less than 2000 mg/m^2, but increases at doses over 2000 mg/m^2 [67]. The threshold for etoposide to induce neoplasms is thus thought to be 2000 mg/m^2 [68]. Prognosis of secondary leukemias caused by etoposide is poor, with most cases arising 2–3 years after initial chemotherapy, and it is thus important to monitor closely for occurrence of secondary leukemia when >2000 mg/m^2 of etoposide is used [69].

There are unfortunately no RCTs comparing different regimens of chemotherapy for MOGCTs. In testicular tumors, the BEP regimen was compared with etoposide, ifosfamide, and cisplatin (VIP therapy), with no significant difference in long-term prognosis reported, although bone marrow suppression was found to be more prominent in the former [70].

Following postoperative BEP chemotherapy, the failure of ovarian function due to toxicity, as well as secondary neoplasms induced by etoposide, should be cared for in particular. Failure of ovarian function is most frequently observed when cyclophosphamide is used in treatment regimens, but BEP has shown a relatively rare rate of failure for ovarian function. Amenorrhea is frequently (62%) observed during BEP chemotherapy, but 91% of patients undergoing this regimen appear to recover menstruation [71]. In general, 80–90% of patients receiving chemotherapy for MOGCTs eventually recover menstruation following treatment [72]. It has been reported that the incidence of infertility, congenital malformation, and spontaneous abortion do not increase after MOGCT chemotherapy [37, 72–75], and there are several reports suggesting that pretreatment with GnRH (gonadotropin-releasing hormone) analogues or oral contraceptives may protect ovarian function during chemotherapy [76–78]. A randomized trial in breast cancer has reported the preservation of ovarian function by GnRH analogues during chemotherapy [79], but there is no consensus regarding the utility of such protection.

The Japan Society of Gynecologic Oncology published the guidelines for the treatment of ovarian tumors [21], and the flow chart of the treatment of MOGCTs is shown in Fig. 10.3.

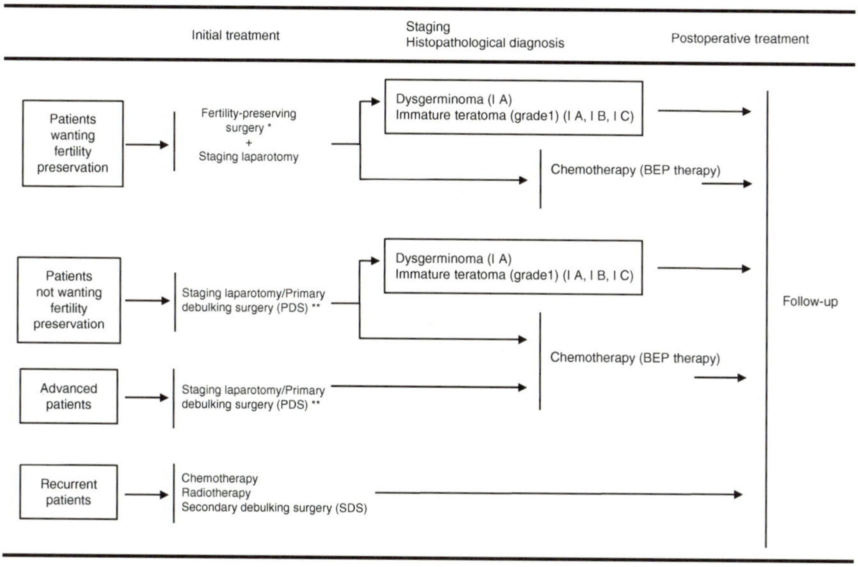

Fig. 10.3 Treatment of malignant ovarian germ cell tumors. *Fertility-preserving surgery—affected-side salpingo-oophorectomy + omentectomy + peritoneal cytology + detailed intra-abdominal examination. **Lymph node dissection (biopsy) can be omitted. Reprint with permission from ref. 21

10.4 Conclusions and Future Directions

Non-epithelial ovarian tumors are rare, and there are few RCTs for the treatment of these tumors. We therefore have limited information in regard to the most appropriate management strategy for these cancers. However, considerable efforts have been made to apply fertility-sparing surgeries for young patients, an approach that has proven to be relatively safe in early-stage tumors. Although pathological diagnosis is occasionally difficult, especially in intraoperative cases, and thus it is not always easy to judge where fertility-sparing surgery may be indicated, it is important that radical surgery be avoided in patients with difficult intraoperative diagnoses. In such cases, fertility-sparing surgery should be performed first, with radical surgery conducted subsequently only if postoperative pathological assessment indicates necessity.

The establishment of BEP chemotherapy has greatly improved outcomes in patients with ovarian germ cell tumors. However, most of the evidence regarding the indications for chemotherapy, as well as the composition of these regimens, has been derived from experience with testicular germ cell tumors, and further evidence from ovarian germ cell tumors is required in the future. Moreover, some issues remain concerning the indication for chemotherapy. Although it is currently standard practice that adjuvant chemotherapy be omitted in patients with Stage IA dysgerminoma and Stage I (Grade 1) immature teratoma, we do not still have conclusive evidence to support this, and the omission of chemotherapy may be extended to more advanced cases. An additional issue is the need for strict compliance of MOGCT chemotherapy regimens to achieve optimal efficacy, something that is completely different from the situation in epithelial ovarian tumors.

An emerging number of molecular studies have revealed some useful biomarkers for MOGCT tumors, but specific biomarkers for each tumor type are limited. The molecular mechanisms through which these tumors arise remain unclear, and we have no information regarding their cells of origin. It is hoped that future progress in these studies will identify the molecular pathways through which these tumors arise and grow, something that is essential for the development of molecularly targeted therapies. Ultimately, it is hoped that such novel molecular approaches can then be combined with effective conventional chemotherapies such as BEP, an approach that has successfully been applied to the treatment of epithelia ovarian tumors.

References

1. Kurman RL, Carcangiu ML, Simon Herrington C, Young RH, editors. WHO classification of tumours of female reproductive organs. 4th ed. Lyon: International Agency for Research on Cancer; 2014.
2. Yamagami W, Aoki D. Annual report of the committee on gynecologic oncology, the Japan society of obstetrics and gynecology. J Obstet Gynaecol Res. 2015;41:1861–9.
3. Saito T, Katabuchi H. Annual report of the committee on gynecologic oncology, Japan society of obstetrics and gynecology: patient annual report for 2013 and treatment annual report for 2008. J Obstet Gynaecol Res. 2016;42:1069–79.
4. Yamagami W, Nagase S, Takahashi F, Ino K, Hachisuga T, Aoki D, Katabuchi H. Clinical statistics of gynecologic cancers in Japan. J Gynecol Oncol. 2017;28:e32. Epub 2017 Feb 10.
5. Colombo N, Parma G, Zanagnolo V, Insinga A. Management of ovarian stromal cell tumors. J Clin Oncol. 2007;25:2944–51.
6. Young RH, Dickersin GR, Scully RE. Juvenile granulosa cell tumor of the ovary. A clinicopathological analysis of 125 cases. Am J Surg Pathol. 1984;8:575–96.
7. Zhang M, Cheung MK, Shin JY, Kapp DS, Husain A, Teng NN, et al. Prognostic factors responsible for survival in sex cord stromal tumors of the ovary–an analysis of 376 women. Gynecol Oncol. 2007;104:396–400.
8. Young RH, Scully RE. Ovarian sertoli-leydig cell tumors. A clinicopathological analysis of 207 cases. Am J Surg Pathol. 1985;9:543–69.
9. Shah SP, Köbel M, Senz J, Morin RD, Clarke BA, Wiegand KC, et al. Mutation of FOXL2 in granulosa-cell tumors of the ovary. N Engl J Med. 2009;360:2719–29.
10. Al-Agha OM, Huwait HF, Chow C, Yang W, Senz J, Kalloger SE, et al. FOXL2 is a sensitive and specific marker for sex cord-stromal tumors of the ovary. Am J Surg Pathol. 2011;35:484–94.
11. Vaz RM, Turner C. Ollier disease (enchondromatosis) associated with ovarian juvenile granulosa cell tumor and precocious pseudopuberty. J Pediatr. 1986;108:945–7.
12. Tanaka Y, Sasaki Y, Nishihira H, Izawa T, Nishi T. Ovarian juvenile granulosa cell tumor associated with Maffucci's syndrome. Am J Clin Pathol. 1992;97:523–7.
13. Amary MF, Damato S, Halai D, Eskandarpour M, Berisha F, Bonar F, et al. Ollier disease and Maffucci syndrome are caused by somatic mosaic mutations of IDH1 and IDH2. Nat Genet. 2011;43:1262–5.
14. Heravi-Moussavi A, Anglesio MS, Cheng SW, Senz J, Yang W, Prentice L, et al. Recurrent somatic DICER1 mutations in nonepithelial ovarian cancers. N Engl J Med. 2012;366:234–42.
15. Ovarian Cancer Guideline (Version 1. 2014). NCCN Clinical Practice Guidelines in Oncology.

16. Brown J, Sood AK, Deavers MT, Milojevic L, Gershenson DM. Patterns of metastasis in sex cord-stromal tumors of the ovary: can routine staging lymphadenectomy be omitted? Gynecol Oncol. 2009;113:86–90.
17. Foulkes WD, Gore M, McCluggage WG. Rare non-epithelial ovarian neoplasms: pathology, genetics and treatment. Gynecol Oncol. 2016;142:190–8.
18. Pecorelli S, Wagenaar HC, Vergote IB, Curran D, Beex LV, Wiltshaw E, et al. Cisplatin (P), vinblastine (V) and bleomycin (B) combination chemotherapy in recurrent or advanced granulosa(−theca) cell tumours of the ovary. An EORTC gynaecological cancer cooperative group study. Eur J Cancer. 1999;35:1331–7.
19. Homesley HD, Bundy BN, Hurteau JA, Roth LM. Bleomycin, etoposide, and cisplatin combination therapy of ovarian granulosa cell tumors and other stromal malignancies: a gynecologic oncology group study. Gynecol Oncol. 1999;72:131–7.
20. Brown J, Shvartsman HS, Deavers MT, Ramondetta LM, Burke TW, Munsell MF, et al. The activity of taxanes compared with bleomycin, etoposide, and cisplatin in the treatment of sex cord-stromal ovarian tumors. Gynecol Oncol. 2005;97:489–96.
21. Komiyama S, Katabuchi H, Mikami M, Nagase S, Okamoto A, Ito K, et al. Japan society of gynecologic oncology guidelines 2015 for the treatment of ovarian cancer including primary peritoneal cancer and fallopian tube cancer. Int J Clin Oncol. 2016;21:435–46.
22. Norris HJ, Zirkin HJ, Benson WL. Immature (malignant) teratoma of the ovary: a clinical and pathologic study of 58 cases. Cancer. 1976;37:2359–72.
23. O'Connor DM, Norris HJ. The influence of grade on the outcome of stage I ovarian immature (malignant) teratomas and the reproducibility of grading. Int J Gynecol Pathol. 1994;13:283–9.
24. Mangili G, Scarfone G, Gadducci A, Sigismondi C, Ferrandina G, Scibilia G, et al. Is adjuvant chemotherapy indicated in stage I pure immature ovarian teratoma (IT)? A multicentre Italian trial in ovarian cancer (MITO-9). Gynecol Oncol. 2010;119:48–52.
25. Kurman RJ, Norris HJ. Malignant germ cell tumors of the ovary. Hum Pathol. 1977;8:551–64.
26. Gershenson DM. Management of ovarian germ cell tumors. J Clin Oncol. 2007;25: 2938–43.
27. Chan JK, Tewari KS, Waller S, Cheung MK, Shin JY, Osann K, et al. The influence of conservative surgical practices for malignant ovarian germ cell tumors. J Surg Oncol. 2008;98:111–6.
28. Murugaesu N, Schmid P, Dancey G, Agarwal R, Holden L, McNeish I, et al. Malignant ovarian germ cell tumors: identification of novel prognostic markers and long-term outcome after multimodality treatment. J Clin Oncol. 2006;24:4862–6.
29. Kumar S, Shah JP, Bryant CS, Imudia AN, Cote ML, Ali-Fehmi R, et al. The prevalence and prognostic impact of lymph node metastasis in malignant germ cell tumors of the ovary. Gynecol Oncol. 2008;110:125–32.
30. Kraggerud SM, Hoei-Hansen CE, Alagaratnam S, Skotheim RI, Abeler VM, Rajpert-De Meyts E, et al. Molecular characteristics of malignant ovarian germ cell tumors and comparison with testicular counterparts: implications for pathogenesis. Endocr Rev. 2013;34:339–76.
31. Atkin NB, Baker MC. I(12p): specific chromosomal marker in seminoma and malignant teratoma of the testis? Cancer Genet Cytogenet. 1983;10:199–204.
32. Fritsch MK, Schneider DT, Schuster AE, Murdoch FE, Perlman EJ. Activation of Wnt/β--catenin signaling in distinct histologic subtypes of human germ cell tumors. Pediatr Dev Pathol. 2006;9:115–31.
33. Eddie SL, Childs AJ, Jabbour HN, Anderson RA. Developmentally regulated IL6-type cytokines signal to germ cells in the human fetal ovary. Mol Hum Reprod. 2012;18:88–95.
34. Schweyer S, Soruri A, Baumhoer D, Peters J, Cattaruzza M, Radzun HJ, et al. Expression of CXC chemokine IP-10 in testicular germ cell tumours. J Pathol. 2002;197:89–97.
35. Palmer RD, Barbosa-Morais NL, Gooding EL, Muralidhar B, Thornton CM, Pett MR, et al. Children's cancer and Leukaemia group. Pediatric malignant germ cell tumors show characteristic transcriptome profiles. Cancer Res. 2008;68:4239–47.
36. Looijenga LH, Hersmus R, Gillis AJ, Pfundt R, Stoop HJ, van Gurp RJ, et al. Genomic and expression profiling of human spermatocytic seminomas: primary spermatocyte as tumorigenic precursor and *DMRT1* as candidate chromosome 9 gene. Cancer Res. 2006;66: 290–302.

37. Fustino N, Rakheja D, Ateek CS, Neumann JC, Amatruda JF. Bone morphogenetic protein signalling activity distinguishes histological subsets of paediatric germ cell tumours. Int J Androl. 2011;34:e218–33.
38. Neumann JC, Chandler GL, Damoulis VA, Fustino NJ, Lillard K, Looijenga L, et al. Mutation in the type IB bone morphogenetic protein receptor *alk6b* impairs germ-cell differentiation and causes germ-cell tumors in zebrafish. Proc Natl Acad Sci U S A. 2011;108:13153–8.
39. Gillis AJ, Stoop HJ, Hersmus R, Oosterhuis JW, Sun Y, Chen C. High-throughput microRNAome analysis in human germ cell tumours. J Pathol. 2007;213:319–28.
40. Murray M, Saini H, van Dongen S, Palmer RD, Muralidhar B, Pett MR, et al. The two most common histological subtypes of malignant germ cell tumour are distinguished by global microRNA profiles, associated with differential transcription factor expression. Mol Cancer. 2010;9:290.
41. Zhang X, Yan Z, Zhang J, Gong L, Li W, Cui J, et al. Combination of hsa-miR-375 and hsa-miR-142–5p as a predictor for recurrence risk in gastric cancer patients following surgical resection. Ann Oncol. 2011;22:2257–66.
42. Hoei-Hansen CE, Kraggerud SM, Abeler VM, Kaern J, Rajpert-De Meyts E, Lothe RA. Ovarian dysgerminomas are characterised by frequent KIT mutations and abundant expression of pluripotency markers. Mol Cancer. 2007;6:12.
43. Chang MC, Vargas SO, Hornick JL, Hirsch MS, Crum CP, Nucci MR. Embryonic stem cell transcription factors and D2–40 (podoplanin) as diagnostic immunohistochemical markers in ovarian germ cell tumors. Int J Gynecol Pathol. 2009;28:347–55.
44. Palmer PE, Wolfe HJ. Immunocytochemical localization of oncodevelopmental proteins in human germ cell and hepatic tumors. J Histochem Cytochem. 1978;26:523–31.
45. Esheba GE, Pate LL, Longacre TA. Oncofetal protein glypican-3 distinguishes yolk sac tumor from clear cell carcinoma of the ovary. Am J Surg Pathol. 2008;32:600–7.
46. Mannisto S, Butzow R, Salonen J, Leminen A, Heikinheimo O, Heikinheimo M. Transcription factors GATA-4 and GATA-6, and their potential downstream effectors in ovarian germ cell tumors. Tumor Biol. 2005;26:265–73.
47. NCI Ovarian Germ Cell Tumors treatment (PDQ) Health Professional Version.
48. Pectasides D, Pectasides E, Kassanos D. Germ cell tumors of the ovary. Cancer Treat Rev. 2008;34:427–41.
49. Williams SD, Blessing JA, DiSaia PJ, Major FJ, Ball HG 3rd, Liao SY. Second-look laparotomy in ovarian germ cell tumors: the gynecologic oncology group experience. Gynecol Oncol. 1994;52:287–91.
50. Gershenson DM. Management of early ovarian cancer: germ cell and sex cord-stromal tumors. Gynecol Oncol. 1994;55:S62–72.
51. Gershenson DM, Miller AM, Champion VL, Monahan PO, Zhao Q, Cella D, et al. Reproductive and sexual function after platinum-based chemotherapy in long-term ovarian germ cell tumor survivors: a gynecologic oncology group study. J Clin Oncol. 2007;25:2792–7.
52. Peccatori F, Bonazzi C, Chiari S, Landoni F, Colombo N, Mangioni C. Surgical management of malignant ovarian germ-cell tumors: 10 years' experience of 129 patients. Obstet Gynecol. 1995;86:367–72.
53. Mahdi H, Swensen RE, Hanna R, Kumar S, Ali-Fehmi R, Semaan A, et al. Prognostic impact of lymphadenectomy in clinically early stage malignant germ cell tumour of the ovary. Br J Cancer. 2011;105:493–7.
54. Beiner ME, Gotlieb WH, Korach Y, Shrim A, Stockheim D, Segal Y, et al. Cystectomy for immature teratoma of the ovary. Gynecol Oncol. 2004;93:381–4.
55. Ovarian Cancer Guideline (Version 1. 2014). NCCM Clinical Practice Guidelines in Oncoloft.
56. Mangili G, Sigismondi C, Lorusso D, Cormio G, Scollo P, Viganò R, et al. Is surgical restaging indicated in apparent stage IA pure ovarian dysgerminoma? The MITO group retrospective experience. Gynecol Oncol. 2011;121:280–4.
57. Williams S, Blessing JA, Liao SY, Ball H, Hanjani P. Adjuvant therapy of ovarian germ cell tumors with cisplatin, etoposide, and bleomycin: a trial of the gynecologic oncology group. J Clin Oncol. 1994;12:701–6.

58. Nichols CR, Catalano PJ, Crawford ED, Vogelzang NJ, Einhorn LH, Loehrer PJ. Randomized comparison of cisplatin and etoposide and either bleomycin or ifosfamide in treatment of advanced disseminated germ cell tumors: an eastern cooperative oncology group, southwest oncology group, and cancer and leukemia group B study. J Clin Oncol. 1998;16:1287–93.
59. Loehrer PJ Sr, Johnson D, Elson P, Einhorn LH, Trump D. Importance of bleomycin in favorable-prognosis disseminated germ cell tumors: an eastern cooperative oncology group trial. J Clin Oncol. 1995;13:470–6.
60. Bajorin DF, Sarosdy MF, Pfister DG, Mazumdar M, Motzer RJ, Scher HI, et al. Randomized trial of etoposide and cisplatin versus etoposide and carboplatin in patients with good-risk germ cell tumors: a multiinstitutional study. J Clin Oncol. 1993;11:598–606.
61. Einhorn LH, Williams SD, Loehrer PJ, Birch R, Drasga R, Omura G, et al. Evaluation of optimal duration of chemotherapy in favorable-prognosis disseminated germ cell tumors: a southeastern cancer study group protocol. J Clin Oncol. 1989;7:387–91.
62. Krege S, Beyer J, Souchon R, Albers P, Albrecht W, Algaba F, et al. European consensus conference on diagnosis and treatment of germ cell cancer: a report of the second meeting of the European germ cell cancer consensus group (EGCCCG): part II. Eur Urol. 2008;53:497–513.
63. Marina NM, Cushing B, Giller R, Cohen L, Lauer SJ, Ablin A, et al. Complete surgical excision is effective treatment for children with immature teratomas with or without malignant elements: a pediatric oncology group/children's cancer group intergroup study. J Clin Oncol. 1999;17:2137–43.
64. Cushing B, Giller R, Ablin A, Cohen L, Cullen J, Hawkins E, et al. Surgical resection alone is effective treatment for ovarian immature teratoma in children and adolescents: a report of the pediatric oncology group and the children's cancer group. Am J Obstet Gynecol. 1999;181:353–8.
65. McKeage MJ, Evans BD, Atkinson C, Perez D, Forgeson GV, Dady PJ. Carbon monoxide diffusing capacity is a poor predictor of clinically significant bleomycin lung. New Zealand clinical oncology group. J Clin Oncol. 1990;8:779–83.
66. Lewis BM, Izbicki R. Routine pulmonary function tests during bleomycin therapy. Tests may be ineffective and potentially misleading. JAMA. 1980;243:347–51.
67. Kollmannsberger C, Hartmann JT, Kanz L, Bokemeyer C. Therapy-related malignancies following treatment of germ cell cancer. Int J Cancer. 1999;83:860–3.
68. Pedersen-Bjergaard J, Daugaard G, Hansen SW, Philip P, Larsen SO, Rørth M. Increased risk of myelodysplasia and leukaemia after etoposide, cisplatin, and bleomycin for germ-cell tumours. Lancet. 1991;338:359–63.
69. Ezoe S. Secondary leukemia associated with the anti-cancer agent, etoposide, a topoisomerase II inhibitor. Int J Environ Res Public Health. 2012;9:2444–53.
70. Hinton S, Catalano PJ, Einhorn LH, Nichols CR, David Crawford E, Vogelzang N, et al. Cisplatin, etoposide and either bleomycin or ifosfamide in the treatment of disseminated germ cell tumors: final analysis of an intergroup trial. Cancer. 2003;97:1869–75.
71. Nicosia SV, Matus-Ridley M, Meadows AT. Gonadal effects of cancer therapy in girls. Cancer. 1985;55:2364–72.
72. Low JJ, Perrin LC, Crandon AJ, Hacker NF. Conservative surgery to preserve ovarian function in patients with malignant ovarian germ cell tumors. A review of 74 cases. J Gynecol Oncol. 2014;25:174–82.
73. Gershenson DM. Menstrual and reproductive function after treatment with combination chemotherapy for malignant ovarian germ cell tumors. J Clin Oncol. 1988;6:270–5.
74. Brewer M, Gershenson DM, Herzog CE, Mitchell MF, Silva EG, Wharton JT. Outcome and reproductive function after chemotherapy for ovarian dysgerminoma. J Clin Oncol. 1999;17:2670–5.
75. Segelov E, Campbell J, Ng M, Tattersall M, Rome R, Free K, et al. Cisplatin-based chemotherapy for ovarian germ cell malignancies: the Australian experience. J Clin Oncol. 1994;12:378–84.
76. Meistrich ML, Shetty G. Hormonal suppression for fertility preservation in males and females. Reproduction. 2008;136:691–701.

77. Blumenfeld Z. GnRH-agonists in fertility preservation. Curr Opin Endocrinol Diabetes Obes. 2008;15:523–8.
78. Weinberg LE, Lurain JR, Singh DK, Schink JC. Survival and reproductive outcomes in women treated for malignant ovarian germ cell tumors. Gynecol Oncol. 2011;121:285–9.
79. McLaren JF, Bates GW. Fertility preservation in women of reproductive age with cancer. Am J Obstet Gynecol. 2012;207:455–62.

Primary Surgical Treatment of Epithelial Ovarian Cancer

11

Mikio Mikami

Abstract

The main purpose of primary surgery for ovarian cancer is to eradicate the tumor completely because the postoperative residual tumor diameter is correlated with the prognosis. Surgery after neoadjuvant chemotherapy should be considered for patients with advanced cancer in whom complete tumor resection cannot be expected because of extensive peritoneal spread as well as patients whose general condition is poor. Recently it is also an acceptable alternative for women with potentially resectable disease who prefer the neoadjuvant approach because neoadjuvant chemotherapy plus subsequent surgery is not inferior to primary surgery in terms of progression-free survival or overall survival. Centralizing the primary care of advanced ovarian cancer to high-volume hospitals also increases the frequency of achieving complete cytoreduction with surgery and significantly improves survival. Although lymphadenectomy is essential for accurate staging of patients, there have been no reports showing therapeutic efficacy of lymphadenectomy. We are waiting for the results of Arbeitsgemeinschaft Gynäkologische Onkologie (AGO) clinical studies to decide the role of lymphadenectomy in advanced ovarian cancer.

Keywords

Primary debulking surgery (PDS) • Interval debulking surgery (IDS) • Neoadjuvant chemotherapy (NAC) • Centralized primary care • Lymphadenectomy • Fertility-preserving surgery

M. Mikami, M.D., Ph.D.
Department of Obstetrics and Gynecology, School of Medicine, Tokai University, Tokyo, Japan
e-mail: mmikami@is.icc.u-tokai.ac.jp

H. Katabuchi (ed.), *Frontiers in Ovarian Cancer Science*, Comprehensive Gynecology and Obstetrics, DOI 10.1007/978-981-10-4160-0_11

11.1 Introduction

The aims of primary surgery for ovarian cancer are (1) to determine the tumor histology and the International Federation of Gynecology and Obstetrics (FIGO) stage, (2) to completely eradicate the tumor, and (3) to obtain information on prognostic factors.

The following surgical methods are employed to achieve these objectives:

1. Standard surgery: bilateral salpingo-oophorectomy + hysterectomy + omentectomy
2. Staging laparotomy: includes sufficient surgical procedures to determine the FIGO stage
3. Exploratory laparotomy: minimal surgery to determine the FIGO stage when it is impossible to remove the tumor completely
4. Debulking surgery: involves removing the tumor as completely as possible
   (a) Primary debulking surgery (PDS) is performed to remove the tumor as completely as possible before other treatment.
   (b) Interval debulking surgery (IDS) is performed to remove the tumor as completely as possible as a secondary procedure after chemotherapy.
   (c) Secondary debulking surgery (SDS) is performed to remove recurrent tumors as completely as possible (including surgery for residual tumors after completion of primary chemotherapy).

The concept of cytoreduction involves removing a malignant tumor as completely as possible, while debulking involves performance of surgical cytoreduction to enhance the effect of chemotherapy by making the tumor volume as small as possible. Thus, "debulking" surgery is similar to "cytoreductive" surgery and is classified into the following three types:

1. Complete surgery: no residual tumor detectable by macroscopic examination
2. Optimal surgery: maximum residual tumor diameter <1 cm
3. Suboptimal surgery: maximum residual tumor diameter ≥1 cm

The completeness of surgery is the most important prognostic factor for patients with ovarian cancer, and the postoperative residual tumor diameter is correlated with the prognosis, especially in patients with advanced cancer [1–4]. Therefore, surgical treatment of this disease should generally involve PDS aimed at complete removal of all lesions. However, performing IDS after several cycles of NAC should be considered for patients with advanced cancer in whom complete tumor resection cannot be expected because of extensive peritoneal dissemination and metastasis, as well as patients with massive ascites, patients whose general condition is poor, and patients with serious complications such as thrombosis. Several randomized trials have recently compared NAC + IDS with PDS to assess the usefulness of NAC for advanced cancer. It is also an acceptable alternative for women with potentially resectable disease who prefer the neoadjuvant approach, as new guidelines indicate that NAC + subsequent surgery is not inferior to surgery in terms of progression-free survival or overall survival [5].

Along with achieving complete tumor resection at primary surgery, it is well known that treatment at a high-volume hospital has a survival benefit for patients with advanced ovarian cancer [6, 7]. Centralizing the primary care of advanced ovarian cancer to high-volume hospitals increases the frequency of achieving complete cytoreduction with PDS, shortens the interval between PDS and initiation of chemotherapy, and significantly improves survival.

The Japan Society of Gynecologic Oncology (JSGO) recently revised its Ovarian Cancer Treatment Guidelines and released the 4th version in 2015 [8]. While the Guidelines state that lymphadenectomy is essential for accurate staging of patients with early ovarian cancer, there have been no reports of randomized controlled trials showing therapeutic efficacy of lymphadenectomy. In patients with advanced disease, lymphadenectomy should also be considered if optimal debulking has been performed, but there is again no evidence of its therapeutic efficacy. We are waiting for the results of AGO (Arbeitsgemeinschaft Gynäkologische Onkologie) clinical studies to decide the role of lymphadenectomy.

Whenever possible, fertility-preserving surgery must be performed without compromising complete tumor removal and staging, taking into consideration the patient's histopathological/clinical status. However, it is difficult to conduct clinical studies on this type of surgery, as we discuss later in this article.

11.2 Centralized Primary Care for Advanced Ovarian Cancer

Ovarian cancer is a complex and often advanced disease that requires multidisciplinary expert surgical and medical management to provide state-of-the-art care, along with counseling, access to clinical trials, and a wealth of experience. Optimum management requires "the skillful and appropriate integration of cancer surgery and chemotherapy and is best carried out in centers in which an experienced and coordinated multidisciplinary team is available". Many studies have shown that outcomes are improved when ovarian cancer is treated in high-volume and/or specialist centers [9–12]. The Swedish study [6] assessed the effects of sweeping, regional, population-based changes to ovarian cancer management in western Sweden by comparison of outcomes between two different periods, which were 2008–2010 (prior to centralization of care for ovarian cancer) versus 2011–2013 (after centralization). This study revealed several important improvements of outcomes, e.g., there was a higher complete cytoreduction rate at primary surgery (37% versus 49%; $p = 0.03$) and a decrease of the interval from surgery to chemotherapy (36 versus 24 days; $p = 0.01$). Despite the two cohorts receiving similar chemotherapy regimens, there was also a slightly higher completion rate of planned chemotherapy with centralized care (88% versus 92%; p: 0.18). The most impressive finding was the increase of the 3-year survival rate in patients with advanced disease undergoing PDS, which rose from 44% to 65% after centralization, along with an estimated 42% decrease of the excess mortality rate ratio (EMRR) (RR: 0.58; 95% CI: 0.42–0.79). Even though use of NAC increased in the second period, when the entire cohort was compared irrespective of primary treatment, the 3-year survival rate still increased from 40% to 61% and EMRR declined (RR: 0.59; 95% CI: 0.45–0.76).

These improvements are consistent with the findings obtained by retrospective studies on the quality of care and outcomes using public databases [9–12]. Thus, management at expert centers improves outcomes, but centralization of care is a long and difficult process which must include professional societies, politicians, clinicians, epidemiologists, payers, and advocates.

11.3 Optimal Surgical Management of Ovarian Cancer Clinically Confined to the Ovary

Even when a lesion is expected to be confined to the ovary, peritoneal dissemination and retroperitoneal lymph node metastasis may be detected by staging laparotomy, resulting in a diagnosis of Stage II-III cancer. Accordingly, even in patients with early ovarian cancer whose disease is expected to be confined to the ovary, it is recommended that not only ipsilateral salpingo-oophorectomy but also contralateral salpingo-oophorectomy and total hysterectomy be performed to confirm the presence or absence of tumor metastasis and infiltration. In addition, intraperitoneal cytologic examination (sampling of ascites or lavage ascites) should also be performed together with omentectomy and peritoneal biopsy at various sites to confirm the presence or absence of intraperitoneal dissemination. Furthermore, taking the possibility of retroperitoneal lymph node metastasis into consideration, dissection or biopsy of the pelvic to para-aortic lymph nodes should be carried out. While this type of staging laparotomy is recommended for histopathological staging and identification of patients who do not require postoperative treatment, there is currently no evidence to indicate whether staging laparotomy itself directly improves the prognosis or not.

Because omental metastases are noted during surgery in 2–7% of patients with a clinical diagnosis of early ovarian cancer, partial omentectomy is also an essential part of management, even in patients with early disease [13].

For accurate staging, it is important to examine various intraperitoneal sites by biopsy. If tumor dissemination is suspected from the results of careful observation during laparotomy, it is recommended that peritoneal biopsy be performed at the pouch of Douglas, vesical peritoneum, right and left lateral pelvic walls, right and left paracolic sulci, and right diaphragm (although biopsy of the diaphragm may be replaced by scraping cytology). If mucinous carcinoma is suspected, appendectomy should be considered for differentiation from primary cancer of the appendix. While the significance of performing appendectomy in ovarian cancer patients has not been established, it has been reported that the incidence of metastasis to a macroscopically normal appendix is 2.8% [14].

11.4 Optimal Surgical Management of Clinical Stage II or More Advanced Ovarian Cancer

The fundamental surgical technique for advanced cancer is primary debulking surgery (PDS), which involves removal of intraperitoneal dissemination and metastases as completely as possible. It has been reported that the diameter of the residual tumor is correlated with the prognosis, and it was recently shown that the prognosis is significantly better after complete surgery than optimal surgery [1–4]. However, it is rare for advanced cancer to be controlled by standard surgical management (bilateral salpingo-oophorectomy + total hysterectomy + omentectomy) alone. There is no standard PDS method for advanced cancer. Tumors are resected as completely as possible for debulking irrespective of the organ affected by dissemination/metastasis. Resection of peritoneal lesions at various sites (including the vesicouterine pouch, the pouch of Douglas, and the paracolic sulci) together with the surrounding peritoneum should be considered for control of dissemination and metastasis. If there is infiltration into the rectum at the pouch of Douglas, infiltration into the sigmoid colon, infiltration/extension of omental lesions into the transverse colon, or infiltration/metastasis affecting the small intestine, partial intestinal resection/reconstruction should be actively considered. If this is done, construction of colostomy may be required, depending on the site of bowel resection. In patients with mucinous carcinoma, appendectomy should be considered in order to detect primary cancer of the appendix [14]. If involvement of the diaphragm is noted, stripping or full-thickness resection should be considered, since the frequency of achieving complete surgery can be increased by resecting diaphragmatic lesions. If infiltration into the spleen is noted, splenectomy should also be considered .The diagnostic significance of retroperitoneal lymph node dissection and biopsy for accurate staging has been established, but the therapeutic significance is not necessarily clear.

Of course, the ability to remove tumors in patients with advanced ovarian cancer irrespective of the organs affected will depend on the skill of the surgeons and the facilities of the treating hospital (Sect. 11.3).

11.5 Neoadjuvant Chemotherapy (NAC) and Interval Debulking Surgery (IDS)

The standard treatment of stage IIIC or IV invasive epithelial ovarian cancer has generally been primary debulking surgery (PDS), followed by chemotherapy, and PDS is still preferred over NAC if there is a high likelihood of achieving residual disease <1 cm in diameter (ideally, no macroscopic disease).

On the other hand, NAC is the preferred treatment option for women with advanced ovarian cancer or related cancers if it is unlikely that PDS can reduce the residual disease to <1 cm in diameter. It is also an alternative approach to the management of potentially resectable disease, since it has been reported that NAC + subsequent surgery is not inferior to surgery with regard to either progression-free survival or overall survival [5]. Thus, women with potentially resectable disease may be offered either NAC or PDS, even if they are fit enough to undergo surgery, as their survival outcomes will be comparable. However, NAC should be the preferred option for women with high surgical risk or those in whom there is little likelihood of achieving residual disease <1 cm in diameter (or no macroscopic disease). The main advantage of NAC + IDS is less perioperative/postoperative morbidity or mortality than PDS, although PDS may achieve superior overall survival in selected patients. Before NAC is commenced, all patients should have histologic confirmation (core biopsy is preferred) of the diagnosis of invasive ovarian cancer. If biopsy cannot be performed, the oncologist should carry out cytologic evaluation. Together with a serum CA-125/carcinoembryonic antigen ratio >25 [5], cytologic evaluation should confirm the primary diagnosis and exclude non-gynecologic cancer. IDS should be performed after a maximum of four NAC cycles in women who respond to treatment or achieve stable disease. In contrast, "patients with progressive disease on NAC have a poor prognosis". For these women, options include switching to an alternative chemotherapy regimen, referral to an appropriate clinical trial, or initiation of best supportive care. Surgery is not advised for these women unless it is required for palliative purposes. Laparoscopy or imaging studies may be performed for more detailed assessment, and whether a patient is eligible for medical or surgical treatment should only be decided in consultation with a gynecologic oncologist.

11.6 Lymph Node Metastasis in the New FIGO Ovarian Cancer Staging System (2014) [15]

Lymph node metastases are found in the majority of patients who undergo lymph node sampling or dissection and in up to 78% of patients with advanced disease. Approximately 9% of patients with tumors that appear to be stage I actually have lymph node metastases, while the corresponding figures for stages II, III, and IV are 36%, 55%, and 88%, respectively. Occasionally, inguinal or supraclavicular (stage IV) lymph node metastasis is the presenting manifestation of ovarian carcinoma. However, less than 10% of ovarian cancers extend beyond the pelvis with exclusively retroperitoneal lymph node involvement. Published evidence indicates that these patients just with lymph node metastasis have a better prognosis than that of patients with involvement of the abdominal peritoneum. The new staging system includes a revision of stage III and assigns patients to stage IIIA1 based on involvement of the retroperitoneal lymph nodes without intraperitoneal dissemination. Stage IIIA1 is further divided into IIIA1 (1) (metastasis ≤10 mm in greatest dimension) and IIIA1 (2) (metastasis >10 mm in greatest dimension), although there are no retrospective data supporting quantification of the size of metastasis. Involvement of retroperitoneal lymph nodes must be proven cytologically or histologically. In the future, we will need to compare outcomes between stage IIIA1 (1) and IIIA1 (2) patients as well as between stage IIIA1 and IIIA2 patients.

11.7 Lymphadenectomy for Early Ovarian Cancer

In 1988, the International Federation of Gynecology and Obstetrics published a surgical staging scheme for ovarian cancer that included pelvic and para-aortic lymph node sampling or lymphadenectomy. However, few studies have shown any benefit of lymphadenectomy in patients with early disease. Although systematic

Table 11.1 Frequency of lymph node metastasis in pT1 disease

Author	Year	Number of patients	Positive rate(%)	Stage (%)			Positive rate(%)	
				Ia	Ib	Ic	PEN	PAN
Sakuragi, et al	2000	78	5.1	3.2	–	6.4	0	5.1
Suzuki, et al	2000	47	10.6	5.6	–	13.8	8.5	4.3
Cass, et al	2001	96	14.5	–	–	–	9.4	7.3
Takeshima, et al	2001	156	12.8	9.3	33.3	15.4	7.1	9.6
Harter, et al	2007	48	6.2	0	25.0	8.0	–	–
Fournier, et al	2009	54	9.3	3.8	0	17.4	–	–
Nomura, et al	2010	60	13.3	28.6	0	9.1	8.3	11.7
Mikami, et al	2014	89	12.3	4	50	17.6	10.1	6.7

PEN pelvic lymphnode, *PAN* paraaortic lymphnodes

lymphadenectomy is necessary for accurate staging and has diagnostic value, it may increase surgical morbidity. Recently, Chan et al. [16] conducted a large-scale, retrospective study that assessed the impact of lymphadenectomy on survival in patients with clinical stage I ovarian cancer, and their findings suggested that lymphadenectomy significantly improved survival. In contrast, a randomized study of systematic lymphadenectomy in patients with pT1 and pT2 ovarian cancer [17] showed that lymphadenectomy had no influence on either progression-free survival or overall survival. Involvement of pelvic nodes has been reported in 5–14% of patients with pT1 disease, and the para-aortic nodes are involved in 4–12% of these patients (Table 11.1.). The chief value of systematic retroperitoneal node dissection may be the upstaging of some patients with clinical stage I cancer, which leads them to receive postoperative chemotherapy. Also, when the initial staging is confirmed to be correct, patients with low-risk disease can avoid undergoing cytotoxic chemotherapy. Therefore, it can be argued that lymphadenectomy is essential to allow accurate staging of the tumor in patients with early ovarian cancer, although there is no supporting evidence from randomized trials.

Accordingly, surgical treatment of ovarian cancer, including systematic lymphadenectomy, should only be performed at institutions that specialize in gynecologic oncology, in order to ensure accurate staging of the tumor.

11.8 Lymphadenectomy for Advanced Ovarian Cancer: Complete Dissection Versus Resection of Bulky Nodes

Primary debulking surgery has been an integral part of treating advanced ovarian cancer. However, it is still unclear whether systematic resection of the retroperitoneal lymph nodes should be part of maximal debulking surgery, and the therapeutic value of systematic lymphadenectomy for women with advanced ovarian cancer remains controversial. Retrospective studies [18] have suggested that systematic lymphadenectomy significantly improves survival in patients undergoing debulking surgery for advanced disease, but no prospective studies have been reported. Panici et al. [19] performed a multicenter randomized clinical trial that revealed significant improvement of progression-free survival by systematic lymphadenectomy, although overall survival was similar between patients receiving systematic lymphadenectomy and those undergoing resection of bulky nodes. They also reported a higher rate of lymph node metastasis in the patients receiving systematic lymphadenectomy than in those having resection of bulky nodes and confirmed that lymph node metastasis is a significant prognostic factor for survival. Furthermore, du Bois [20] reviewed three prospective randomized trials of platinum/taxane-based chemotherapy for advanced ovarian cancer and concluded that lymphadenectomy might mainly benefit patients with advanced disease who underwent complete intraperitoneal debulking. However, this conclusion needs to be confirmed by performing a further prospective randomized trial. In these three trials, 24.8% of patients who underwent pelvic and para-aortic lymphadenectomy without suspected intraoperative lymph node involvement had histologically positive nodes, whereas the rate was 17.1% in patients who underwent partial retroperitoneal lymphadenectomy. This suggests that almost one third of positive nodes are not detectable clinically and may also be missed by partial lymphadenectomy. A prospective randomized trial comparing complete intraperitoneal tumor resection with or without sampling of suspicious lymph nodes in patients with advanced ovarian cancer (Lymphadenectomy In Ovarian Neoplasms [Lion] trial) is underway, and the results will hopefully shed new light on this important issue. Accordingly, systemic pelvic and para-aortic lymphadenectomy should be considered in patients who are fit to receive optimal debulking surgery.

11.9 Can Interval Debulking Surgery (IDS) Be Recommended After Primary Debulking Surgery (PDS) with a Suboptimal Outcome?

The usefulness of interval debulking surgery (IDS) during chemotherapy has been investigated for patients in whom the maximum residual tumor diameter could not be decreased to ≤1 cm by suboptimal primary surgery. Conflicting results have been obtained, with improvement of the prognosis in one study [21] and no benefit in another study [22], so there is no consensus as to whether IDS is useful for improving the prognosis of these patients. Study European Organization for Research and Treatment of Cancer-Gyne Cancer Group (EORTC-GCG) [21] enrolled 425 patients with Stage IIb-IV advanced ovarian cancer in whom the maximum tumor diameter was ≥1 cm at primary surgery, and tumor reduction (complete or partial response) was achieved in 319 patients by 3 cycles of combination chemotherapy with cyclophosphamide + cisplatin. These 319 patients were subjected to randomized comparison of the influence of IDS on the prognosis, revealing that overall survival was 33% higher in the IDS group compared with the non-IDS group. In Study GOG152 [22], the usefulness of IDS was assessed in 550 Stage III-IV ovarian cancer patients with suboptimal primary debulking surgery. A total of 448 patients received 3 cycles of post-PDS chemotherapy with paclitaxel + cisplatin and were randomized to two groups that were treated by chemotherapy alone or IDS followed by chemotherapy. As a result, both progression-free survival and overall survival showed no significant difference between the two groups. These two randomized comparative trials yielded different results, presumably because there was a higher percentage of Stage IV patients and the residual tumor diameter was larger after primary surgery in Study EORTC-GCG, while a higher percentage of patients received PDS from gynecologic oncologists, and the residual tumor diameter was smaller in the Gynecologic Oncology Group (GOG) study. In other words, it seems likely that IDS is more closely related to improvement of the prognosis in patients with a larger residual tumor diameter after primary surgery.

11.10 Optimal Management for Preservation of Fertility

There are histopathological and clinical requirements to consider with regard to preserving fertility in patients with ovarian cancer. Histopathologically, preserving fertility is indicated for patients with Stage Ia Grade 1 or 2 serous carcinoma, mucinous carcinoma, or endometrioid carcinoma (non-clear), while it can be considered for non-clear Stage Ic (localized to one ovary with negative in ascites cytology) Grade 1 or 2 or Stage Ia clear cell carcinoma.

After fertility-preserving surgery, the recurrence rate of ovarian cancer was 5.2%, 20%, and ≥50% for Stage Ia patients with Grade 1, 2, and 3 disease, respectively, while it was 8%, 21%, and 33% for Stage Ic patients with the respective grades. These results are considered to confirm the above histopathological conditions for preserving fertility [23, 24]. However, fertility preservation should be selected with great care, because investigation of 29 Stage Ic patients revealed that the recurrence rate was higher in patients with positive ascites cytology or patients with infiltration into the capsule [25]. Because it is impossible for rapid intraoperative histopathological examination to evaluate all of the necessary factors, including the histologic type and differentiation, it is necessary to await the results of accurate postoperative histopathological diagnosis.

Importance must also be attached to the following clinical factors. (1) The patient has a strong desire for pregnancy and is of childbearing age. (2) The patient and her family fully understand the nature of ovarian cancer and fertility-preserving surgery, as well as the risk of recurrence. (3) The patient agrees to receive strict long-term follow-up after surgery. (4) The patient can undergo careful intraperitoneal exploration by a skillful gynecologic oncologist. Prior to surgery, it must also be explained fully that preservation of fertility might be impossible and reoperation (2-stage surgery) might be needed, depending on the results of postoperative histopathological examination. Because recurrence even 10 years postoperatively has been reported, it is also necessary to discuss possible completion of surgery after delivery [26].

For fertility-preserving surgery, the basic procedure includes ipsilateral salpingo-oophorectomy and omentectomy. Endometrial curettage must also be considered to exclude concurrent endometrial cancer [27, 28]. Accurate staging is required when selecting patients who can be considered for fertility-preserving surgery. Omission of any of the procedures in staging laparotomy can only be considered when very careful macroscopic observation and palpation reveal nothing abnormal. Microscopic metastasis to the contralateral ovary has been reported to be rare in patients with Grade 1 ovarian cancer in whom macroscopic observation reveals no infiltration of the capsule surface, capsule disruption, or peritoneal dissemination. To avoid infertility due to decreased ovarian reserve and postoperative adhesions, it is permissible to omit biopsy of a macroscopically normal contralateral ovary. Concerning retroperitoneal lymph node dissection, it has been reported that the frequency of metastasis is low if the patient has mucinous carcinoma or endometrioid carcinoma and if there is no intrapelvic invasion or peritoneal dissemination [27]. Because fertility may be disturbed by postoperative adhesions due to lymph node dissection, it is permissible to limit examination to biopsy or lower levels if the clinical probability of metastasis is low.

Since the prognosis of the disease after recurrence is generally poor [29], very careful attention to management and providing adequate information for patients are essential.

11.11 Surgery for Elderly Patients

It is thought that maximal debulking surgery should also be performed in elderly patients with the aim of achieving complete resection, although the age range corresponding to "elderly" is not well defined. It is important to plan surgery by taking the patient's general condition, nutritional status, and complications into consideration. Caution must be exercised when performing surgical treatment on elderly patients because the incidence of intraoperative complications is higher and perioperative complications are also more frequent due to cardiac dysfunction [30]. The 30-day mortality rate after ovarian cancer surgery gradually increases with age from <70 years old to 70–79 years and then >80 years, with the causes of death including postoperative infection, hemorrhage, respiratory failure, heart failure, and thromboembolism. The incidence of perioperative complications increases as surgery becomes more complex due to addition of partial bowel resection, diaphragmatic resection, and/or splenectomy to the standard procedure of bilateral salpingo-oophorectomy + total hysterectomy + omentectomy. The best surgical procedure should be selected by considering the patient's age, general condition, nutritional status, and tumor stage at the time of diagnosis. The general condition is evaluated by determining the performance status (PS) (Table 11.2) and by using the American Society of Anesthesiologists (ASA) physical status classification (Table 11.3). Special care must be taken when the general condition corresponds to ASA Class 3 or higher (equivalent to a PS of 3 or higher) and the nutritional status is poor (serum albumin <3.0 g/dL), as well as when surgery is performed for Stage III or IV cancer [30]. In these patients, NAC should be performed before surgery is considered. After improvement of the general condition and the nutritional status, complete surgery can be performed as IDS [31]. However, performing NAC also requires care in the elderly because of the risk of complications such as thrombosis.

Table 11.2 ECOG performance status. Reuse from http://ecog-acrin.org/resources/ecog-performance-status, with permission

Developed by the Eastern Cooperative Oncology Group, Robert L. Comis, MD, Group Chair.[a]	
Grade	ECOG performance status
0	Fully active, able to carry on all pre-disease performance without restriction
1	Restricted in physically strenuous activity but ambulatory and able to carry out work of a light or sedentary nature, e.g., light house work, office work
2	Ambulatory and capable of all selfcare but unable to carry out any work activities, up and about more than 50% of waking hours
3	Capable of only limited selfcare, confined to bed or chair more than 50% of waking hours
4	Completely disabled, cannot carry on any selfcare; totally confined to bed or chair
5	Dead

[a]Oken M, Creech R, Tormey D, et al. Toxicity and response criteria of the Eastern Cooperative Oncology Group. *Am J Clin Oncol*. 1982;5:649–655

Table 11.3 ASA physical status classification system. Reuse from https://www.asahq.org/resources/clinical-information/asa-physical-status-classification-system with permission

Last approved by the ASA House of Delegates on October 15, 2014		
Current definitions (NO CHANGE) and Examples (NEW)		
ASA PS Classification	Definition	Examples, including, but not limited to:
ASA I	A normal healthy patient	Healthy, non-smoking, no or minimal alcohol use
ASA II	A patient with mild systemic disease	Mild diseases only without substantive functional limitations. Examples include (but not limited to): current smoker, social alcohol drinker, pregnancy, obesity (30 < BMI < 40), well-controlled DM/HTN, mild lung disease
ASA III	A patient with severe systemic disease	Substantive functional limitations; One or more moderate to severe diseases. Examples include (but not limited to): poorly controlled DM or HTN, COPD, morbid obesity (BMI ≥40), active hepatitis, alcohol dependence or abuse, implanted pacemaker, moderate reduction of ejection fraction, ESRD undergoing regularly scheduled dialysis, premature infant PCA < 60 weeks, history (>3 months) of MI, CVA, TIA, or CAD/stents.
ASA IV	A patient with severe systemic disease that is a constant threat to life	Examples include (but not limited to): recent (<3 months) MI, CVA, TIA, or CAD/stents, ongoing cardiac ischemia or severe valve dysfunction, severe reduction of ejection fraction, sepsis, DIC, ARD or ESRD not undergoing regularly scheduled dialysis
ASA V	A moribund patient who is not expected to survive without the operation	Examples include (but not limited to): ruptured abdominal/thoracic aneurysm, massive trauma, intracranial bleed with mass effect, ischemic bowel in the face of significant cardiac pathology or multiple organ/system dysfunction
ASA VI	A declared brain-dead patient ASA VI whose organs are being removed for donor purposes	

11.12 Is Laparoscope-Assisted Surgery Possible?

The survival rate of patients with early ovarian cancer may be similar between after laparoscope-assisted staging surgery and laparotomy if these procedures are performed by skillful gynecologic oncologists [32, 33]. Laparoscopy is useful for observing intraperitoneal lesions and for staging in patients with advanced ovarian cancer or patients with incomplete primary surgery [33, 34]. Many studies have demonstrated that the upstaging rate is similar with these two procedures, and carbon dioxide pneumoperitoneum is considered to have no adverse influence on the survival of patients with advanced ovarian cancer and intraperitoneal metastases. However, it was reported that the incidence of tumor capsule rupture is higher with laparoscopy than laparotomy [35] and metastasis has occurred at the site of trocar insertion, so it cannot be concluded that laparoscope-assisted surgery is superior to laparotomy. Furthermore, although laparoscope-assisted surgery is considered to be a useful alternative to laparotomy for performing intraperitoneal observation/tissue sampling in patients with advanced ovarian cancer, it is not currently recommended for tumor debulking surgery. Only a few randomized trials of laparoscope-assisted surgery for ovarian cancer have been conducted, so there is little scientific evidence regarding its usefulness, and the indications for this technique are very limited.

Characteristically, rapid histopathological diagnosis is required during ovarian cancer surgery to determine whether the operative field should be extended or not. Because tumor capsule disruption may occur (possible iatrogenic upstaging) during surgery and because exploratory laparotomy with or without combined resection may be required for advanced cancer patients, it is relatively difficult to employ laparoscope-assisted surgery as an alternative to standard laparotomy. These factors also make it difficult to perform large-scale clinical studies for comparison of laparoscopy with laparotomy, and there have been no randomized comparison trials evaluating laparoscopic surgery for ovarian cancer. While the safety and efficacy of laparoscopic procedures have been reported in selected patients, there are still many problems to be solved such as lack of sufficient data to demonstrate a comparable survival rate. Therefore, it is still unclear whether laparoscope-assisted procedures can be introduced as primary standard surgery for ovarian cancer.

Conclusion

The completeness of surgery is the most important prognostic factor for patients with ovarian cancer, and the postoperative residual tumor diameter is correlated with the prognosis, especially in patients with advanced cancer. Increased use of NAC in women with advanced stage ovarian cancer has contributed to improved quality of life and reduced perioperative morbidity. However, questions remain about how to identify which patients are most likely to benefit from NAC. The creative strategies should be needed to triage patients between PDS and NAC. To shed light on these points, researchers should be exploring tumor markers and molecular pathways associated with invasive metastatic behavior.

References

1. Winter WE 3rd, Maxwell GL, Tian C, Sundborg MJ, Rose GS, Rose PG, et al. Tumor residual after surgical cytoreduction in prediction of clinical outcome in stage IV epithelial ovarian cancer: a gynecologic oncology group study. J Clin Oncol. 2008;26:83–9.
2. Winter WE 3rd, Maxwell GL, Tian C, Carlson JW, Ozols RF, Rose PG, et al. Prognostic factors for stage III epithelial ovarian cancer: a gynecologic oncology group study. J Clin Oncol. 2007;25:3621–7.
3. Chi DS, Eisenhauser EL, Lang J, Huh J, Haddad L, Abu-Rustum NR, et al. What is the optimal goal of primary cytoreductive surgery for bulky stage IIIC epithelial ovarian carcinoma(EOC)? Gynecol Oncol. 2006;103:559–64.
4. Eisenhauer EL, Abu-Rustum NR, Sonoda Y, Aghajanian C, Barakat RR, Chi DS. The effect of maximal surgical cytoreduction on sensitivity to platinum-taxane chemotherapy and subsequent survival in patients with advanced ovarian cancer. Gynecol Oncol. 2008;108:276–81.
5. Wright AA, Bohlke K, Armstrong DK, Bookman MA, Cliby WA, Coleman RL, Dizon DS, Kash JJ, Meyer LA, Moore KN, Olawaiye AB, Oldham J, Salani R, Sparacio D, Tew WP, Vergote I, Edelson MI. Neoadjuvant chemotherapy for newly diagnosed, advanced ovarian cancer: society of gynecologic oncology and American society of clinical oncology clinical practice guideline. J Clin Oncol. 2016;34:3460–73.
6. Dahm-Kähler P, Palmqvist C, Staf C, Holmberg E, Johannesson L. Centralized primary care of advanced ovarian cancer improves complete cytoreduction and survival - a population-based cohort study. Gynecol Oncol. 2016;142:211–6.
7. Aletti GD, Cliby WA. Time for centralizing patients with ovarian cancer: what are we waiting for? Gynecol Oncol. 2016;142:209–10.
8. Komiyama S, Katabuchi H, Mikami M, Nagase S, Okamoto A, Ito K, Morishige K, Suzuki N, Kaneuchi M, Yaegashi N, Udagawa Y, Yoshikawa H. Japan society of gynecologic oncology guidelines 2015 for the treatment of ovarian cancer including primary peritoneal cancer and fallopian tube cancer. Int J Clin Oncol. 2016;21:435–46.
9. Kumpulainen S, Sankila R, Leminen A, Kuoppala T, Komulainen M, Puistola U, et al. The effect of hospital operative volume, residual tumor and first-line chemotherapy on survival of ovarian cancer — a prospective nation-wide study in Finland. Gynecol Oncol. 2009;115:199–203.
10. Tingulstad S, Skjeldestad FE, Hagen B. The effect of centralization of primary surgery on survival in ovarian cancer patients. Obstet Gynecol. 2003;102:499–505.
11. du Bois A, Rochon J, Pfisterer J, Hoskins WJ. Variations in institutional infrastructure, physician specialization and experience, and outcome in ovarian cancer: a systematic review. Gynecol Oncol. 2009;112:422–36.
12. Bristow RE, Palis BE, Chi DS, Cliby WA. The national cancer database report on advanced-stage epithelial ovarian cancer: impact of hospital surgical case volume on overall survival and surgical treatment paradigm. Gynecol Oncol. 2010;118:262–7.
13. Arie AB, McNally L, Kapp DS, Teng NN. The omentum and omentectomy in epithelial ovarian cancer: a reappraisal: part II--the role of omentectomy in the staging and treatment of apparent early stage epithelial ovarian cancer. Gynecol Oncol. 2013;131:784–90.
14. Ayhan A, Gultekin M, Taskiran C, Salman MC, Celik NY, Yuce K, Usubutun A, Kucukali T. Routine appendectomy in epithelial ovarian carcinoma: is it necessary? Obstet Gynecol. 2005;105:719–24.
15. Prat J. FIGO committee on gynecologic oncology. Staging classification for cancer of the ovary, fallopian tube, and peritoneum. Int J Gynaecol Obstet. 2014;124:1–5.
16. Chan JK, Munro EG, Cheung MK, Husain A, Teng NN, Berek JS, et al. Association of lymphadenectomy and survival in stage I ovarian cancer patients. Obstet Gynecol. 2007;109:12–9.
17. Maggioni A, Benedetti Panici P, Dell'Anna T, Landoni F, Lissoni A, Pellegrino A, et al. Randomised study of systematic lymphadenectomy in patients with epithelial ovarian cancer macroscopically confined to the pelvis. Br J Cancer. 2006;95:699–704.

18. Chan JK, Urban R, Hu JM, Shin JY, Husain A, Teng NN, et al. The potential therapeutic role of lymph node resection in epithelial ovarian cancer: a study of 13918 patients. Br J Cancer. 2007;96:1817–22.
19. Panici PB, Maggioni A, Hacker N, Landoni F, Ackermann S, Campagnutta E, et al. Systematic aortic and pelvic lymphadenectomy versus resection of bulky nodes only in optimally debulked advanced ovarian cancer: a randomized clinical trial. J Natl Cancer Inst. 2005;97:560–6.
20. du Bois A, Reuss A, Harter P, Pujade-Lauraine E, Ray-Coquard I, Pfisterer J, et al. Potential role of lymphadenectomy in advanced ovarian cancer: a combined exploratory analysis of three prospectively randomized phase III multicenter trials. J Clin Oncol. 2010;28:1733–9.
21. van der Burg ME, van Lent M, Buyse M, Kobierska A, Colombo N, Favalli G, Lacave AJ, Nardi M, Renard J, Pecorelli S. The effect of debulking surgery after induction chemotherapy on the prognosis in advanced epithelial ovarian cancer. Gynecological cancer cooperative group of the European organization for research and treatment of cancer. N Engl J Med. 1995;332:629–34.
22. Rose PG, Nerenstone S, Brady MF, Clarke-Pearson D, Olt G, Rubin SC, Moore DH, Small JM. Gynecologic oncology group. Secondary surgical cytoreduction for advanced ovarian carcinoma. N Engl J Med. 2004;351:2489–97.
23. Satoh T, Hatae M, Watanabe Y, Yaegashi N, Ishiko O, Kodama S, Yamaguchi S, Ochiai K, Takano M, Yokota H, Kawakami Y, Nishimura S, Ogishima D, Nakagawa S, Kobayashi H, Shiozawa T, Nakanishi T, Kamura T, Konishi I, Yoshikawa H. Outcomes of fertility-sparing surgery for stage I epithelial ovarian cancer: a proposal for patient selection. J Clin Oncol. 2010;28:1727–32.
24. Anchezar JP, Sardi J, Soderini A. Long-term follow-up results of fertility sparing surgery in patients with epithelial ovarian cancer. J Surg Oncol. 2009;100:55–8.
25. Kajiyama H, Shibata K, Suzuki S, Ino K, Nawa A, Kawai M, Nagasaka T, Kikkawa F. Fertility-sparing surgery in young women with invasive epithelial ovarian cancer. Eur J Surg Oncol. 2010;36:404–8.
26. Moore MM, Tewari K, Rose GS, Fruehauf JP, DiSaia PJ. Long-term consequences following conservative management of epithelial ovarian cancer in an infertile patient. Gynecol Oncol. 1999;73:452–4.
27. Morice P, Joulie F, Camatte S, Atallah D, Rouzier R, Pautier P, Pomel C, Lhommé C, Duvillard P, Castaigne D. Lymph node involvement in epithelial ovarian cancer: analysis of 276 pelvic and paraaortic lymphadenectomies and surgical implications. J Am Coll Surg. 2003;197:198–205.
28. Morice P, Denschlag D, Rodolakis A, Reed N, Schneider A, Kesic V, Colombo N. Fertility task force of the European society of gynecologic oncology. Recommendations of the fertility task force of the European society of gynecologic oncology about the conservative management of ovarian malignant tumors. Int J Gynecol Cancer. 2011;21:951–63.
29. Marpeau O, Schilder J, Zafrani Y, Uzan C, Gouy S, Lhommé C, Morice P. Prognosis of patients who relapse after fertility-sparing surgery in epithelial ovarian cancer. Ann Surg Oncol. 2008;15:478–783.
30. Langstraat C, Aletti GD, Cliby WA. Morbidity, mortality and overall survival in elderly women undergoing primary surgical debulking for ovarian cancer: a delicate balance requiring individualization. Gynecol Oncol. 2011;123:187–91.
31. Glasgow MA, Yu H, Rutherford TJ, Azodi M, Silasi DA, Santin AD, Schwartz PE. Neoadjuvant chemotherapy (NACT) is an effective way of managing elderly women with advanced stage ovarian cancer (FIGO stage IIIC and IV). J Surg Oncol. 2013;107:195–200.
32. Ghezzi F, Malzoni M, Vizza E, Cromi A, Perone C, Corrado G, Uccella S, Cosentino F, Mancini E, Franchi M. Laparoscopic staging of early ovarian cancer: results of a multi-institutional cohort study. Ann Surg Oncol. 2012;19:1589–94.

33. Nezhat FR, Ezzati M, Chuang L, Shamshirsaz AA, Rahaman J, Gretz H. Laparoscopic management of early ovarian and fallopian tube cancers: surgical and survival outcome. Am J Obstet Gynecol. 2009;200:83.e1–6.
34. Chereau E, Lavoue V, Ballester M, Coutant C, Selle F, Cortez A, Daraï E, Leveque J, Rouzier R. External validation of a laparoscopic-based score to evaluate resectability for patients with advanced ovarian cancer undergoing interval debulking surgery. Anticancer Res. 2011;31:4469–74.
35. Smorgick N, Barel O, Halperin R, Schneider D, Pansky M. Laparoscopic removal of adnexal cysts: is it possible to decrease inadvertent intraoperative rupture rate? Am J Obstet Gynecol. 2009;200:237.e1–3.

Primary Chemotherapy and Targeted Molecular Therapy of Epithelial Ovarian Cancer

12

Satoru Nagase, Tsuyoshi Ohta, and Manabu Seino

Abstract

The use of paclitaxel in addition to cisplatin resulted in the improvement of ovarian cancer treatment. Based on the results of several randomized clinical trials (RCTs), the combination of paclitaxel and carboplatin administered every 3 weeks intravenously (IV) or a dose-dense regimen of weekly paclitaxel plus carboplatin demonstrates high clinical benefit and has become the standard primary chemotherapy. However, ovarian cancer remains the gynecological cancer with the highest mortality rate despite the establishment of highly effective chemotherapeutic regimens. One strategy to obtain further chemotherapeutic efficacy in the primary treatment of advanced ovarian cancer is neoadjuvant chemotherapy (NAC), and another is intraperitoneal (IP) chemotherapy. NAC is gaining acceptance in cases in which complete resection is not possible with only primary debulking surgery. IP therapy has been reported to be superior to conventional IV chemotherapy; on the other hand, there are complications specific to IP therapy. Several RCTs are currently underway to address these issues. In recent years, molecularly targeted drugs have been widely used in cancer treatment, and they currently play major roles in the treatment of ovarian cancer. In this article, the molecularly targeted therapy used in initial chemotherapy and subsequent maintenance therapy for ovarian cancer will be discussed.

Keywords

Dose-dense TC • Neoadjuvant chemotherapy • Intraperitoneal chemotherapy • Bevacizumab • Olaparib

S. Nagase, M.D., Ph.D. (✉) • T. Ohta, M.D., Ph.D. • M. Seino, M.D., Ph.D.
Department of Obstetrics & Gynecology, Faculty of Medicine, Yamagata University, 2-2-2 Iida-nishi, Yamagata 990-9585, Japan
e-mail: nagases@med.id.yamagata-u.ac.jp

H. Katabuchi (ed.), *Frontiers in Ovarian Cancer Science*, Comprehensive Gynecology and Obstetrics, DOI 10.1007/978-981-10-4160-0_12

12.1 Introduction

Ovarian cancer is recognized as one of the first solid malignant tumors that is highly sensitive to chemotherapy. After initial surgery with an attempt at maximal debulking, the mainstay of treatment is chemotherapy. The platinum-based chemotherapy was established as a standard regimen based on the results of several randomized clinical trials (RCTs) over the last 30 years, and more effective regimen has been groped along the introduction of molecular targeted agents.

This chapter focuses on the first-line chemotherapy for epithelial ovarian cancer and will discuss the history and current status including neoadjuvant chemotherapy, intraperitoneal chemotherapy, and the impact on the targeted molecular therapy.

12.2 The History of Primary Chemotherapy

The early agents utilized in the treatment of ovarian cancer were predominantly the alkylating agents, melphalan and cyclophosphamide. Investigators attempted to combine one or more drugs, such as doxorubicin, 5-fluorouracil, and methotrexate, with alkylating agents. Response rates were usually reported to be in the range of 20–60%; however, the impact on overall survival (OS) was quite modest [1, 2].

The most important development in the management of advanced ovarian cancer was the introduction of cisplatin in the early 1980s. Cisplatin increased response rates to the 50–80% range and quickly became the major component of first-line therapy for ovarian cancer. The Gynecologic Oncology Group (GOG) 047 trial demonstrated the usefulness of concomitant therapy with cyclophosphamide, doxorubicin, and cisplatin (CAP) [3]. A subsequent meta-analysis showed that cyclophosphamide and cisplatin (CP) therapy is as effective as CAP and has fewer side effects [4]. As a result, CP therapy became the standard of care.

With the advent of paclitaxel in the 1990s, standard chemotherapy regimens have changed greatly. Paclitaxel is a compound extracted from the Pacific yew tree. Its novel mechanism of action involves binding to tubulin and inhibiting the disassembly of microtubules, thereby resulting in the inhibition of completion of the mitotic process and thus the inhibition of cell division. Comparison of CP therapy with paclitaxel plus cisplatin (TP) therapy revealed significantly improved complete response rates and survival rates with TP therapy. Thus, TP therapy became the standard treatment regimen [5, 6].

The introduction of carboplatin also led to important modifications in ovarian cancer treatment. Carboplatin does not require a large amount of hydration and can be easily administered in an outpatient setting. Several studies demonstrated that cisplatin and carboplatin were equally efficacious, and carboplatin had a more favorable toxicity profile [7, 8]. Subsequently, phase III randomized trials directly comparing cisplatin plus paclitaxel and a carboplatin-paclitaxel combination (TC) were conducted. One study performed in 2000 showed that a regimen of paclitaxel 175 mg/m^2 administered intravenously (IV) as a 3-h infusion followed by carboplatin (area under the plasma concentration-time curve [AUC] of 5) was feasible for outpatients with ovarian cancer, and had a better toxicity profile than paclitaxel followed by cisplatin 75 mg/m^2 [9]. In 2003, a phase III randomized trial conducted by the Arbeitsgemeinschaft Gynäkologische Onkologie Ovarian Cancer Study Group (AGO-OVAR) directly compared TP with TC in patients with International Federation of Gynecology and Obstetrics (FIGO) stage IIB-IV tumors who had undergone optimal debulking surgery [10]. This study showed that two platinum agents (carboplatin; AUC 6, cisplatin; 75 mg/m^2) in combination with paclitaxel (185 mg/m^2) were equivalent in efficacy; however, the TC regimen was associated with better tolerability and quality of life scores. Another phase III trial conducted by a GOG randomly assigned patients with optimally debulked stage III tumors to receive either cisplatin 75 mg/m^2 plus a 24-h infusion of paclitaxel 135 mg/m^2 or IV carboplatin AUC 7.5 plus paclitaxel 175 mg/m2 over 3 h [11]. This GOG158 study also demonstrated that the TC regimen resulted in less toxicity, was easier to administer, and was not inferior, in comparison to the TP regimen. Based on these studies, paclitaxel (175–180 mg/m^2 over 3 h) and carboplatin (AUC 5–6) administered IV every 3 weeks became the standard primary chemotherapy regimen for both early and advanced ovarian cancer [12–14].

One strategy to achieve further efficacy in the primary treatment of advanced ovarian cancer might be the addition of non-cross-resistant drugs to combination therapy with paclitaxel and carboplatin. From past reports, topotecan, a topoisomerase I inhibitor; pegylated liposomal doxorubicin (PLD), in which a polyethylene glycol layer surrounds a doxorubicin-containing liposome; and gemcitabine have been considered as additional active agents. Most notably, a phase III randomized study demonstrated that treatment with topotecan (1.5 mg/m^2/day for 5 days every 21 days) achieved comparable efficacy and survival to that of paclitaxel (175 mg/m^2/day as a 3-h infusion every 21 days) in the setting of recurrent ovarian cancer, with manageable and noncumulative hematological toxicity [15]. PLD (50 mg/m^2 every 28 days) was found to significantly prolong the survival compared with topotecan (1.5 mg/m^2 per day for 5 days every 21 days) in patients with recurrent and refractory epithelial ovarian cancer [16]. GOG 182/the International Collaborative Ovarian Neoplasm (ICON) 5 conducted multiple international phase III trials to evaluate whether incorporation of an additional cytotoxic agent, specifically gemcitabine, PLD, or topotecan, improved OS and progression-free survival (PFS). Unfortunately, the addition of a third drug to the platinum-taxane regimen was not found to yield improvements in PFS or OS compared with standard paclitaxel and carboplatin regimens [17]. Anthracyclines are also among the candidates for incorporation as a third drug. Epirubicin, a doxorubicin analog, has shown activity as a form of second-line chemotherapy, and it has been shown by a phase I/II study that the addition of epirubicin to TC is feasible [18, 19]. The AGO-OVAR performed a prospective randomized phase III study comparing a regimen of carboplatin (AUC 5) plus paclitaxel (175 mg/m^2) with the same regimen plus epirubicin (60 mg/m^2) (TEC); however, TEC did not show any clinical benefit [20].

A regimen that was able to extend the duration of survival longer than TC therapy did not appear for a while. In 2009, a randomized multicenter phase III trial conducted by a Japanese GOG (JGOG) reported that dose-dense weekly paclitaxel

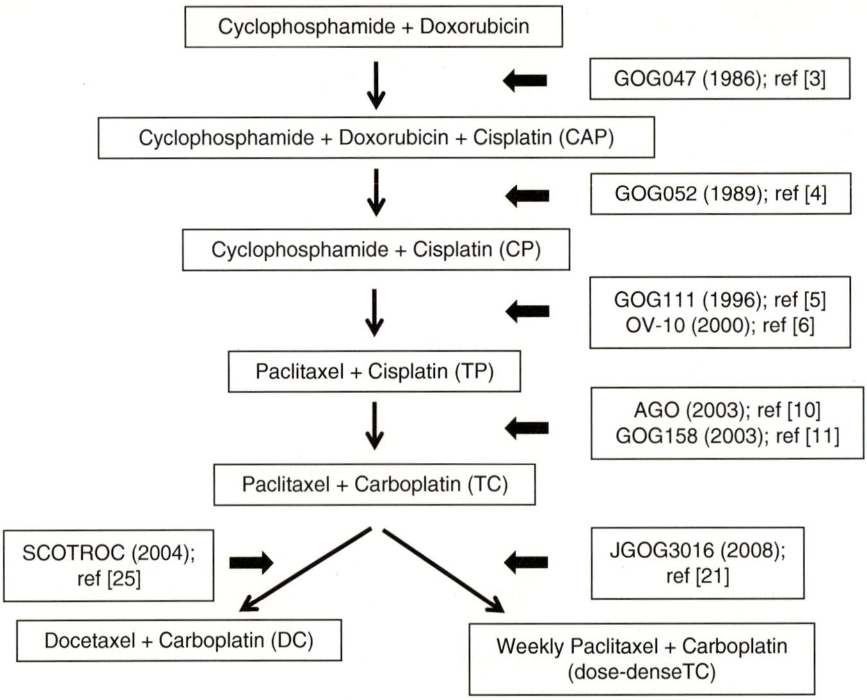

Fig. 12.1 The history of primary chemotherapy for epithelial ovarian cancer

(80 mg/m^2; 1-h intravenous infusion given on days 1, 8, and 15) plus carboplatin (AUC 6) improved survival compared with paclitaxel (180 mg/m^2; 3-h IV infusion on day 1) plus carboplatin (AUC 6) in patients with stage II-IV cancer, although the dose-dense TC regimen was associated with significantly higher rates of grade 3–4 anemia [21]. The updated data in 2013 showed that the median OS was 100.5 months (95% confidence interval [CI] 65.2–∞) in the dose-dense treatment group and 62.2 months (95% CI 52.1–82.6) in the conventional treatment group (hazard ratio [HR] 0.79, 95% CI 0.63–0.99; $p = 0.039$) [22]. Thus, this dose-dense TC regimen has been recognized as one of the standard primary chemotherapy regimens (Fig. 12.1).

In contrast to paclitaxel, fractionated weekly dosing of carboplatin remains a challenging regimen. The Multicentre Italian Trials in Ovarian Cancer (MITO) aimed to assess whether a weekly schedule of carboplatin plus paclitaxel was more effective than the same drugs given every 21 days (MITO-7) [23]. Patients with FIGO stage IC-IV ovarian cancer were randomly assigned to receive either carboplatin (AUC 6) plus paclitaxel (175 mg/m^2) every 21 days for six cycles or carboplatin (AUC 2) or carboplatin (AUC 2) plus paclitaxel (60 mg/m^2) every week for 18 weeks. Although the weekly schedule had lower toxicity and was better tolerated than the standard schedule, it did not appear to be associated with better PFS.

12.3 An Alternative Primary Chemotherapy

Docetaxel, a semisynthetic side-chain analogue of paclitaxel, was shown to be an active drug when delivered in the setting of platinum-resistant disease by a phase II trial [24]. One study by Scottish Randomized Trial in Ovarian Cancer (SCOTROC) directly compared carboplatin (AUC 5) plus paclitaxel (175 mg/m^2) every 21 days with carboplatin (AUC 5) plus docetaxel (75 mg/m^2). In this study, docetaxel-carboplatin was associated with a statistically higher incidence of grade 3–4 neutropenia, while the paclitaxel-carboplatin regimen resulted in a greater incidence of grade 3–4 peripheral neuropathy. However, the two regimens yielded similar efficacy in terms of PFS and response [25]. Thus, docetaxel (75 mg/m^2) plus carboplatin (AUC 5) represents an alternative first-line chemotherapy regimen [12–14] (Fig. 12.1).

PLD plus carboplatin (PLD-C) is one of the options for patients who have difficulty taking taxane agents. According to the MITO-2 trial that evaluated whether PLD-C (carboplatin AUC 5, PLD 30 mg/m^2) administered every 21 days was superior in terms of PFS to the standard TC regimen, there was no difference in response rate, PFS, or OS between the two regimens [26]. In view of the different toxicities (more hematologic adverse effects but less neurotoxicity and alopecia), PLD-C might be considered an alternative to standard therapy in some cases.

12.4 Adjuvant Chemotherapy for Early-Stage Ovarian Cancer

The use of adjuvant chemotherapy and its role in stage I ovarian cancer remains controversial. Several studies have been reported in which patients did not receive adjuvant chemotherapy after surgery. One prospective study enrolled 67 eligible patients with stage I ovarian cancer following accurate surgical staging. With a median follow-up time of 4 years, only one patient with clear cell carcinoma (CCC) experienced recurrence in the stage Ia and Ib group. The results of this study suggested that patients determined to have stage Ia or Ib cancer by accurate staging laparotomy and with histological grade 1 or 2 could be followed without adjuvant chemotherapy [27]. In another prospective randomized trial, 81 patients with histological grade 1 or 2 tumors and with stage Ia and Ib cancer on the basis of surgical resection plus comprehensive staging were assigned to receive either no chemotherapy or melphalan. As there were no significant differences between the two groups, this study concluded that adjuvant chemotherapy for patients with localized ovarian cancer who underwent comprehensive surgical staging could be omitted [28].

In 2003, two randomized controlled studies to evaluate the efficacy of adjuvant chemotherapy for early ovarian cancer were reported [29, 30]. In the ACTION1 trial, patients with ovarian cancer with stages Ia and Ib, grade II or III tumor; all grade of stages Ic-IIa; and all CCC, were randomly assigned to either observation or platinum-based chemotherapy following surgery [31]. This study showed that adjuvant chemotherapy statistically significantly improved the recurrence-free survival when all patients were taken into account; however, it was not effective in optimally staged patients. The ICON1 trial, in which patients with FIGO stage I disease constituted 93% of study subjects, also demonstrated that adjuvant chemotherapy with a platinum-based regimen improved survival and delayed recurrence [30]. The combined analysis of these two randomized clinical trials showed that OS at 5 years was 82% in the chemotherapy arm and 74% in the observation arm (HR = 0.67) and concluded that platinum-based adjuvant chemotherapy improved OS and recurrence-free survival at 5 years [31].

A meta-analysis that included five randomized controlled trials involving 1277 women with early-stage ovarian cancer indicated that women who received adjuvant platinum-based chemotherapy had better OS and PFS than those who did not (HR 0.71 and 0.65, respectively). In particular, women who were suboptimally staged or those who had high-risk disease received the greatest benefit from adjuvant chemotherapy. On the other hand, a benefit of adjuvant chemotherapy for women with adequate surgical staging and women with low- or intermediate-risk disease remained uncertain [32]. Taking these findings together, it has been generally accepted that adjuvant chemotherapy can be omitted in patients with stage IA or IB with grade 1 tumors.

12.5 Treatment Strategy by Histologic Subtype

It is currently unclear how to define treatment strategy by histologic subtype of ovarian cancer. TC have been recommended as primary chemotherapeutic agents for ovarian cancer based on the results of prior clinical studies [9, 10]. However, almost all patients enrolled in large randomized controlled trials of ovarian cancer have high-grade serous carcinoma, and the number of enrolled patients with CCC or mucinous carcinoma is limited. Several studies have demonstrated that CCC and mucinous carcinoma are less sensitive to platinum-based chemotherapy, and the median survival time of patients with these subtypes in advanced stages is significantly lower than patients with high-grade serous carcinoma [33, 34].

An in vitro study suggested that irinotecan (CPT-11) may be an effective agent for the treatment with CCC [35]. The JGOG and GCIG conducted the first randomized phase III trial of patients with CCC that compared irinotecan and cisplatin (CPT-P) with TC [36]. The JGOG3017/GCIG trial found that CPT-P provides no significant survival benefit to patients with CCC compared with TC. Treatment with existing anticancer agents has limitations for improving the prognosis of CCC. Therefore, another clinical trial using mTOR inhibitors (temsirolimus) is ongoing in patients with CCC, based on evidence that CCC expresses high levels of mTOR [37]. Mucinous carcinoma also demonstrates poor response to TC, and it has been suggested that mucinous carcinoma is more likely to be metastatic tumors from gastrointestinal cancer such as gastric and colon cancer than a primary ovarian tumor [38]. S-1 plus oxaliplatin has been assessed by clinical trial in patients with advanced gastric cancer. Thus, an oxaliplatin plus S-1 regimen is one of the treatment options for patients with mucinous carcinoma in ovary. Phase II clinical trials of oxaliplatin and S-1 for treating cases of advanced and recurrent mucinous ovarian cancer reported a 13% response rate and a 68% disease control rate (Shimada M, et al. Japan Society of Gynecologic and Obstetrics Annual Meeting 2013 abstract (unpublished date)).

Recently, The Cancer Genomic Atlas has revealed the genomic profiles of ovarian carcinoma [39], and the specific gene mutations in each histologic subtype are known [40]. Moreover, we can identify drug targets for those gene mutations by using the publicly available Genomics of Drug Sensitivity in Cancer drug database [41]. Over the past half century, ovarian cancer has been recognized as a single disease in clinical studies. However, the necessity of defining a treatment strategy by histological subtype has become a global consensus in ovarian cancer.

12.6 Neoadjuvant Chemotherapy

In patients diagnosed with ovarian cancer, the attempt is made to provide treatment with initial debulking surgery followed by chemotherapy. In cases in which the cancer has progressed so far that optimal surgery cannot be performed during the initial procedure, the goal is to minimize complications during the perisurgical stage and to improve complete excision rates as far as possible during this initial surgery. NAC may be considered to achieve these objectives.

Before 2010, most research regarding whether NAC contributes to improved prognosis following initial surgery was based on retrospective observational studies and involved differences in patient characteristics such as performance status (PS) and age. In a few non-randomized prospective studies, optimal surgery rates were found to improve [42, 43], perisurgical complications decreased [43–45] quality of life improved [46], and OS improved [42]. Two meta-analyses have compared prognosis based on whether surgery or NAC came first. One study showed poorer prognosis in the NAC group [47], while the other showed that although survival rates were equivalent, a greater percentage of patients received optimal surgery after NAC, and thus this treatment approach may be effective in improving prognosis [48].

The first prospective randomized study was reported in 2010 (EORTC 55971). In this study, 670 patients with stage IIIc to stage IV ovarian cancer, fallopian tube cancer, or peritoneal carcinoma were allocated to either a treatment group in which primary debulking surgery (PDS) was followed by at least six courses of the initial chemotherapy or another treatment group in which three courses of NAC preceded interval debulking surgery (IDS) that was then followed by a minimum of three additional courses of postsurgical chemotherapy. This was a noninferiority study in which the goal was to verify that the outcomes in the NAC group were not inferior to those in the PDS group; however, the median OS time was equal in both groups, with an OS of 29 months in the PDS group and 30 months in the NAC group [49]. When postoperative and perioperative complications and death rates were compared, the rates were significantly higher in the PDS group (severe hemorrhage

7.4% and deaths 2.5% vs. severe hemorrhage 4.1% and deaths 0.7% in the NAC group). This study concluded that NAC should be considered in cases in which complete resection is not possible with PDS alone. Furthermore, the authors stated that the most important prognostic factor in both groups is whether all macroscopic lesions can be completely resected during surgery.

The CHORUS study results, published in 2015, found NAC to be an acceptable form of standard therapy [50]. In this study, 552 patients believed to have stage III or stage IV ovarian cancer were allocated to either an NAC or a PDS group. Median survival times in the PDS and NAC groups were 22.6 months and 24.1 months, respectively, with an HR of 0.87, proving that NAC was noninferior. However, the median surgical time was very short in both groups at only 120 min, and the low optimal cytoreduction rates in the PDS group were mentioned as a factor.

Recently, the Japan Clinical Oncology Group published results comparing PDS to IDS in a phase III noninferiority trial (JCOG 0602). A total of 301 patients with Stage III and Stage IV ovarian cancer, fallopian tube cancer, or peritoneal carcinoma were allocated to either a PDS or an IDS group. The PDS group received eight courses of TC therapy after PDS, while IDS was performed after four courses of TC therapy, followed by four postsurgical courses of TC. In this study, surgical invasiveness was evaluated in addition to survival times. In the NAC group, there were fewer incidents requiring intestinal resection or resection of other organs due to complications. Moreover, a lower incidence of grade 3 or 4 postsurgical complications, smaller hemorrhage volumes, and albumin infusion requirements were noted in the NAC group. In this study, although surgical invasiveness was more limited in the NAC group, a similar survival time was achieved, suggesting that NAC may potentially become established as a standard form of therapy [51].

A growing body of evidence supports the use of NAC therapy in Stage IIIC and Stage IV ovarian cancer. In the future, it may be important to select an appropriate patient population in which NAC therapy is most likely to be effective. The objective of surgery in ovarian cancer is the complete resection of macroscopic lesions, and the clinician will need to choose between NAC and PDS from this perspective. Gastrointestinal resection and resection of other involved organs may become an issue in patient populations such as the elderly, those with low PS, or those in a poor nutritional state in which surgical invasiveness is an important consideration; NAC therapy is believed to be more appropriate in these patient groups [52–54] Evidence also suggests that patients with Stage IV cancer will benefit from NAC [55, 56].

12.7 Intraperitoneal Chemotherapy

As described above, current standard chemotherapy in ovarian cancer calls for IV administration of paclitaxel and carboplatin. However, most recurrent cases of ovarian cancer involve dissemination in the peritoneal cavity. Because direct IP administration allows more effective infiltration of cancer by antineoplastic drugs, researchers have investigated the efficacy of IP administration of cisplatin [57]. Since 1994, several randomized trials have been conducted on IP therapy [58–64] and significant improvements in survival rates were reported in three of those studies. In a review of reports in which taxanes were combined with platinum formulations (the current standard therapy), it was revealed that patients in the GOG114/SWOG9227 study comprised 462 cases with Stage III disease in which the residual tumor load after the initial surgery was ≤1 cm in diameter [63]. Patients were allocated into either an IV group treated with six courses of 135 mg/m^2 of IV paclitaxel +75 mg/m^2 of IV cisplatin or an IP group that received two courses of IV carboplatin (AUC 9) followed by six courses of 135 mg/m^2 IV paclitaxel +100 mg/m^2 of cisplatin IP. A significant increase in PFS was noted in the IP group compared to the IV group (28 months vs. 22 months, respectively), with increased OS of 63 months vs. 52 months. However, patients in the IP group received a higher dose of carboplatin for a greater number of courses, which was believed to be responsible for the increase in PFS, and since the IP group experienced a higher rate of toxicity, this form of administration could not be recommended as standard therapy. The GOG172 study compared 415 patients with Stage III cancer allocated into either an IV group treated with six courses of IV paclitaxel 135 mg/m^2 + IV cisplatin 75 mg/m^2 or an IP group administered 135 mg/m^2 IV paclitaxel (Day 1) + 75 mg/m^2 IP cisplatin (Day 2) + 60 mg/m^2 IP paclitaxel (Day 8) [64]. In the IP group, significant increases were noted in both PFS (19 months vs. 24 months) and OS (49 months vs. 67 months); however, the cisplatin dose was higher in the IP group and an additional dose of paclitaxel was administered on Day 8, so it may be difficult to compare the superiority or inferiority of these treatments directly.

Based on these comparative studies, the US National Cancer Institute (NCI) and GOG conducted a meta-analysis and found that the risk of death decreased 21.5% with IP therapy vs. IV therapy. They announced in January 2006 that patients with ovarian cancer with optimally debulked FIGO Stage III ovarian cancer should receive counseling regarding the clinical benefit associated with combined IV and IP administration of chemotherapy [65, 66]. Long-term follow-up results from the GOG172 and GOG114 studies were reported in 2015 [67]. In these studies, the median duration of follow-up observation was 10.7 years, and the median survival time in the IV group was 51.4 months, whereas the median survival time in the IP group was 61.8 months. This indicates that there was a 23% reduction in risk of death in the IP group. This report strongly supports the efficacy of IP treatment.

However, it was pointed out that IP therapy involves higher toxicity and a lower completion rate. Furthermore, comparative studies to date are not direct comparisons of the administration methods, and a major issue is that carboplatin, the current standard treatment, was not used in the above studies.

A larger, Phase III clinical study on IP administration is currently underway to resolve these issues in study design. One phase II/III study known as the JGOG3019 (iPocc trial) involves PDS patients with Stage II to Stage IV disease. This study compares a dose-dense TC therapy group (paclitaxel 80 mg/m^2 [Days 1, 8, and 15] + carboplatin AUC 6 [Day 1]) against a group receiving paclitaxel 80 mg/m^2 IP or IV + carboplatin AUC 6 IP administration and should allow direct assessment of the efficacy of IP administration [68]. The GOG conducted the GOG252 study, in which concurrent bevacizumab and maintenance therapy were added to all study arms. GOG252 involved women with Stage II-III epithelial ovarian, fallopian tube, or primary peritoneal carcinoma. All patients underwent optimal surgical debulking to 1 cm or less residual disease. In this study, three arms were compared: dose-dense TC chemotherapy as the standard treatment, IP carboplatin alone, and the experimental arm in the GOG172 study as the investigational treatment group. Furthermore, the National Cancer Institute of Canada (NCIC) conducted a phase II/III clinical study in patients who underwent optimal surgery after NAC [69]. A three-arm study was designed as a Phase II clinical study in which arm one received IV paclitaxel 135 mg/m^2 (Day 1) + IV carboplatin AUC 5 to 6 (Day 2) + IV paclitaxel 60 mg/m^2 (Day 8). Arm two consisted of the experimental arm of the GOG172 study, while arm three received 135 mg/m^2 IV paclitaxel (Day 1) + IP carboplatin AUC 5–6 (Day 2) + paclitaxel 60 mg/m^2 IP (Day 8). The most superior form of IP therapy in the Phase II study was then compared to arm one in a Phase III clinical study. This study compared IP administration of cisplatin against carboplatin to determine which was more effective and also allowed assessment of whether IP therapy was more effective than IV administration.

Although it has been reported that the effect of IP therapy is superior to that of conventional TC therapy, there are also complications specific to this treatment, such as the risk of infection from catheter use, catheter occlusion, adhesions, and peritoneal irritation due to local exposure to antineoplastic agents. If the results of the Phase III studies described above become available, the risks and benefits of IP therapy may become clearer, allowing clinicians to establish appropriate indications and administration methods. IP therapy would then become an effective treatment method for advanced ovarian carcinoma.

12.8 Targeted Molecular Therapy

In recent years, molecularly targeted drugs have become widely used in cancer treatment and have played major roles in the treatment of ovarian cancer. The molecularly targeted drugs that have been reported to be effective in chemotherapy for ovarian cancer can be broadly classified into the following two groups: anti-angiogenic target agents and poly (ADP-ribose) polymerase (PARP) inhibitors. Bevacizumab is a widely used anti-vascular endothelial growth factor (VEGF) human monoclonal antibody that belongs in the former category. Olaparib is the most common example of the latter and is closely dependent on the presence of BRCA mutations. In this section, we will discuss molecularly targeted therapy used in initial chemotherapy and subsequent maintenance therapy.

12.8.1 Anti-Angiogenetic Target Therapies

Neovascularization plays a vital role in the progression of dissemination and metastases, as well as the production of ascites in ovarian cancer. VEGF and vascular endothelial growth factor receptor (VEGFR) are strongly expressed in ovarian cancer, and it has been reported that VEGF expression correlates with ovarian cancer progression and the development of ascites [70]. The most widely used molecularly targeted therapy worldwide against ovarian cancer is a monoclonal antibody against VEGF called bevacizumab (BEV). BEV is a drug that has been shown to be effective against other cancers such as colon cancer, lung cancer, and breast cancer, in addition to ovarian cancer.

In a clinical study conducted by GOG using BEV as the initial therapy (GOG218), patients with FIGO stage III to stage IV ovarian cancer were divided into three treatment arms. With this study design, arm one comprised six courses of TC therapy (administered every 3 weeks), arm two included six courses of TC therapy with BEV 15 mg per kilogram administered concurrently from the second course, and arm three was composed of six courses of TC therapy with BEV administered from the second course until the 15th month. The study results showed a significant increase in PFS (3.8 months) in arm three compared to the control arm; however, there were no differences in OS [71]. In addition, ICON 7 was a randomized study conducted in patients with Stage I to stage IV ovarian cancer in which TC therapy was compared to combined treatment with BEV + maintenance treatment. In this study, concurrent BEV was administered from the second course of TC chemotherapy at a dose of 7.5 mg/kg and continued for 12 courses after conclusion of the TC regimen. Compared to the control group, the TC + BEV group showed a significant increase in PFS (1.7 months) [72]. In addition, in cases of platinum-resistant recurrent ovarian cancer, a synergistic effect was confirmed with the addition of BEV [73]. Based on the above findings, added effects of BEV were confirmed both during initial therapy and recurrent therapy for ovarian cancer; however, both outcomes were merely increases in PFS, and thus far, no increases in OS have been observed.

Characteristic serious adverse events associated with BEV include gastrointestinal perforation, thromboembolism, hypertension, delayed wound healing, hemorrhage, proteinuria, and fistula. There was a high incidence of gastrointestinal perforation (11%; 5/44 cases) during the Phase II study in patients with ovarian cancer, resulting in premature discontinuation of the study. However, a retrospective analysis revealed that the significant risk factor for gastrointestinal perforation was the treatment history rather than any of the three treatment regimens [74]. In the GOG 218 study, patients with intestinal obstruction or a history of radiation therapy to the abdomen or pelvis were excluded from the study, and the incidence of gastrointestinal bleeding and perforation was 3.4% in the BEV administration group, which was higher than the 1.7% in the placebo group [71]. While BEV can be an effective drug that inhibits the production of ascites and alleviates symptoms that could markedly decrease the quality of life of patients with ovarian cancer, it can also cause serious adverse events such as gastrointestinal perforation. During the administration of BEV, more consideration should be given to the selection criteria and exclusion criteria in clinical trials to carefully select patients and monitor for adverse events.

Nintedanib is a tyrosine kinase inhibitor (TKI) that inhibits VEGFR, fibroblast growth factor receptor (FGFR), and platelet-derived growth factor receptor

(PDGFR). In a Phase III clinical study, nintedanib was reported to have an additive effect on TC therapy in patients with Stage IIb to Stage IV ovarian cancer [75]. Patients in the nintedanib administration group ingested 200 mg of nintedanib for a maximum of 120 weeks. Compared to the placebo group, patients in the nintedanib group showed a significant increase in PFS (17.2 months vs. 16.6 months, HR = 0.84).

Pazopanib is a TKI that inhibits VEGFR, PDGFR, c-kit, and c-fms. Patients with Stage II–Stage IV ovarian cancer were investigated in an RCT to examine the effectiveness of maintenance therapy with pazopanib. When 800 mg of pazopanib was ingested for a maximum of 2 years, PFS was found to increase significantly compared to the placebo group (17.9 months vs. 12.3 months, HR = 0.77) [76]. However, the incidence of discontinuation of treatment on the basis of serious adverse events such as hypertension, neutropenia, liver dysfunction, and diarrhea was much higher in the pazopanib treatment group at 33.3% compared to the 5.6% observed in the control group. Regarding maintenance therapy with pazopanib, it has been reported to adversely affect OS in East Asian patients compared to non-East Asian patients [77].

12.8.2 Poly-Ribose Polymerase Inhibitor

The other effective molecular target is believed to be PARP. Genes can be damaged by a variety of factors, and PARP is a DNA-binding protein that detects and binds to sites of DNA damage (single-strand breaks, SSB), activating the base excision repair pathway. In humans, the PARP subfamily has 17 types; however, most of the DNA repair activity is handled by PARP-1, which has been widely studied [78]. PARP inhibitors express antitumor activity by inhibiting SSB DNA repair, so when these drugs were first developed, they were believed to potentiate the effects of chemotherapy. Subsequently, it was discovered that cell lines with BRCA 1/2 gene deletions were found to be 100- to 1000-fold more sensitive to PARP inhibitors compared to cell lines without BRCA mutations [79, 80]. PARP inhibitors were known to induce cell death in a manner known as synthetic lethality in cells with BRCA 1/2 gene dysfunction, drawing attention to PARP inhibitors as potential drugs with activity against ovarian cancer.

Olaparib was the first PARP inhibitor introduced into clinical use. The results of a randomized double-blind Phase II study were reported in patients with platinum-sensitive recurrent ovarian cancer or fallopian tube cancer or primary peritoneal carcinoma [81]. This study evaluated the effectiveness of maintenance therapy with olaparib. In a group that received 400 mg of olaparib for 8 weeks, PFS increased significantly in the olaparib group compared to the placebo group (8.4 months vs. 4.8 months, HR = 0.35). Furthermore, when patients were divided into a group with BRCA genetic abnormalities vs. those without genetic abnormalities to compare the efficacy of olaparib, a marked increase in PFS was noted in the group with BRCA genetic mutations (11.2 months vs. 4.3 months, HR = 0.18) [82]. Updated results were reported in 2016, revealing a statistically significant difference in PFS in the olaparib group compared to placebo (HR 0–35). Maximum effects were confirmed in the group with BRCA gene mutations (HR = 0.18) [83]. Based on the above findings, olaparib is an effective treatment for patients with advanced ovarian cancer with BRCA gene mutations and has been approved by the Food and Drug Administration (FDA), drawing attention to its use as a new therapeutic agent.

Veliparib, another PARP inhibitor, was shown to be useful in a Phase II study in patients with BRCA gene mutations and recurrent epithelial ovarian cancers. Complete responses were seen in two cases, partial responses in 11 cases, and stable disease in 24 cases. Anemia and decreased white blood cell counts were noted as adverse events in a large percentage of patients; however, this accompanying toxicity was within acceptable limits [84]. Patients with FIGO Stage III/IV high-grade serous ovarian cancer, fallopian tube cancer, or peritoneal carcinoma are currently participating in a phase III RCT to validate the advantages of concomitant veliparib with TC therapy or maintenance therapy.

Conclusion

Chemotherapeutic management as well as surgery constitute the pillar of treatment to ovarian cancer. The combination of paclitaxel and carboplatin demonstrates high clinical benefit and has been widely utilized as the standard treatment regimen. One option to obtain further chemotherapeutic efficacy in the primary treatment of advanced ovarian cancer is NAC, and another is IP chemotherapy. Selection of patients for NAC needs to be balanced by an individualized assessment of perioperative risks, possibility of resecting all macroscopic disease, although NAC appears to be gaining popularity. On the other hand, even though IP therapy has been reported to be superior to conventional IV chemotherapy, the choice of IP therapy needs to be careful because of IP therapy-specific complications.

Molecularly targeted drugs have played major roles in the treatment of ovarian cancer. Well-tolerated TC regimen is now supplemented by concurrent and maintenance bevacizumab in patients with FIGO stage III to stage IV ovarian cancer. As expanding knowledge of the molecular pathway of ovarian carcinogenesis, several candidates are under clinical investigation and are likely to change the way we treat ovarian cancer in the future.

References

1. Piver S, Barlow JJ, Chung WS, Lee FT, Vongtama V. Primary treatment of advanced ovarian adenocarcinoma, stages III and IV. Natl Cancer Inst Monogr. 1975;42:177–82.
2. Fisher RI, Young RC. Advances in the staging and treatment of ovarian cancer. Cancer. 1977;39:967–72.
3. Omura G, Blessing JA, Ehrlich CE, Miller A, Yordan E, Creasman WT, Homesley HD. A randomized trial of cyclophosphamide and doxorubicin with or without cisplatin in advanced ovarian carcinoma. Cancer. 1986;57:1725–30.

4. Omura GA, Bundy BN, Berek JS, Curry S, Delgado G, Mortel R. Randomized trial of cyclophosphamide plus cisplatin with or without doxorubicin in ovarian carcinoma: a Gynecologic Oncology Group Study. J Clin Oncol. 1989;7:457–65.
5. McGuire WP, Hoskins WJ, Brady MF, Kucera PR, Partridge EE, Look KY, et al. Cyclophosphamide and cisplatin versus paclitaxel and cisplatin: a phase III randomized trial in patients with suboptimal stage III/IV ovarian cancer (from the Gynecologic Oncology Group). Semin Oncol. 1996;23:40–7.
6. Piccart MJ, Bertelsen K, James K, Cassidy J, Mangioni C, Simonsen E, et al. Randomized intergroup trial of cisplatin-paclitaxel versus cisplatin-cyclophosphamide in women with advanced epithelial ovarian cancer: three-year results. J Natl Cancer Inst. 2000;92:699–708.
7. Alberts DS, Green S, Hannigan EV, O'Toole R, Stock-Novack D, Anderson P, et al. Improved therapeutic index of carboplatin plus cyclophosphamide versus cisplatin plus cyclophosphamide: final report by the Southwest Oncology Group of a phase III randomized trial in stages III and IV ovarian cancer. J Clin Oncol. 1992;10:706–17.
8. Swenerton K, Jeffrey J, Stuart G, Roy M, Krepart G, Carmichael J, et al. Cisplatin-cyclophosphamide versus carboplatin-cyclophosphamide in advanced ovarian cancer: a randomized phase III study of the National Cancer Institute of Canada Clinical Trials Group. J Clin Oncol. 1992;10:718–26.
9. Neijt JP, Engelholm SA, Tuxen MK, Sorensen PG, Hansen M, Sessa C, et al. Exploratory phase III study of paclitaxel and cisplatin versus paclitaxel and carboplatin in advanced ovarian cancer. J Clin Oncol. 2000;18:3084–92.
10. du Bois A, Lück HJ, Meier W, Adams HP, Möbus V, Costa S, et al. A randomized clinical trial of cisplatin/paclitaxel versus carboplatin/paclitaxel as first-line treatment of ovarian cancer. J Natl Cancer Inst. 2003;95:1320–9.
11. Ozols RF, Bundy BN, Greer BE, Fowler JM, Clarke-Pearson D, Burger RA, et al. Phase III trial of carboplatin and paclitaxel compared with cisplatin and paclitaxel in patients with optimally resected stage III ovarian cancer: a Gynecologic Oncology Group study. J Clin Oncol. 2003;21:3194–200.
12. Ovarian Cancer (Version 1. 2016) NCCN Clinical Practice Guidelines in Oncology https://www.nccn.org/professionals/physician_gls/f_guidelines.asp#ovarian
13. Komiyama S, Katabuchi H, Mikami M, Nagase S, Okamoto A, Ito K, Morishige K, Suzuki N, Kaneuchi M, Yaegashi N, Udagawa Y, Yoshikawa H. Japan Society of Gynecologic Oncology guidelines 2015 for the treatment of ovarian cancer including primary peritoneal cancer and fallopian tube cancer. Int J Clin Oncol. 2016;21:435–46.
14. Ledermann JA, Raja FA, Fotopoulou C, Gonzalez-Martin A, Colombo N, Sessa C, ESMO Guidelines Working Group. Newly diagnosed and relapsed epithelial ovarian carcinoma: ESMO Clinical Practice Guidelines for diagnosis, treatment and follow-up. Ann Oncol. 2013;24(Suppl 6):vi24–32.
15. ten Bokkel HW, Lane SR, Ross GA, International Topotecan Study Group. Long-term survival in a phase III, randomised study of topotecan versus paclitaxel in advanced epithelial ovarian carcinoma. Ann Oncol. 2004;15:100–3.
16. Gordon AN, Tonda M, Sun S, Rackoff W, Doxil Study 30–49 Investigators. Long-term survival advantage for women treated with pegylated liposomal doxorubicin compared with topotecan in a phase 3 randomized study of recurrent and refractory epithelial ovarian cancer. Gynecol Oncol. 2004;95:1–8.
17. Bookman MA, Brady MF, McGuire WP, Harper PG, Alberts DS, Friedlander M, et al. Evaluation of new platinum-based treatment regimens in advanced-stage ovarian cancer: a Phase III Trial of the Gynecologic Cancer Intergroup. J Clin Oncol. 2009;27:1419–25.
18. Vermorken JB, Kobierska A, van der Burg ME, Chevallier B, Zanaboni F, ten Bokkel Huinink WW, et al. High-dose epirubicin in platinum-pretreated patients with ovarian carcinoma: the EORTC-GCCG experience. Eur J Gynaecol Oncol. 1995;16:433–8.
19. du Bois A, Lück HJ, Bauknecht T, Meier W, Richter B, Kuhn W, et al. First-line chemotherapy with epirubicin, paclitaxel, and carboplatin for advanced ovarian cancer: a phase I/II study

of the Arbeitsgemeinschaft Gynäkologische Onkologie Ovarian Cancer Study Group. J Clin Oncol. 1999;17:46–51.

20. du Bois A, Weber B, Rochon J, Meier W, Goupil A, Olbricht S, et al. Addition of epirubicin as a third drug to carboplatin-paclitaxel in first-line treatment of advanced ovarian cancer: a prospectively randomized gynecologic cancer intergroup trial by the Arbeitsgemeinschaft Gynaekologische Onkologie Ovarian Cancer Study Group and the Groupe d'Investigateurs Nationaux pour l'Etude des Cancers Ovariens. J Clin Oncol. 2006;24:1127–35.
21. Katsumata N, Yasuda M, Takahashi F, Isonishi S, Jobo T, Aoki D, et al. Dose-dense paclitaxel once a week in combination with carboplatin every 3 weeks for advanced ovarian cancer: a phase 3, open-label, randomised controlled trial. Lancet. 2009;374:1331–8.
22. Katsumata N, Yasuda M, Isonishi S, Takahashi F, Michimae H, Kimura E, et al. Long-term results of dose-dense paclitaxel and carboplatin versus conventional paclitaxel and carboplatin for treatment of advanced epithelial ovarian, fallopian tube, or primary peritoneal cancer (JGOG 3016): a randomised, controlled, open-label trial. Lancet Oncol. 2013;14:1020–6.
23. Pignata S, Scambia G, Katsaros D, Gallo C, Pujade-Lauraine E, De Placido S, et al. Carboplatin plus paclitaxel once a week versus every 3 weeks in patients with advanced ovarian cancer (MITO-7): a randomised, multicentre, open-label, phase 3 trial. Lancet Oncol. 2014;15:396–405.
24. Markman M, Zanotti K, Webster K, Peterson G, Kulp B, Belinson J. Phase 2 trial of single agent docetaxel in platinum and paclitaxel-refractory ovarian cancer, fallopian tube cancer, and primary carcinoma of the peritoneum. Gynecol Oncol. 2003;91:573–6.
25. Vasey PA, Jayson GC, Gordon A, Gabra H, Coleman R, Atkinson R, et al. Phase III randomized trial of docetaxel-carboplatin versus paclitaxel-carboplatin as first-line chemotherapy for ovarian carcinoma. J Natl Cancer Inst. 2004;96:1682–91.
26. Pignata S, Scambia G, Ferrandina G, Savarese A, Sorio R, Breda E, et al. Carboplatin plus paclitaxel versus carboplatin plus pegylated liposomal doxorubicin as first-line treatment for patients with ovarian cancer: the MITO-2 randomized phase III trial. J Clin Oncol. 2011;29:3628–35.
27. Monga M, Carmichael JA, Shelley WE, Kirk ME, Krepart GV, Jeffrey JF, Pater JL. Surgery without adjuvant chemotherapy for early epithelial ovarian carcinoma after comprehensive surgical staging. Gynecol Oncol. 1991;43:195–7.
28. Young RC, Walton LA, Ellenberg SS, Homesley HD, Wilbanks GD, Decker DG, et al. Adjuvant therapy in stage I and stage II epithelial ovarian cancer. Results of two prospective randomized trials. N Engl J Med. 1990;322:1021–7.
29. Trimbos JB, Vergote I, Bolis G, Vermorken JB, Mangioni C, Madronal C, et al. Impact of adjuvant chemotherapy and surgical staging in early-stage ovarian carcinoma: European Organisation for Research and Treatment of Cancer-Adjuvant ChemoTherapy in Ovarian Neoplasm trial. Natl Cancer Inst. 2003;95:113–25.
30. Colombo N, Guthrie D, Chiari S, Parmar M, Qian W, Swart AM, et al. International Collaborative Ovarian Neoplasm trial 1: a randomized trial of adjuvant chemotherapy in women with early-stage ovarian cancer. J Natl Cancer Inst. 2003;95:125–32.
31. Trimbos JB, Parmar M, Vergote I, Guthrie D, Bolis G, Colombo N, et al. International Collaborative Ovarian Neoplasm trial 1 and adjuvant ChemoTherapy in Ovarian Neoplasm trial : two parallel randomized phase III trials of adjuvant chemotherapy in patients with early -stage ovarian carcinoma. Natl Cancer Inst. 2003;95:105–12.
32. Winter-Roach BA, Kitchener HC, Lawrie TA. Adjuvant (post-surgery) chemotherapy for early stage epithelial ovarian cancer. Cochrane Database Syst Rev. 2012;3:CD004706. Review. Update in: Cochrane Database Syst Rev. 2015; (12): CD004706
33. Sugiyama T, Kamura T, Kigawa J, Terakawa N, Kikuchi Y, Kita T, et al. Clinical characteristics of clear cell carcinoma of the ovary: a distinct histologic type with poor prognosis and resistance to platinum-based chemotherapy. Cancer. 2000;88:2584–9.

34. Hess V, A'Hern R, Nasiri N, King DM, Blake PR, Barton DP, et al. Mucinous epithelial ovarian cancer: a separate entity requiring specific treatment. J Clin Oncol. 2004;22:1040–4.
35. Itamochi H, Kigawa J, Sultana H, Iba T, Akeshima R, Kamazawa S, et al. Sensitivity to anticancer agents and resistance mechanisms in clear cell carcinoma of the ovary. Jpn J Cancer Res. 2002;93:723–8.
36. Sugiyama T, Okamoto A, Enomoto T, Hamano T, Aotani E, Terao Y, et al. Randomized Phase III Trial of Irinotecan Plus Cisplatin Compared With Paclitaxel Plus Carboplatin As First-Line Chemotherapy for Ovarian Clear Cell Carcinoma:JGOG3017/GCIG Trial. J Clin Oncol. 2016;34:2881–7.
37. Temsirolimus, Carboplatin, and Paclitaxel as First-Line Therapy in Treating Patients With Newly Diagnosis Stage III/IV Clear Cell Ovarian Cancer (NCT01195429). http://clinicaltrials.gov/show/NCT01196429
38. Seidman JD, Kurman RJ, Ronnett BM. Primary and metastatic mucinous adenocarcinomas in the ovaries: incidence in routine practice with a new approach to improve intraoperative diagnosis. Am J Surg Pathol. 2003;27:985–93.
39. Cancer Genome Atlas Research Network. Integrated genomic analyses of ovarian carcinoma. Nature. 2011;474:609–15.
40. Jarboe EA, Folkins AK, Drapkin R, Ince TA, Agoston ES, Crum CP. Tubal and ovarian pathways to pelvic epithelial cancer: a pathological perspective. Histopathology. 2009;55:619.
41. Yang W, Soares J, Greninger P, Edelman EJ, Lightfoot H, Forbes S, et al. Genomics of drug Sensitivity in cancer (GDSC): a resource for therapeutic biomarker discovery in cancer cells. Nucleic Acids Res. 2013;41(Database issue):D955–61.
42. Kuhn W, Rutke S, Spathe K, Schmalfeldt B, Florack G, von Hundelshausen B, et al. Neoadjuvant chemotherapy followed by tumor debulking prolongs survival for patients with poor prognosis in International Federation of Gynecology and Obstetrics stage IIIc ovarian carcinoma. Cancer. 2001;92:2585–91.
43. Lee SJ, Kim BG, Lee JW, Park CS, Lee JH, Bae DS. Preliminary results of neoadjuvant chemo therapy with paclitaxel and cisplatin in patients with advanced epithelial ovarian cancer who are inadequate for optimum primary surgery. J Obsret Gynaecol Res. 2006;32:99–106.
44. Hegazy MA, Hegazi RA, Elshafei MA, Setit AE, Elshamy MR, Eltaroongy M, et al. Neoadjuvant chemotherapy versus primary surgery in advanced ovarian carcinoma. World J Surg Oncol. 2005;3:57.
45. Giannopoulos T, Butler-Ylanuel S, Taylor A, Ngeh N, Thomas H. Clinical outcomes of neoadjuvant chemotherapy and primary debulking surgery in advanced ovarian carcinoma. Eur J Gynaecol Oncol. 2006;27:25–8.
46. Chan YM, Ng TY, Ngan HY, Wong LC. Quality of life in women treated with neoadjuvant chemotherapy for advanced ovarian cancer: a prospective longitudinal study. Gynecol Oncol. 2003;88:9–16.
47. Bristow RE, Chi DS. Platinum-based neoadjuvant chemotherapy and interval surgical cytoreduction for advanced ovarian cancer: a meta-analysis. Gynecol Oncol. 2006;103:1070–6.
48. Kang S, Nam BH. Does neoadjuvant chemotherapy increase optimal cytoreduction rate in advanced ovarian cancer ? Meta-analysis of 21 studies. Ann Surg Oncol. 2009;16:2315–20.
49. Vergote I, Tropé CG, Amant F, Kristensen GB, Ehlen T, Johnson N, et al. Neoadjuvant chemotherapy or primary surgery in stage IIIC or IV ovarian cancer. N Engl J Med. 2010;363:943–53.
50. Kehoe S, Hook J, Nankivell M, Jayson GC, Kitchener H, Lopes T, et al. Primary chemotherapy versus primary surgery for newly diagnosed advanced ovarian cancer (CHORUS): an open-label, randomised, controlled, non-inferiority trial. Lancet. 2015;386:249–57.
51. Onda T, Satoh T, Saito T, Kasamatsu T, Nakanishi T, Nakamura K, et al. Comparison of treatment invasiveness between upfront debulking surgery versus interval debulking surgery following neoadjuvant chemotherapy for stage III/IV ovarian, tubal, and peritoneal cancers in a phase III randomised trial: Japan Clinical Oncology Group Study JCOG0602. Eur J Cancer. 2016;64:22–31.

52. Aletti GD, Eisenhauer EL, Santillan A, Axtell A, Aletti G, Holschneider C, et al. Identification of patient groups at highest risk from traditional approach to ovarian cancer treatment. Gynecol Oncol. 2011;120:23–8.
53. Wright JD, Lewin SN, Deutsch I, Burke WM, Sun X, Neugut AI, et al. Defining the limits of radical cytoreductive surgery for ovarian cancer. Gynecol Oncol. 2011;123:467–73.
54. Thrall MM, Goff BA, Symons RG, Flum DR, Gray HJ. Thirty-day mortality after primary cytoreductive surgery for advanced ovarian cancer in the elderly. Obstet Gynecol. 2011;118:537–47.
55. Thrall MM, Gray HJ, Symons RG, Weiss NS, Flum DR, Goff BA. Neoadjuvant chemotherapy in the Medicare cohort with advanced ovarian cancer. Gynecol Oncol. 2011;123:461–6.
56. Rauh-Hain JA, Rodriguez N, Growdon WB, Goodman AK, Boruta DM 2nd, Horowitz NS, et al. Primary debulking surgery versus neoadjuvant chemotherapy in stage IV ovarian cancer. Ann Surg Oncol. 2012;19:959–65.
57. Howell SB, Pfeifle CL, Wung WE, Olshen RA, Lucas WE, Yon JL, et al. Intraperitoneal cisplatin with systemic thiosulfate protection. Ann Intern Med. 1982;97:845–51.
58. Braly PS, McClay EF, Saltzstein SL, Plaxe SC, Kim S, et al. A comparison of intravenous versus intraperitoneal chemotherapy for the initial treatment of ovarian cancer. Gynecol Oncol. 1994;54:338–44.
59. Alberts DS, Liu PY, Hannigan EV, O'Toole R, Williams SD, Young JA, et al. Intraperitoneal cisplatin plus intravenous cyclophosphamide versus intravenous cisplatin plus intravenous cyclophosphamide for stage III ovarian cancer. N Engl J Med. 1996;335:1950–5.
60. Polyzos A, Tasvaris N, Kosmas C, Giannikos L, Katsikas M, Kalahanis N, et al. A comparative study of intraperitoneal carboplatin versus intravenous carboplatin with intravenous cyclophosphamide in both arms as initial chemotherapy for stage III ovarian cancer. Oncology. 1999;56:291–6.
61. Gadducci A, Carnino F, Chiara S, Brunetti I, Tanganelli L, Romanini A, et al. Intraperitoneal versus intravenous cisplatin in combination with intravenous cyclophosphamide and epidoxorubicin in optimally cytoreduced advanced epithelial ovarian cancer : a randomized trial of the Gruppo Oncologica Nord Ovest. Gynecol Oncol. 2000;76:157–62.
62. Yen MS, Juang CM, Lai CR, Chao GC, Ng HT, Yuan CC. Intraperitoneal cisplatin-based chemotherapy vs. intravenous cisplatin-based chemotherapy for stage III optimally cytoreduced epithelial ovarian cancer. Int J Gynaecol Obstet. 2001;72:55–60.
63. Markman M, Bundy BN, Alberts DS, Fowler JM, Clark-Pearson DL, Carson LF, et al. Phase III trial of standard-dose intravenous cisplatin plus paclitaxel versus moderately high-dose carboplatin followed by intravenous paclitaxel and intraperitoneal cisplatin in small-volume stage III ovarian carcinoma: an intergroup study of the Gynecologic Oncology Group, Southwestern Oncology Group, and Eastern Cooperative Oncology Group. J Clin Oncol. 2001;19:1101–7.
64. Armstrong DK, Bundy B, Wenzel L, Huang HQ, Baergen R, Lele S, et al. Intraperitoneal cisplatin and paclitaxel in ovarian cancer. N Engl J Med. 2006;354:34–43.
65. NCI Clinical Announcement on Intraperitoneal Chemotherapy in Ovarian Cancer. 2006. https://ctep.cancer.gov/highlights/20060105_ovarian.htm
66. Alberts DS, Markman M, Muggia F, Ozols RF, Eldermire E, Bookman MA, et al. Proceedings of a GOG workshop on intraperitoneal therapy for ovarian cancer. Gynecol Oncol. 2006;103:783–92.
67. Tewari D, Java JJ, Salani R, Armstrong DK, Markman M, Herzog T, et al. Long-term survival advantage and prognostic factors associated with intraperitoneal chemotherapy treatment in advanced ovarian cancer: a gynecologic oncology group study. J Clin Oncol. 2015;33:1460–6.
68. Fujiwara K, Aotani E, Hamano T, Nagao S, Yoshikawa H, Sugiyama T, et al. A randomized phase II/III trial of 3 weekly intraperitoneal versus intravenous carboplatin in combination with intravenous weekly dose-dense paclitaxel for newly diagnosed ovarian, fallopian tube and primary peritoneal cancer. Jpn J Clin Oncol. 2011;41:278–82.

69. Mackay HJ, Provencheur D, Heywood M, Tu D, Eisenhauer EA, Oza AM, et al. Phase II/III study of intraperitoneal chemotherapy after neoadjuvant chemotherapy for ovarian cancer: ncic ctg ov.21. Curr Oncol. 2011;18:84–90.
70. Graybill W, Sood AK, Monk BJ, Coleman RL. State of the science: emerging therapeutic strategies for targeting angiogenesis in ovarian cancer. Gynecol Oncol. 2015;138:223–6.
71. Burger RA, Brady MF, Bookman MA, Fleming GF, Monk BJ, Huang H, et al. Incorporation of bevacizumab in the primary treatment of ovarian cancer. N Engl J Med. 2011;365:2473–83.
72. Perren TJ, Swart AM, Pfisterer J, Ledermann JA, Pujade-Lauraine E, Kristensen G, et al. A phase 3 trial of bevacizumab in ovarian cancer. N Engl J Med. 2011;365:2484–96.
73. Pujade-Lauraine E, Hilpert F, Weber B, Reuss A, Poveda A, Kristensen G, et al. Bevacizumab combined with chemotherapy for platinum-resistant recurrent ovarian cancer : the AURELIA open-label randomized phase III trial. J Clin Oncol. 2014;32:1302–8.
74. Cannistra SA, Matulonis UA, Penson RT, Hambleton J, Dupont J, Mackey H, et al. Phase II study of bevacizumab in patients with platinum-resistant ovarian cancer or peritoneal serous cancer. J Clin Oncol. 2007;25:5180–6.
75. du Bois A, Kristensen G, Ray-Coquard I, Reuss A, Pignata S, Colombo N, et al. Standard first-line chemotherapy with or without nintedanib for advanced ovarian cancer (AGO-OVAR 12): a randomised, double-blind, placebo-controlled phase 3 trial. Lancet Oncol. 2016;17:78–89.
76. du Bois A, Floquet A, Kim JW, Rau J, del Campo JM, Friedlander M, et al. Incorporation of pazopanib in maintenance therapy of ovarian cancer. J Clin Oncol. 2014;32:3374–82.
77. Kim MK, Seong SJ, Kim JW, Bae DS, Jeon S, Kwon SH, et al. Management of endometrial hyperplasia: a survey of members of the Korean Gynecologic Oncology Group. Int J Gynecol Cancer. 2015;25:1277–84.
78. Amé JC, Rolli V, Schreiber V, Niedergang C, Apiou F, Decker P, et al. PARP-2, a novel mammalian DNA damage-dependent poly(ADP-ribose) polymerase. J Biol Chem. 1999;274:17860–8.
79. Bryant HE, Schultz N, Thomas HD, Parker KM, Flower D, Lopez E, et al. Specific killing of BRCA2-deficient tumours with inhibitors of poly(ADP-ribose) polymerase. Nature. 2005;434:913–7.
80. Farmer H, McCabe N, Lord CJ, Tutt AN, Johnson DA, Richardson TB, et al. Targeting the DNA repair defect in BRCA mutant cells as a therapeutic strategy. Nature. 2005;434:917–21.
81. Ledermann J, Harter P, Gourley C, Friedlander M, Vergote I, Rustin G, et al. Olaparib maintenance therapy in platinum-sensitive relapsed ovarian cancer. N Engl J Med. 2012;366:1382–92.
82. Ledermann J, Harter P, Gourley C, Friedlander M, Vergote I, Rustin G, et al. Olaparib maintenance therapy in patients with platinum-sensitive relapsed serous ovarian cancer: a preplanned retrospective analysis of outcomes by BRCA status in a randomized phase 2 trial. Lancet Oncol. 2014;15:852–61.
83. Ledermann JA, Harter P, Gourley C, Friedlander M, Vergote I, Rustin G, et al. Overall survival in patients with platinum-sensitive recurrent serous ovarian cancer receiving olaparib maintenance monotherapy: an updated analysis from a randomised, placebo-controlled, double-blind, phase 2 trial. Lancet Oncol. 2016;17:1579–1589.
84. Coleman RL, Sill MW, Bell-McGuinn K, Aghajanian C, Gray HJ, Tewari KS, et al. A phase II evaluation of the potent, highly selective PARP inhibitor veliparib in the treatment of persistent or recurrent epithelial ovarian, fallopian tube, or primary peritoneal cancer in patients who carry a germline BRCA1 or BRCA2 mutation - an NRG Oncology/Gynecologic Oncology Group study. Gynecol Oncol. 2015;137:386–91.

Immunology and Immunotherapy in Ovarian Cancer

13

Masaki Mandai, Junzo Hamanishi, Kaoru Abiko, Noriomi Matsumura, Tsukasa Baba, and Ikuo Konishi

Abstract

With a substantial success of immune checkpoint inhibitor such as anti-CTLA-4 antibodies and anti-PD-L1/PD-1 antibodies, cancer immunotherapy is now drawing a broad attention. In ovarian cancer, several trials have already shown a promising result of anti-PD-L1/PD-1 therapy. In addition, basic research using ovarian cancer cell line has demonstrated a rationale of immune checkpoint inhibition against ovarian cancer. Nevertheless, given the extraordinary cost of using these drugs and relatively low response rate, it is still unclear whether immunotherapy can be widely applied and used for the treatment of ovarian cancer. In order to promote immunotherapy, development of effective biomarkers that can predict response of immune checkpoint inhibitors is most important. At the same time, appropriate handling of immunotherapy-specific adverse effects, that has also been noted in clinical trials, is another important issue. If we could solve these problems, immunotherapy will serve as a major treatment modality for ovarian cancer in the future.

Keywords

Ovarian cancer • Immunotherapy • PD-1 • Immune checkpoint

M. Mandai, M.D., Ph.D. (✉) • J. Hamanishi, M.D., Ph.D. • K. Abiko, M.D., Ph.D.
T. Baba, M.D., Ph.D.
Department of Gynecology and Obstetrics, Kyoto University Graduate School of Medicine, Kyoto, Japan
e-mail: mandai@kuhp.kyoto-u.ac.jp

N. Matsumura, M.D., Ph.D.
Department of Obstetrics and Gynecology, Faculty of Medicine, Kinki University, Osakasayama, Japan

I. Konishi, M.D., Ph.D.
National Kyoto Medical Center, Kyoto, Japan

H. Katabuchi (ed.), *Frontiers in Ovarian Cancer Science*, Comprehensive Gynecology and Obstetrics, DOI 10.1007/978-981-10-4160-0_13

13.1 Introduction

Ovarian cancer is the leading cause of mortality from gynecological malignancies. Because ovarian cancer is generally diagnosed at late stages, it is commonly spread into the peritoneal cavity at the time of diagnosis. Therefore, treating advanced disease is the main focus of ovarian cancer therapies. During the past two decades, the standard medical treatment for ovarian cancer has been surgical cytoreduction and cytotoxic chemotherapy, especially the combination of carboplatin and paclitaxel. The effective combination of thorough debulking surgery and recent development of chemotherapies has significantly improved the outcomes of patients with ovarian cancer. Nevertheless, achieving a complete cure remains difficult. Recently, in addition to conventional cytotoxic chemotherapeutic reagents, novel molecular targeted drugs have been employed in many malignant tumors, including ovarian cancer. Prospective studies have demonstrated that bevacizumab, an antiangiogenic reagent that acts against vascular endothelial growth factor (VEGF), is clinically effective in ovarian cancer in both adjuvant and recurrent settings [1, 2]. The "Japan Society of Gynecologic Oncology guidelines 2015 for the treatment of ovarian cancer including primary peritoneal cancer and fallopian tube cancer" recommends bevacizumab as a molecular targeting drug to be considered to use in combination with chemotherapy in these settings [3]. Olaparib, an inhibitor of the enzyme poly ADP ribose polymerase (PARP), has also been reported to be promising in treating BRCA-positive ovarian cancer [4].

Cancer immunotherapy has been expected to be a promising modality for solid tumors. Since ovarian cancer biology is deeply associated with microenvironment in the abdominal cavity, altering the intraperitoneal environment is thought to be useful as a treatment strategy. As described below, the immune microenvironment in the abdominal cavity also significantly affects ovarian cancer progression. Therefore, several immunotherapy clinical trials for ovarian cancer have been conducted. However, the results were not as effective as expected [5]. Very recently, a novel type of immunotherapy that targets the CD28/CTLA-4 family, especially the programmed cell death ligand-1 (PD-L1)/programmed cell death-1 (PD-1) signaling pathway, has been introduced and was found to be surprisingly effective in many solid tumors, including malignant melanoma and lung cancer [6, 7]. This class of drugs is known as immune checkpoint inhibitors and is creating a new frontier in cancer treatment.

13.2 Before Immune Checkpoint Inhibition: Conventional Immunotherapies Against Ovarian Cancer

More than 50 clinical trials (including phase III trials) of immunotherapy for ovarian cancer have been conducted thus far. There are many immune therapies, which generally can be classified into four types (Table 13.1). One is to activate the host's own anticancer immunity by some means (Table 13.2). The so-called cancer vaccine belongs to this category, which consists of therapies such as the peptide vaccine

Table 13.1 Classification of conventional immunotherapy

Specificity activation	Non-specific (activate systemic immunity, relatively old)	Specific (target cancer cells or cancer-specific antigens, relatively old)
Active immunization (to elicit immunity in vivo)	Biological response modifier	Cancer vaccine Dendritic cell therapy
Passive immunotherapy (to elicit immunity in vitro)	Lymphokine-activated killer cell therapy Natural killer cell therapy	Cancer specific-antibodies

Table 13.2 Clinical trials for ovarian cancer—active immunotherapy

Therapy	Immune response	Clinical response	Report
FR-specific gene-modified T-cell therapy	FR-specific IFN-γ production	No objective response	Kershaw, Clin Cancer Res, 2006; 12:6106
HER2-/MUC1-derived peptide sensitized DC vaccine	Specific IFN-γ-producing T cell, specific CTL activity in 2/3	2/3 SD	Brossart P, Blood, 2000; 96:3102
HER2-derived peptide vaccine	specific IFN-γ-producing T cell in 1/1	PD	Murray, Clin Cancer Res, 2002; 8:3407
HER2-derived peptide vaccine	Immune response in ELISPOT in 1/2	PD in 2/2	Knutson, Clin Cancer Res, 2002; 8:1014
NY-SO-1-derived peptide vaccine	specific antibody in 10/13, peptide specific T cell in 3/5	CR in 1 (at least)	Odunsi, Pro NAS, 2007; 104:12,837
NY-SO-1derived peptide vaccine	Peptide-specific T cell in 7/9	Remission-free in 3/9	Diefenbach, Clin Cancer Res, 2008; 14:2740
P53-derived peptide vaccine	Peptide-specific T cell in 20/20	SD in 2/20	Leffers, Int J Cancer, 2009; 125:2104
P53-derived peptide vaccine	Immune response in tetramer assay in 9/13	Median OS, 40.8M	Rahma, Cancer Immunol immunother, 2012; 61:373
P53-derived peptide sensitized DC vaccine	Immune response in tetramer assay in 5/6	Median OS, 29.6M	Rahma, Cancer Immunol immunother, 2012; 61:373
P53-derived peptide vaccine + low-dose cyclophosphamide	Immune response in ELISPOT in 9/10	SD in 2/10	Vermeij, Int J Cancer, 2012; 131:E670
Mannan-MUC1 fusion protein sensitized DC vaccine	Specific IFN-γ-producing T cell in 9/10	SD > 10Y in 2/10	Loveland, Clin Cancer Res, 2006; 12:869

(continued)

Table 13.2 (continued)

Therapy	Immune response	Clinical response	Report
MUC1-specific Th1-type CD4+ effector cell therapy	MUC1-specific CTL in all	CR in 1/4	Dobrzanski, Cancer Immunol Immunother, 2012; 61:839
WT-1 peptide vaccine	Delayed cutaneous hypersensitivity in 5/6	SD in 2/6	Ohno, Anticancer Res, 2009; 29:4779
Anti-CA-125 idiotypic antibody (ACA125, abagovomab)	Specific anti-anti-idiotypic antibody in 28/42	Significant prognostic improvement in patient with immune response	Wagner, Clin Cancer Res, 2001; 7:1154
Anti-CA-125 idiotypic antibody (ACA125, abagovomab)	Specific anti-anti-idiotypic antibody in 81/119	Significant prognostic improvement in patient with immune response	Reinartz, Clin Cancer Res, 2004; 10:1580
Tumor cell sensitized DC vaccine	Specific IFN-γ-producing T cell in 2/6	>SD response in 4/6	Hernando, Cancer Immunol Immunother, 2002; 51:45

and dendritic cell therapies. The peptide vaccine is the most popular because it is relatively easy to produce. Cancer antigens including HER2/new, p53, MUC1, NY-ESO-1, and WT-1 have also been used to target ovarian cancer. While dendritic cell therapy theoretically has potent vaccine efficacy, the process of its ex vivo amplification and efficient antigen stimulation is technically difficult and not suitable for large-scale production. Another category of immunotherapy is "passive immunotherapy," which primarily comprises antibody therapies (Table 13.3). Developing therapeutic antibodies is expensive and time consuming because of strict quality control requirements. However, once developed, these antibodies are suitable for large-scale production. Therefore, this category is now regarded as the most important among immunotherapies. Among the available immunotherapies, antibodies that target ovarian cancers include the anti-CA-125 antibody, anti-folate receptor antibody, and double antibodies against EpCAM and CD3.

13.2.1 Active Immunotherapy for Ovarian Cancer (Table 13.2)

13.2.1.1 Immunotherapy that Targets MUC1

MUC1 is highly expressed in many ovarian cancers and has been a primary target candidate for immunotherapy. Dobrzanski and colleagues conducted phase I and phase II studies by using a Th1 type of self-replenishing CD4+ T cells producing IL-10 and IFN-γ to combat recurrent ovarian cancer [8]. One of the four cases showed remission, and another showed a tumor-bearing survival of 16 weeks; however, the remaining two cases died of cancer within 3–5 months. T cells from

Table 13.3 Clinical trials for ovarian cancer—passive immunotherapy

Therapy	Case	Clinical response	Report
Anti-CA-125 Ab (B43.13; oregovomab)	32	>SD response in six with Ab2-positive case	Baum, Cancer, 1994; 73(3 Suppl):1121
Anti-CA-125 Ab (B43.13; oregovomab)	20 (recurrent)	Significant prognostic improvement in patient with immune response	Gordon, Gynecol Oncol, 2004; 94: 340
Anti-CA-125 Ab (B43.13; oregovomab)	145 (post-remission)	No PFS improvement, but significant prognostic improvement in patient with immune response	Berek, J Clin Oncol, 2004; 22:3507
Anti-CA-125 Ab (B43.13; oregovomab)	373 (post-remission)	No PFS improvement	Berek, J Clin Oncol, 2009; 27:418
Anti-CA-125 Ab (B43.13; oregovomab)	40 (stage III/IV)		Braly, J Immunother, 2009; 32:54
Anti-FrαAb (MORAb-003; farletuzumab)	25 (recurrent, refractory)	SD in 9, CA-125 decrease in 2	Konner, Clin Cancer Res, 2010; 16:5288
Anti-EpCAM x anti-CD3 Ab (catumaxomab)	23 (with ascites)	No need of abdominocentesis in 22/23	Burges, Clin Cancer Res, 2007; 13:3899
Anti-EpCAM x anti-CD3 Ab (catumaxomab)	129 (with ascites)	Prolonged duration to next abdominocentesis	Heiss, Int J Cancer, 2010; 127:2209
Anti-EpCAM x anti-CD3 Ab (catumaxomab)	45 (recurrent, refractory)	PR in 1, SD in 7	Baumann, Gynecol Oncol, 2011; 123:27

long-term survivors showed IFN-γ production and an increase in the number of memory cells and TNF family ligands. Moreover, the therapy was likely to contribute to the survival of ovarian cancer patients by affecting the percentage of the regulatory T-cell subsets and by improving the number of memory CD4+ T cells.

13.2.1.2 Vaccine Therapy with p53 Peptide

Genetic aberrations of p53 and abnormal accumulation of p53 protein have been observed in the majority of serous ovarian cancers. In a cohort of stage III, stage IV, and recurrent ovarian cancer patients with no obvious disease, Rahma et al. compared one group directly administered with p53(264–272) peptide (group A) and another group administered with dendritic cells expressing the p53(264–272) peptide (group B) in a phase II study in the USA [10] and observed a tumor immune response in 69% of the group A patients and 83% of the group B patients. Progression-free survival (PFS) was 4.2 months and 8.7 months, respectively. Because there was no significant difference, they concluded that simple subcutaneous administration may be sufficient.

On the other hand, a Dutch research group conducted a phase II study for recurrent ovarian cancer by using a vaccine comprising a long-chain peptide of p53 (p53-synthetic long peptide, p53-SLP). Only two of the 20 cases showed stable disease, and they did not show a p53-specific immune response. The researchers concluded that there was no obvious effect of p53 peptide on improving the subsequent chemosensitivity or PFS [9, 10].

13.2.1.3 Immunotherapy Targeting HER2-Derived Peptide

Since HER2 is known to be highly expressed in many ovarian cancers, it is considered a good immunotherapy target. However, there was no significant clinical effect observed with by a vaccine using p369–p377 (Table 13.2). Although the trial or similar attempts using the DC vaccine are ongoing, a clinically useful vaccine has not been developed.

13.2.1.4 Vaccine Therapy Targeting WT-1

WT-1 is known to be expressed in more than half of serous ovarian cancers. A phase II trial use a WT-1 peptide as a vaccine against ovarian cancer has been performed in Japan. In 12 cases of treatment-resistant ovarian cancer, SD was noted in three cases, and the remaining nine cases were PD [11].

13.2.1.5 Active Immunotherapy Targeting CA-125

Because CA-125 is a specific protein that is expressed in a majority of ovarian cancers, it has been considered to be a good immunotherapy target. Aside from oregovomab (which will be discussed later), another potential immunotherapy for CA-125 includes the use of an anti-idiotypic antibody against the anti-CA-125 antibody ACA-125 (abagovomab). Since ACA-125 is structurally similar to CA-125, it was expected that abagovomab would elicit antitumor immunity against CA-125 if administered as a vaccine. Wagner et al. reported that in 42 patients with recurrent ovarian cancer, the immune response after administration of abagovomab (which was measured as the production of Ab3) was correlated with improved prognosis [12]. Reinartz et al. also reported that in 119 patients with ovarian cancer, individuals with a good immune response showed a significantly better outcome [13].

13.2.2 Passive Immunotherapy for Ovarian Cancer (Table 13.3)

13.2.2.1 Passive Immunotherapy with Anti-CA-125 Antibody

Large-scale development of the immunotherapy reagent oregovomab, a mouse monoclonal antibody B43.13 against CA-125, has been produced. The initial exploratory study showed that among the patients administered oregovomab, patients in whom anti-idiotypic antibodies (Ab2) and T-cell immunity have been induced showed a better tendency of prognosis and elicited the expected immunotherapeutic response to oregovomab (Table 13.3). Then, Berek et al. conducted a randomized phase II trial in which oregovomab was administered as a maintenance therapy to 145 patients with recurrent ovarian cancer after postoperative TC therapy.

This study showed that the PFS of patients with increased Ab2 levels was 18.8 months, while that of the cases with a weak immune reaction was 6.1 months; the PFS of the placebo group was 10.3 months [14]. Unfortunately, a phase III trial with 373 cases failed to reproduce the results of the phase II study [15]. Thus, a single use of oregovomab did not show an apparent clinical effect. However, another research group indicated that based on the results of a randomized phase II study of 40 cases of ovarian cancer, the combination of paclitaxel/carboplatin chemotherapy with oregovomab may augment antitumor immunity [16].

13.2.2.2 Immunotherapy with an Antibody Against the Folate Receptor

Elevated expression of folate receptor α, which is thought to be involved in cancer growth, has been shown in ovarian cancer as well as in many other cancers. A treatment effect with anti-folate receptor antibodies against ovarian cancer has been reported in expiratory clinical trials (Table 13.3). In 2007, MORAb-003 (farletuzumab), a humanized antibody against folate receptor, was developed by Morphotek, Inc. In the phase I study for platinum-resistant ovarian cancer, 36% of patients maintained SD [17]. Furthermore, phase II trials for platinum-sensitive and platinum-resistant ovarian cancer have been reported. Currently, a phase III trial using the combination of chemotherapy and farletuzumab is underway [18].

13.2.2.3 Immunotherapy Using Antibodies Against EpCAM and CD3

Another promising passive immunotherapy for ovarian cancer targets epithelial cell surface antigen (EpCAM). Catumaxomab is a double antibody against both EpCAM and CD3. Heiss et al. examined the inhibitory effect of catumaxomab on cancerous ascites and showed that the period to next puncture was significantly extended in the administration group [19]. Furthermore, Baumann et al. reported the clinical effect of catumaxomab in ovarian cancer [20] (Table 13.3).

13.2.3 Problems Toward the Development and Clinical Application of Immunotherapy

As described above, there have been continuous attempts to develop immunotherapy for ovarian cancer, and recently, clinical efficacy has been shown in some instances. However, despite a long history of immunotherapy against solid cancers, the effect of cancer immunotherapy has been limited because there are several problems in its development. Every time new knowledge of tumor immunity was discovered in the basic fields, the new idea of immunotherapy was usually evaluated in preclinical trials with animal experiments similar to the process of evaluating other anticancer reagents. In this step, in vivo mouse models play an important role as an immunotherapy model, but there is inherent problem with the use of mouse models as the evaluation system. The use of established cancer cell lines along with pure mouse strains is thought to mimic the immune reaction of human immunity. This experimental system has been established using cancer cell lines from a wide variety of organs. The effect of the immunotherapies is validated in animal models as the preclinical phase and is eventually administered to actual cancer patients in clinical trials. However, in most cases, only a small percentage of the patients show efficacy despite a marked effect in the animal experiments. One of the reasons is that the immune reaction is a highly complex biological phenomenon compared to chemotherapy agents. In the case of chemotherapy agents, a mouse model system using transplanted tumor has much in common with human cancers, and the effectiveness of a therapy in animal experiments may predict clinical efficacy. In contrast, animal models of cancer immunotherapy are only a simplified model of the true complex tumor immunity in humans, and there is a large gap between them. For example, an established murine cell line often grows rapidly in vivo, but human cancers can maintain a state of dormancy for years. Such differences may influence the evaluation of tumor immunity.

Second, the evaluation method in clinical trials is also challenging regarding the clinical efficacy of immunotherapy. With chemotherapy agents, evaluating the tumor size may be associated with long-term efficacy. However, in case of immunotherapy, an initial antitumor effect does not necessarily correspond to the final clinical efficacy. Compared to conventional chemotherapies, immunotherapy requires a longer time interval to elicit an antitumor effect. However, we are unaware of the exact signaling mechanisms in the immune system, and we do not have a reliable method to predict the final effect of immunotherapy. Similar to other molecularly targeted drugs, it is important to develop effective predictive biomarkers in order to efficiently implement immunotherapy.

13.3 Immune Checkpoint Inhibition in Ovarian Cancer

Several years ago, a novel immunotherapy attracted a great deal of attention. A therapy using an anti-PD-1 antibody, which inhibits the binding of PD-L1 to PD-1, was used for malignant melanoma, renal cancer, and lung cancer. The first trial showed that the antibody had a high antitumor effect not only in melanoma and renal cancer (which have high immunogenicity) but also in lung cancer, which is not considered to be immunogenic [21, 22].

13.3.1 Basic Mechanism of Function of Immune Checkpoint Molecules

Generally, an immune reaction to antigens (including cancers) is initiated with antigen recognition by antigen-presenting cells (APCs) such as dendritic cells (cognitive phase). Following antigen recognition, dendritic cells migrate to lymph nodes and present specific antigens to T cells via MHC class II molecules. As a result, T cells, including CD8-positive cytotoxic T cells, recognize the existence of cancer and become activated in a tumor-specific manner via the T-cell receptor (TCR). This

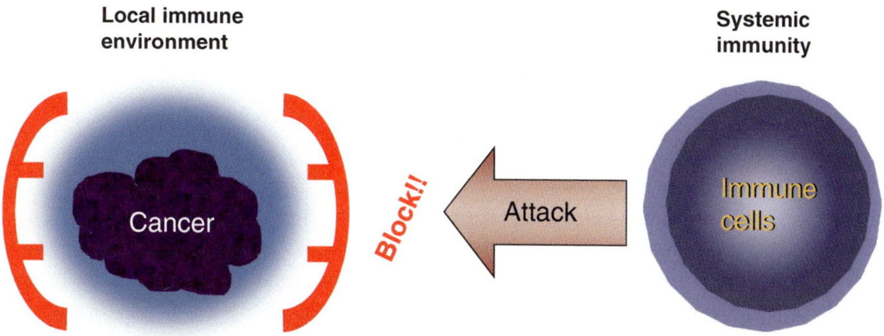

Fig. 13.1 Tumor immune escape hypothesis. This hypothesis is proposed to explain why systemic immunotherapy has not been successful. According to the hypothesis, by using unknown mechanism, e.g., expressing some immunoinhibitory molecules, tumor cells keep their local immune environment in immunosuppressive state. Therefore, even if we can successfully elicit potent systemic antitumor immunity, it does not effectively reach tumor cells

interaction between the MHCs on APCs and TCRs on T cells is called the "first signal." At the same time, a "second signal" is sent via interaction of specific molecules known as immune checkpoint molecules. If this interaction occurs between B7 and CD28, active immunity is initiated. In contrast, if the interaction occurs between B7 and CTLA-4 (cytotoxic T lymphocyte-associated protein 4), there is inhibition of the immune response [23].

This type of pro-/anti-immune mechanism also exists in local immunity when T cells recognize their targets (effector phase). During this phase, the interaction between PD-1 on T cells and PD-L1 on target cells is thought to result in the attenuation of the immune response. Therefore, if tumor cells express PD-L1, there is a reduction in the immune attack by T cells [24] (Fig. 13.1).

These immunoinhibitory molecules are considered to serve as cancer immune escape machinery; thus, inhibition of these signals is expected to be a target for potent immunotherapies (Fig. 13.1).

13.3.2 Immune Checkpoint Inhibition as a Cancer Immunotherapy

In 1999, clinical trials using the anti-CTLA-4 antibodies ipilimumab and tremelimumab were initiated [25, 26]. Ipilimumab is a humanized IgG1-type anti-CTLA-4 antibody and is currently used clinically to treat malignant melanoma. On the other hand, antibodies against PD-1/PD-L1 have been used in various cancers [6, 21, 22]. Nivolumab is a current treatment for malignant melanoma and lung cancer in Japan and the USA, and pembrolizumab has also been approved for use against these cancers in the USA. In addition, the anti-PD-L1 antibody atezolizumab is administered to treat urothelial cancer. At present, many immune checkpoint inhibitors are being developed and are expected to have clinical applications in the near future.

13.3.3 Rationale of Immune Checkpoint Inhibition in Ovarian Cancer

Failure of conventional cancer immunotherapies has brought forth the idea of an immune escape mechanism in tumors. According to this theory, cancer cells actively alter and attenuate their local micro-immune environment by expressing immunosuppressive molecules (Fig. 13.2a). Thus, simply strengthening the immunity of the whole body is insufficient to achieve a therapeutic effect due to the local immune escape mechanism (Fig. 13.1). We and other researchers have shown that the local immune environment, especially tumor infiltration of CD8+ T cells, is closely associated with outcome of patients with ovarian cancer [27–29]. Furthermore, we showed that PD-L1 expression in ovarian cancer is a prognostic factor for ovarian cancer, and its expression is negatively associated with CD8+ T-cell infiltration, suggesting that the expression of PD-L1 in tumor cells plays a major role in the suppression of local immunity [29].

In addition, we performed an in vivo study. When PD-L1 expression was knocked down in PD-L1-high mouse ovarian cancer cells, the cells became less immunogenic; moreover, in a mouse xenograft model, the tumor grew more rapidly, leading to shorter survival [30, 31].

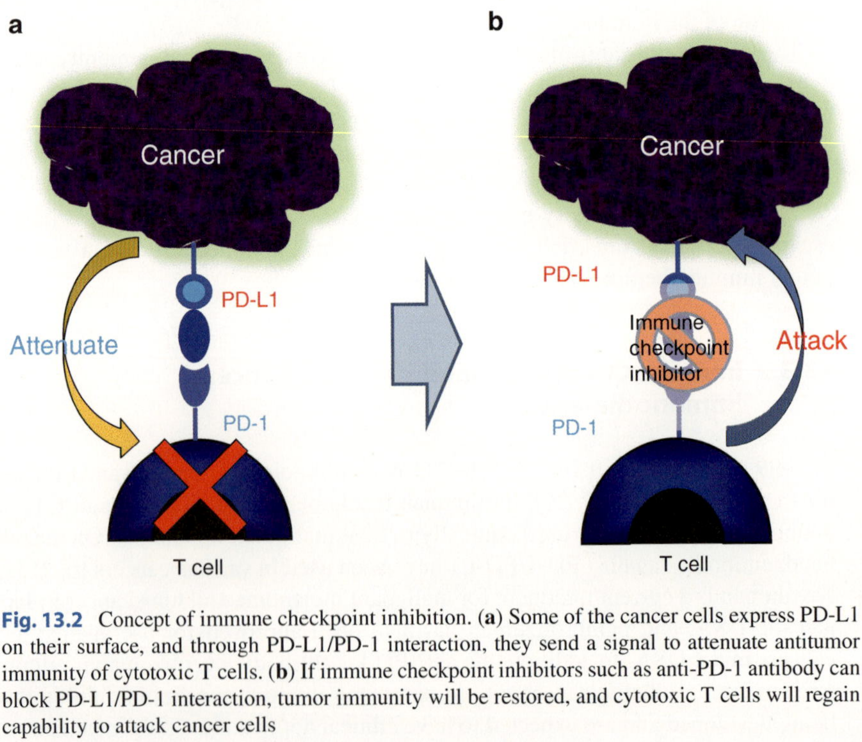

Fig. 13.2 Concept of immune checkpoint inhibition. (**a**) Some of the cancer cells express PD-L1 on their surface, and through PD-L1/PD-1 interaction, they send a signal to attenuate antitumor immunity of cytotoxic T cells. (**b**) If immune checkpoint inhibitors such as anti-PD-1 antibody can block PD-L1/PD-1 interaction, tumor immunity will be restored, and cytotoxic T cells will regain capability to attack cancer cells

Matsuzaki et al. reported that tumor-infiltrating NY-ESO-1-specific CD8+ T cells are negatively regulated by LAG-3 and PD-1 in human ovarian cancer [32]. Expression of LAG-3 and PD-1 on CD8+ T cells was upregulated by IL-10, IL-6, and tumor-derived antigen-presenting cells. Dual blockade of LAG-3 and PD-1 during T-cell priming efficiently augmented the proliferation of and cytokine production by NY-ESO-1-specific CD8+ T cells. Krempski et al. reported that tumor-infiltrating programmed death receptor-1+ dendritic cells mediate immunosuppression in ovarian cancer [33]. PD-1 blockade in mice bearing ovarian cancer cells substantially reduced the tumor burden and increased the effector Ag-specific T-cell responses. Thus, multiple basic/preclinical studies convinced us that inhibition of PD-L1/PD-1 signaling in ovarian cancer could be an effective treatment strategy (Fig. 13.2b).

13.3.4 Clinical Application of Immune Checkpoint Inhibitors in Ovarian Cancer (Table 13.4)

13.3.4.1 Clinical Trials Using Anti-PD-1 Antibodies

In 2010, we initiated the first clinical trial of nivolumab, a humanized anti-PD-1 antibody, for ovarian cancer. It was a principal investigator-initiated, phase II trial in patients with platinum-resistant refractory ovarian cancer [34]. A total of 20 patients were included, and they received one of two doses every 2 weeks up to 1 year: 1 mg/kg for ten patients and 3 mg/kg for ten patients. Among the 20 patients, the best overall response rate was 15% (2 CR and 1 PR), and the disease control rate was 45%. The

Table 13.4 Clinical trials for ovarian cancer—immune checkpoint inhibitor

Target	Antibody	Code name	Phase	Trial identifier	Company
CTLA-4	Ipilimumab	YervoyR, MDX-010	I, II	NCT01611558	Bristol–Myers Squibb
	Tremelimumab	Ticilimumab, CP-675,206	I	NCT01975831	MedImmune/ AstraZeneca
PD-1	Nivolumab	OpdivoR, BMS-936558, MDX1106	II	UMIN000005714	Bristol–Myers Squibb/Ono
	Pembrolizumab	KeytrudaR MK-3475, lambrolizumab	I	NCT02054806	Merck
	Pidilizumab	CT-011	I	NCT01386502	Cure Tech
	MEDI0680	AMP-514	I	NCT02013804	Amplimmune/ GlaxoSmithKline
PD-L1	MS-936559	MDX1105	I	NCT00729664	Bristol–Myers Squibb
	Atezolizumab	MPDL3280A	I	NCT02174172	Roche/Genentech
	Durvalumab	MEDI4736	I	NCT01693562	MedImmune/ AstraZeneca
	Avelumab	MSB0010718C	I	NCT01772004	Merck Serono/ Pfizer

median overall survival was 20.0 months, and the median PFS was 3.5 months at the end of trial. Two patients with CR showed no evidence of disease for over 1 year.

A phase Ib clinical trial of pembrolizumab, another humanized anti-PD-1 antibody, was conducted as part of the KEYNOTE-028 trial, which included 26 patients with recurrent ovarian cancer. In the interim analysis, response rate was 11.5% (1 CR and 2 PR), and the disease control rate was 34.6% [35].

13.3.4.2 Clinical Trials Using Anti-PD-L1 Antibodies

Avelumab is a human anti-PD-L1 antibody with naïve Fc receptor. A phase I trial for 75 patients with recurrent ovarian cancer was conducted [36]. The overall response rate was 10.7% (0 CR and 8 PR), and the disease control rate was 54.7%. Another phase I trial using a different human anti-PD-L1 antibody, BMS-936599, included 17 ovarian cancer patients, and the response rate was 6.9% (0 CR, 1 PR) [22].

In addition to these trials, many trials testing anti-PD-1 and anti-PD-L1 antibodies for ovarian cancer are ongoing, as shown in Table 13.1.

13.4 Problems with Current Trials of Immunotherapy

There is no doubt that immunotherapy has great potential and is a promising approach for future cancer treatments, including ovarian cancer, but there are also many issues to be addressed.

13.4.1 Biomarker to Predict Efficacy of Immune Checkpoint Inhibitors

Considering the extraordinarily high cost of immune checkpoint inhibitors, identifying the ideal patient who would most benefit from this treatment is mandatory. For this purpose, a search for effective biomarkers to identify patients who are expected to have favorable response is necessary. In ovarian cancer, clear cell histology is often associated with a chemoresistant phenotype. However, at least several cases in early trial have shown that a clear cell histology has a good response to immune checkpoint inhibitors [34]. Thus, the histology of ovarian cancers may not predict the response of these drugs.

The first biomarker candidate is the expression of PD-L1 on tumor cells. Studies have reported that PD-L1 expression on ovarian cancer cells is associated with worse prognosis [6, 29]. Moreover, several clinical trials studying melanoma and non-squamous cell lung cancer showed that PD-L1 expression was correlated with an antitumor response upon anti-PD-1 antibody treatment [6]. By contrast, PD-L1 expression was not shown to be predictive of a response in other trials, including a phase II ovarian cancer trial [34]. These conflicting data may be ascribed to the different anti-PD-L1 antibodies used to evaluate PD-L1 expression. However, it may also be possible that PD-L1 expression cannot serve as a predictive factor in some cancers. Further studies that either use multiple antibodies or standardize the evaluation methods are necessary.

Another promising candidate of predictive biomarkers is the so-called mutation burden of cancer cells. It is well known that the frequency of mutations is high in melanoma and lung cancer, in which immune checkpoint inhibition is effective. It was reported that in colorectal cancer patients, the treatment response was significantly better in patients with deficiencies in DNA mismatch repair [37]. There is currently no data on whether mutation burden could also serve as a predictive marker in ovarian cancer; however, BRCA gene mutations in ovarian cancer are associated with hypermutations within the tumors and clinically associated with a favorable outcome [38]. Therefore, BCRA may be a good candidate as a predictive biomarker of immune checkpoint inhibition.

13.4.2 How to Combine Novel Immunotherapies with Other Treatments

A realistic issue in the application of immunotherapies for clinical practice is how to combine them with other treatments, including conventional chemotherapy or molecularly targeted therapies. In ovarian cancer, the response rate of first-line chemotherapy is relatively high, and chemotherapy is thought to maintain its status as the primary treatment for ovarian cancer. Therefore, it is important to know whether a combination of chemotherapy and immunotherapy is more effective. By using a mouse model, we have shown that some chemotherapy reagents induce PD-L1 expression on cancer cells, and the combination of chemotherapy and anti-PD-L1 antibodies increases the efficacy of treatment, possibly by inducing a cytotoxic immune reaction after chemotherapy [39]. A phase II clinical trial of the combination of paclitaxel/carboplatin chemotherapy with pembrolizumab in ovarian cancer is ongoing (NCT02520154).

Other combinations of immunotherapy with radiation therapy, molecularly targeted reagents, and other cancer immunotherapies have also been considered. Preclinical studies indicated that radiotherapy can enhance the efficacy of the blockade of CTLA-4 and PD-1 [40, 41]. In addition, several clinical cases and retrospective studies suggest that radiotherapy may enhance the efficacy of the immune checkpoint blockade [42], and there are prospective trials underway to address this possibility. Molecularly targeted therapy is another emerging treatment for various cancers. A combination of this therapy with immune checkpoint inhibition is currently under investigation, but early reports indicate issues with adverse effects [43]. Several trials such as the combination of an anti-CTLA-4 antibody with a PARP inhibitor (NCT02571725) or an anti-PD-L1 antibody with bevacizumab (NCT02659384) are ongoing. Finally, one of the most promising combination strategies is the combination of two different immunotherapies. Concomitant CTLA-4 and PD-1 blockades in patients with melanoma resulted in a highly durable response rate and an impressive overall survival [44]. A phase II trial of the combination treatment of an anti-PD-L1 antibody and an anti-CTLA-4 antibody for ovarian cancer is underway (NCT02261220).

13.4.3 Handling Immune-Specific Adverse Events

With increasing data regarding immune checkpoint inhibition for various cancers, it is becoming clear that there are adverse effects specific to immunotherapy. Immune-specific adverse effects likely arise from general immunologic enhancement and thus include dermatological, gastrointestinal, hepatic, endocrine, and other less common inflammatory events [44, 45]. The most clinically relevant events are diarrhea/colitis, endocrinopathies affecting the pituitary, adrenal, and thyroid glands and pneumonitis. Treatments of these adverse effects generally involve temporary immunosuppression with corticosteroids, tumor necrosis factor-α antagonists, mycophenolate mofetil, or other agents [46]. However, no standard treatment strategy has been established. In addition, early detection and initiation of treatment against adverse reactions are believed to be important.

13.5 Conclusion: Future Directions

Immunotherapy, especially immune checkpoint inhibition targeting PD-1/PD-L1, has been shown to improve the outcome of patients with a variety of malignancies. Ovarian cancer is obviously another malignancy that should be examined to determine the efficacy of immune checkpoint inhibitors; presently, many clinical trials addressing this question are ongoing. One of the advantages of immunotherapies is their durability. Once the patient is responsive to immunotherapy, the patient is often cured instead of simply prolonging survival. However, there are still many obstacles to be solved in order to apply immunotherapy for the clinical management of ovarian cancer. First, considering the high cost of these drugs, we should attempt to find an effective biomarker (companion marker) to select patients. Second, we should become more familiar with immune-specific adverse effects, which are significantly different from those of chemotherapy. Third, we should pursue the best way to implement immunotherapies, especially regarding combinations with other treatments. To address these three problems, it is necessary to more thoroughly understand the biological consequences of immunotherapy in human cancers, including the use of basic research. Further understanding of the mechanisms involved in immunological manipulation may lead us to personalized and more finely tuned immunotherapy in the future (Fig. 13.3).

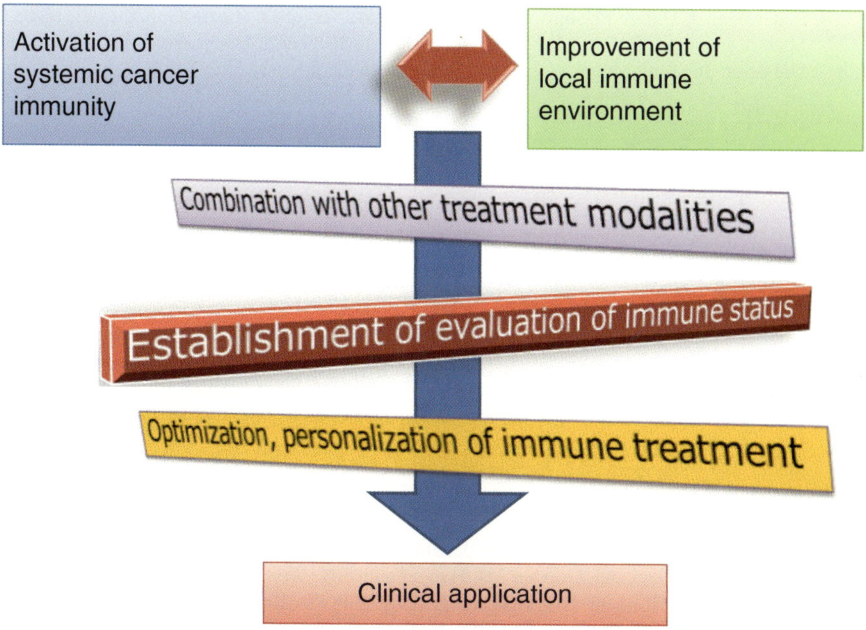

Fig. 13.3 Future direction of the cancer immunotherapy. Firstly, to obtain effective cancer immunotherapy, improvement of both systemic and local immunities is mandatory. Then, further combination with other cancer treatments including chemotherapy should be optimized. Establishment of evaluation method of tumor immunity is also important, which should lead to optimization and personalization of immunotherapy. As a result, we can apply immunotherapy in future daily practice

References

1. Burger RA, Brady MF, Bookman MA, Fleming GF, Monk BJ, Huang H, Mannel RS, Homesley HD, Fowler J, Greer BE, Boente M, Birrer MJ, Liang SX, Gynecologic Oncology Group. Incorporation of bevacizumab in the primary treatment of ovarian cancer. N Engl J Med. 2011;365:2473–83.
2. Poveda AM, Selle F, Hilpert F, Reuss A, Savarese A, Vergote I, Witteveen P, Bamias A, Scotto N, Mitchell L, Pujade-Lauraine E. Bevacizumab combined with weekly paclitaxel, pegylated liposomal doxorubicin, or topotecan in platinum-resistant recurrent ovarian cancer: analysis by chemotherapy cohort of the randomized phase III AURELIA trial. J Clin Oncol. 2015;33:3836–8.
3. Komiyama S, Katabuchi H, Mikami M, Nagase S, Okamoto A, Ito K, Morishige K, Nao Suzuki N, Kaneuchi M, Yaegashi N, Udagawa Y, Yoshikawa H, Japan Society of Gynecologic Oncology guidelines 2015 for the treatment of ovarian cancer including primary peritoneal cancer and fallopian tube cancer. Int J Clin Oncol 2016; 21:435–446.

4. Ledermann J, Harter P, Gourley C, Friedlander M, Vergote I, Rustin G, Scott CL, Meier W, Shapira-Frommer R, Safra T, Matei D, Fielding A, Spencer S, Dougherty B, Orr M, Hodgson D, Barrett JC, Matulonis U. Olaparib maintenance therapy in patients with platinum-sensitive relapsed serous ovarian cancer: a preplanned retrospective analysis of outcomes by BRCA status in a randomised phase 2 trial. Lancet Oncol. 2014;15:852–61.
5. Fujii S, Takayama T, Asakura M, Aki K, Fujimoto K, Shimizu K. Dendritic cell-based cancer immunotherapies. Arch Immunol Ther Exp. 2009;57:189–98.
6. Hamanishi J, Mandai M, Matsumura N, Abiko K, Baba T, Konishi I. PD-1/PD-L1 blockade in cancer treatment: perspectives and issues. Int J Clin Oncol. 2016;21:462–73.
7. Mandai M, Hamanishi J, Abiko K, Matsumura N, Baba T, Konishi I. Anti-PD-L1/PD-1 immune therapies in ovarian cancer: basic mechanism and future clinical application. Int J Clin Oncol. 2016;21:456–61.
8. Dobrzanski MJ, Rewers-Felkins KA, Samad KA, Quinlin IS, Phillips CA, Robinson W, Dobrzanski DJ, Wright SE. Immunotherapy with IL-10- and IFN-γ-producing CD4 effector cells modulate "natural" and "inducible" CD4 TReg cell subpopulation levels: observations in four cases of patients with ovarian cancer. Cancer Immunol Immunother. 2012;61:839–54.
9. Rahma OE, Ashtar E, Czystowska M, Szajnik ME, Wieckowski E, Bernstein S, Herrin VE, Shams MA, Steinberg SM, Merino M, Gooding W, Visus C, Deleo AB, Wolf JK, Bell JG, Berzofsky JA, Whiteside TL, Khleif SN. A gynecologic oncology group phase II trial of two p53 peptide vaccine approaches: subcutaneous injection and intravenous pulsed dendritic cells in high recurrence risk ovarian cancer patients. Cancer Immunol Immunother. 2012;61:373–84.
10. Leffers N, Lambeck AJ, Gooden MJ, Hoogeboom BN, Wolf R, Hamming IE, Hepkema BG, Willemse PH, Molmans BH, Hollema H, Drijfhout JW, Sluiter WJ, Valentijn AR, Fathers LM, Oostendorp J, van der Zee AG, Melief CJ, van der Burg SH, Daemen T, Nijman HW. Immunization with a P53 synthetic long peptide vaccine induces P53-specific immune responses in ovarian cancer patients, a phase II trial. Int J Cancer. 2009;125:2104–13.
11. Ohno S, Kyo S, Myojo S, Dohi S, Ishizaki J, Miyamoto K, Morita S, Sakamoto J, Enomoto T, Kimura T, Oka Y, Tsuboi A, Sugiyama H, Inoue M. Wilms' tumor 1 (WT1) peptide immunotherapy for gynecological malignancy. Anticancer Res. 2009;29:4779–84.
12. Wagner U, Köhler S, Reinartz S, Giffels P, Huober J, Renke K, Schlebusch H, Biersack HJ, Möbus V, Kreienberg R, Bauknecht T, Krebs D, Wallwiener D. Immunological consolidation of ovarian carcinoma recurrences with monoclonal anti-idiotype antibody ACA125: immune responses and survival in palliative treatment. Clin Cancer Res. 2001;7:1154–62.
13. Reinartz S, Köhler S, Schlebusch H, Krista K, Giffels P, Renke K, Huober J, Möbus V, Kreienberg R, DuBois A, Sabbatini P, Wagner U. Vaccination of patients with advanced ovarian carcinoma with the anti-idiotype ACA125: immunological response and survival (phase Ib/II). Clin Cancer Res. 2004;10:1580–7.
14. Berek JS, Taylor PT, Gordon A, Cunningham MJ, Finkler N, Orr J Jr, Rivkin S, Schultes BC, Whiteside TL, Nicodemus CF. Randomized, placebo-controlled study of oregovomab for consolidation of clinical remission in patients with advanced ovarian cancer. J Clin Oncol. 2004;22:3507–16.
15. Berek J, Taylor P, McGuire W, Smith LM, Schultes B, Nicodemus CF. Oregovomab maintenance monoimmunotherapy does not improve outcomes in advanced ovarian cancer. J Clin Oncol. 2009;27:418–25.
16. Braly P, Nicodemus CF, Chu C, Collins Y, Edwards R, Gordon A, McGuire W, Schoonmaker C, Whiteside T, Smith LM, Method M. The immune adjuvant properties of front-line carboplatin-paclitaxel: a randomized phase 2 study of alternative schedules of intravenous oregovomab chemoimmunotherapy in advanced ovarian cancer. J Immunother. 2009;32:54–65.
17. Konner JA, Bell-McGuinn KM, Sabbatini P, Hensley ML, Tew WP, Pandit-Taskar N, Vander Els N, Phillips MD, Schweizer C, Weil SC, Larson SM, Old LJ. Farletuzumab, a humanized monoclonal antibody against folate receptor alpha, in epithelial ovarian cancer: a phase I study. Clin Cancer Res. 2010;16:5288–95.

18. Jelovac D, Armstrong DK. Role of farletuzumab in epithelial ovarian carcinoma. Curr Pharm Des. 2012;18:3812–5.
19. Heiss MM, Murawa P, Koralewski P, Kutarska E, Kolesnik OO, Ivanchenko VV, Dudnichenko AS, Aleknaviciene B, Razbadauskas A, Gore M, Ganea-Motan E, Ciuleanu T, Wimberger P, Schmittel A, Schmalfeldt B, Burges A, Bokemeyer C, Lindhofer H, Lahr A, Parsons SL. The trifunctional antibody catumaxomab for the treatment of malignant ascites due to epithelial cancer: results of a prospective randomized phase II/III trial. Int J Cancer. 2010;127:2209–21.
20. Baumann K, Pfisterer J, Wimberger P, Burchardi N, Kurzeder C, du Bois A, Loibl S, Sehouli J, Huober J, Schmalfeldt B, Vergote I, Lück HJ, Wagner U. Intraperitoneal treatment with the trifunctional bispecific antibody Catumaxomab in patients with platinum-resistant epithelial ovarian cancer: a phase IIa study of the AGO Study Group. Gynecol Oncol. 2011;123:27–32.
21. Topalian SL, Hodi FS, Brahmer JR, Gettinger SN, Smith DC, McDermott DF, Powderly JD, Carvajal RD, Sosman JA, Atkins MB, Leming PD, Spigel DR, Antonia SJ, Horn L, Drake CG, Pardoll DM, Chen L, Sharfman WH, Anders RA, Taube JM, McMiller TL, Xu H, Korman AJ, Jure-Kunkel M, Agrawal S, McDonald D, Kollia GD, Gupta A, Wigginton JM, Sznol M. Safety, activity, and immune correlates of anti-PD-1 antibody in cancer. N Engl J Med. 2012;366:2443–54.
22. Brahmer JR, Tykodi SS, Chow LQ, Hwu WJ, Topalian SL, Hwu P, Drake CG, Camacho LH, Kauh J, Odunsi K, Pitot HC, Hamid O, Bhatia S, Martins R, Eaton K, Chen S, Salay TM, Alaparthy S, Grosso JF, Korman AJ, Parker SM, Agrawal S, Goldberg SM, Pardoll DM, Gupta A, Wigginton JM. Safety and activity of anti-PD-L1 antibody in patients with advanced cancer. N Engl J Med. 2012;366:2455–65.
23. Chen L, Flies DB. Molecular mechanisms of T cell co-stimulation and co-inhibition. Nat Rev Immunol. 2013;13:227–42.
24. Hamanishi J, Mandai M, Konishi I. Immune checkpoint inhibition in ovarian cancer. Int Immunol. 2016;28:339–48.
25. Hodi FS, O'Day SJ, McDermott DF, Weber RW, Sosman JA, Haanen JB, Gonzalez R, Robert C, Schadendorf D, Hassel JC, Akerley W, van den Eertwegh AJ, Lutzky J, Lorigan P, Vaubel JM, Linette GP, Hogg D, Ottensmeier CH, Lebbé C, Peschel C, Quirt I, Clark JI, Wolchok JD, Weber JS, Tian J, Yellin MJ, Nichol GM, Hoos A, Urba WJ. Improved survival with ipilimumab in patients with metastatic melanoma. N Engl J Med. 2010;363:711–23.
26. Calabrò L, Morra A, Fonsatti E, Cutaia O, Fazio C, Annesi D, Lenoci M, Amato G, Danielli R, Altomonte M, Giannarelli D, Di Giacomo AM, Maio M. Efficacy and safety of an intensified schedule of tremelimumab for chemotherapy-resistant malignant mesothelioma: an open-label, single-arm, phase 2 study. Lancet Respir Med. 2015;3:301–9.
27. Zhang L, Conejo-Garcia JR, Katsaros D, Gimotty PA, Massobrio M, Regnani G, Makrigiannakis A, Gray H, Schlienger K, Liebman MN, Rubin SC, Coukos G. Intratumoral T cells, recurrence, and survival in epithelial ovarian cancer. N Engl J Med. 2003;348:203–13.
28. Sato E, Olson SH, Ahn J, Bundy B, Nishikawa H, Qian F, Jungbluth AA, Frosina D, Gnjatic S, Ambrosone C, Kepner J, Odunsi T, Ritter G, Lele S, Chen YT, Ohtani H, Old LJ, Odunsi K. Intraepithelial CD8+ tumor-infiltrating lymphocytes and a high CD8+/regulatory T cell ratio are associated with favorable prognosis in ovarian cancer. Proc Natl Acad Sci U S A. 2005;102:18538–43.
29. Hamanishi J, Mandai M, Iwasaki M, Okazaki T, Tanaka Y, Yamaguchi K, Higuchi T, Yagi H, Takakura K, Minato N, Honjo T, Fujii S. Programmed cell death 1 ligand 1 and tumor-infiltrating CD8+ T lymphocytes are prognostic factors of human ovarian cancer. Proc Natl Acad Sci U S A. 2007;104:3360–5.
30. Abiko K, Mandai M, Hamanishi J, Yoshioka Y, Matsumura N, Baba T, Yamaguchi K, Murakami R, Yamamoto A, Kharma B, Kosaka K, Konishi I. PD-L1 on tumor cells is induced in ascites and promotes peritoneal dissemination of ovarian cancer through CTL dysfunction. Clin Cancer Res. 2013;19:1363–74.

31. Abiko K, Matsumura N, Hamanishi J, Horikawa N, Murakami R, Yamaguchi K, Yoshioka Y, Baba T, Konishi I, Mandai M. IFN-γ from lymphocytes induces PD-L1 expression and promotes progression of ovarian cancer. Br J Cancer. 2015;112:1501–9.
32. Matsuzaki J, Gnjatic S, Mhawech-Fauceglia P, Beck A, Miller A, Tsuji T, Eppolito C, Qian F, Lele S, Shrikant P, Old LJ, Odunsi K. Tumor-infiltrating NY-ESO-1-specific CD8+ T cells are negatively regulated by LAG-3 and PD-1 in human ovarian cancer. Proc Natl Acad Sci U S A. 2010;107:7875–80.
33. Krempski J, Karyampudi L, Behrens MD, Erskine CL, Hartmann L, Dong H, Goode EL, Kalli KR, Knutson KL. Tumor-infiltrating programmed death receptor-1+ dendritic cells mediate immune suppression in ovarian cancer. J Immunol. 2011;186:6905–13.
34. Hamanishi J, Mandai M, Ikeda T, Minami M, Kawaguchi A, Murayama T, Kanai M, Mori Y, Matsumoto S, Chikuma S, Matsumura N, Abiko K, Baba T, Yamaguchi K, Ueda A, Hosoe Y, Morita S, Yokode M, Shimizu A, Honjo T, Konishi I. Safety and antitumor activity of anti-PD-1 antibody, nivolumab, in patients with platinum-resistant ovarian cancer. J Clin Oncol. 2015;33:4015–22.
35. Varga A, Piha-Paul SA, Ott PA, et al. Antitumor activity and safety of pembrolizumab in patients with PD-L1 positive advanced ovarian cancer: interim result from a phase Ib study. J Clin Oncol. 2015;33(Suppl.): Abstract no. 5510.
36. Dsis ML, Patel MR, Pant S et al. Avelumab (MSB0010718C), an anti-PD-L1 antibody, in patient with previously treated, recurrent or refractory ovarian cancer: a phase Ib, open-label expansion trial. J Clin Oncol. 2015;33(Suppl.): Abstract no. 5509.
37. Le DT, Uram JN, Wang H, Bartlett BR, Kemberling H, Eyring AD, Skora AD, Luber BS, Azad NS, Laheru D, Biedrzycki B, Donehower RC, Zaheer A, Fisher GA, Crocenzi TS, Lee JJ, Duffy SM, Goldberg RM, de la Chapelle A, Koshiji M, Bhaijee F, Huebner T, Hruban RH, Wood LD, Cuka N, Pardoll DM, Papadopoulos N, Kinzler KW, Zhou S, Cornish TC, Taube JM, Anders RA, Eshleman JR, Vogelstein B, Diaz LA Jr. PD-1 blockade in tumors with mismatch-repair deficiency. N Engl J Med. 2015;372:2509–20.
38. Birkbak NJ, Kochupurakkal B, Izarzugaza JM, Eklund AC, Li Y, Liu J, Szallasi Z, Matulonis UA, Richardson AL, Iglehart JD, Wang ZC. Tumor mutation burden forecasts outcome in ovarian cancer with BRCA1 or BRCA2 mutations. PLoS One. 2013;8:e80023.
39. Peng J, Hamanishi J, Matsumura N, Abiko K, Murat K, Baba T, Yamaguchi K, Horikawa N, Hosoe Y, Murphy SK, Konishi I, Mandai M. Chemotherapy induces programmed cell death-ligand 1 overexpression via the nuclear factor-κB to foster an immunosuppressive tumor microenvironment in ovarian cancer. Cancer Res. 2015;75:5034–45.
40. Demaria S, Kawashima N, Yang AM, et al. Immune-mediated inhibition of metastases after treatment with local radiation and CTLA-4 blockade in a mouse model of breast cancer. Clin Cancer Res. 2005;11:728–34.
41. Deng L, Liang H, Burnette B, et al. Irradiation and anti-PD-L1 treatment synergistically promote antitumor immunity in mice. J Clin Invest. 2014;124:687–95.
42. Grimaldi AM, Simeone E, Giannarelli D, et al. Abscopal effects of radiotherapy on advanced melanoma patients who progressed after ipilimumab immunotherapy. Oncoimmunology. 2014;3:e28780.
43. Ribas A, Hodi FS, Callahan M, et al. Hepatotoxicity with combination of vemurafenib and ipilimumab. N Engl J Med. 2013;368:1365–6.
44. Wolchok JD, Kluger H, Callahan MK, et al. Nivolumab plus ipilimumab in advanced melanoma. N Engl J Med. 2013;369:122–33.
45. Marrone KA, Ying W, Naidoo J. Immune-related adverse events from immune checkpoint inhibitors. Clin Pharmacol Ther. 2016;100:242–51.
46. Champiat S, Lambotte O, Barreau E, Belkhir R, Berdelou A, Carbonnel F, Cauquil C, Chanson P, Collins M, Durrbach A, Ederhy S, Feuillet S, François H, Lazarovici J, Le Pavec J, De Martin E, Mateus C, Michot JM, Samuel D, Soria JC, Robert C, Eggermont A, Marabelle A. Management of immune checkpoint blockade dysimmune toxicities: a collaborative position paper. Ann Oncol. 2016;27:559–74.

Treatment of Recurrent Epithelial Ovarian Cancer

14

Shintaro Yanazume and Hiroaki Kobayashi

Abstract

Recurrent ovarian cancer (ROC) treatment is drawing attention and treatment strategies appear to be changing. Although an average response rate of 70% was achieved in initial treatment through aggressive operations leading to optimal resection followed by chemotherapy, most patients in advanced disease stages recurred within 2 years. Multiple-line clinical trials, including newly proposed targeted therapies, are ongoing and are steadily proving positive survival outcomes. Thus, the role of secondary cytoreductive surgery is being reassessed accordingly. The goal of treatment in ROC is prolonged survival without decreasing quality of life. In the near future, there may be a chance to expect the treatment leading to complete cure in ROC. However, the financial burden of continually increasing prices suffers patients with the expectancy of life prolongation. Besides costs, treatment choices of ROC should consider complex factors such as platinum agent efficacy, germline mutation, drug toxicities, disease spread, and treatment convenience. Finally, treatment of recurrence should be individually tailored to each patient with the intention of securing a high quality of life.

Keywords

Recurrent ovarian cancer • Platinum-sensitive relapse • Platinum-resistant relapse

14.1 Introduction

Although initial multimodality therapy for advanced stages of ovarian cancer is commonly effective, 55% of patients recurred within 2 years, and over 70% relapsed within 5 years [1]. The 5-year overall survival (OS) rates for patients with ovarian

S. Yanazume, M.D., Ph.D. • H. Kobayashi, M.D., Ph.D. (✉)
Department of Obstetrics and Gynecology, Faculty of Medicine, Kagoshima University,
8-35-1 Sakuragaoka, Kagoshima 890-8520, Japan
e-mail: hirokoba@m2.kufm.kagoshima-u.ac.jp

H. Katabuchi (ed.), *Frontiers in Ovarian Cancer Science*, Comprehensive Gynecology and Obstetrics, DOI 10.1007/978-981-10-4160-0_14

cancer were 48.1% for stage III and 29.4% for stage IV [2]. Ovarian cancer recurrence was incapable of being cured; therefore the treatment goals were possibly prolonged survival, improved quality of life (QOL), and controlled the cancer-related symptoms [3]. The proper treatment should be determined by evaluating several factors including symptom, extent and location of the disease, the number of metastasis, treatment toxicity, and treatment convenience. Recently, the treatment strategy should be generally tailored depending on factors such as BRCA mutation when using the poly(ADP-ribose) polymerase inhibitor (PARPi) in high-grade serous ovarian cancer (HGSOC).

An outline of ROC treatment strategy is described in Fig. 14.1, which was a modified Japanese version of Japan Society of Gynecologic Oncology guidelines 2015 for the treatment of ovarian cancer. Chemotherapy is the main treatment for ROC and is composed of some commonly used cytotoxic agents including cisplatin, carboplatin, paclitaxel, docetaxel, irinotecan, topotecan, gemcitabine, liposomal doxorubicin, and etoposide. Recently, antiangiogenic agents, PARPi, and immune checkpoint inhibitors are attracting the most attention. Second-line chemotherapy offers a significant benefit in treating ROC, but lower response rates (RR) and shorter clinical remission than first-line chemotherapy have been reported. Its benefit depends on the initial RR and progression-free survival (PFS) after completion of a platinum-containing prior regimen. In regard to the selection of the effective chemotherapy, the interval between the completion of the previous platinum regimen and the start of treatment, "platinum-free interval" (PFI), is the most reliable predictor. Recurrence with the PFI under 6 months is classified as "platinum resistant," PFI within 6–12 months are classified as "partially platinum sensitive," and PFI over 12 months are classified as "fully platinum sensitive." Each RR is ≤10%, 27–33%, and 44–84%, respectively, whereas PFS is <6 months in platinum resistant and 6–13 months in sensitive groups [4–8]. The 5-year survival for ovarian cancer significantly increased from 36% during 1975–1977 to 45% during 2004–2010 [9]. Recent improvement in multiple lines of chemotherapy, surgical procedures, and supportive care has increased survival rate in ROC (Table 14.1). In some clinical trials for ROC, PFS is set as a primary endpoint because the results of OS data are likely to be affected by confounding factors involving multiple and effective post-progression therapy [10].

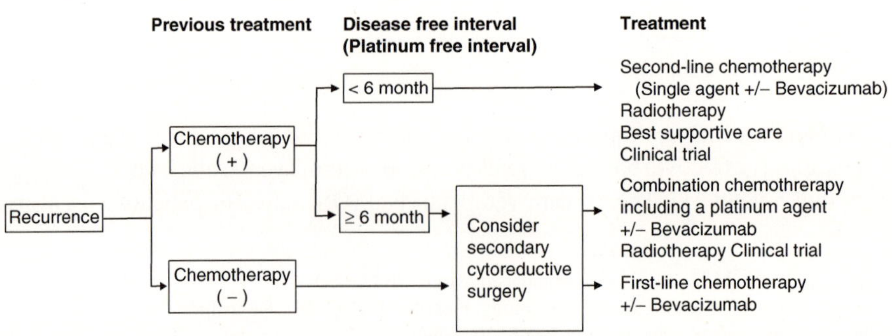

Fig. 14.1 Treatment strategy of recurrent epithelial ovarian cancer

14.2 Platinum-Sensitive Recurrent Ovarian Cancer

14.2.1 Chemotherapy for Platinum-Sensitive Disease

Several reports are proving the significance of secondary debulking surgery (SDS) in patients with sensitive recurrence (≥6 months) [11, 12], and the National Comprehensive Cancer Network (NCCN) guidelines of ovarian cancer [13] provide the possible benefit of SDS for the patient before considering the selection of chemotherapeutic agent. Platinum-based combination chemotherapy is superior in the patients with recurrence ≥6 months after first-line chemotherapy, and combination therapy including a platinum agent is strongly recommended in guidelines [7, 13–15]. Currently, the most commonly recommended regimens for platinum-sensitive patients are paclitaxel plus carboplatin (TC), gemcitabine plus carboplatin (GC), and pegylated liposomal doxorubicin plus carboplatin (PLD-C) [7, 8, 14, 16].

A phase III trial of ICON4 and AGO-OVAR-2.2 proved paclitaxel plus platinum agent improved OS (hazard ratio (HR) 0.82; 95% CI 0.69–0.97, $p = 0.02$) and PFS (HR 0.76, $p = 0.0004$) better than conventional platinum-based therapy with a median follow-up of 42 months. The 2-year OS rate of the paclitaxel group significantly improved 7% over the conventional treatment groups (57% vs. 50%), and median survival increased an average of 5 months (29 vs. 24 months). The 1-year PFS rate also improved with a significance of 10% (50% vs. 40%) and a median PFS increase of 3 months (13 vs. 10 months) in the paclitaxel regimen [7]. A comparison between the administration of TC versus carboplatin in platinum-sensitive ROC patients showed a significant difference in the RR in favor of the TC group (75.6% vs. 50%) of the phase II trial in 78 patients [14]. Although mucositis, alopecia, myalgia/arthralgia, and peripheral neuropathy were more frequent in the paclitaxel-containing group, no significant differences were observed in grades 3–4 hematological toxicity. The median time to progression was superior in the combination group (49.1 vs. 33.7 weeks, $p = 0.021$).

Another phase III randomized controlled trial (RCT) study by Gynecologic Cancer InterGroup (GCIG) compared the use of carboplatin alone versus GC in platinum-sensitive ROC [8]. With a median follow-up of 17 months, GC treatment significantly improves the median PFS (8.6 vs. 5.8 months; HR 0.72, $p = 0.0032$) of patients. The RR for the GC was higher than carboplatin (47.2% vs. 30.9%, $p = 0.0016$), and patients treated with GC showed significant improvement in symptomatic participants such as abdominal pain. OS was not precisely analyzed due to a lack of statistical power.

A large number of 975 patients joined the phase III RCT of CARIPSO [16, 17], the purpose of which was the evaluation for the efficacy and safety of the combination of PLD with carboplatin (CD) compared with standard TC against platinum-sensitive ROC. PFS for the CD was statistically superior to the TC arm (HR, 0.821; $p = 0.005$); median PFS was 11.3 versus 9.4 months, respectively. However, in the final analysis of OS, median survival times were 30.7 months in the CD and 33.0 months in the TC (HR, 0.99; $p = 0.005$). Non-prolonged OS probably originated in the fact that 90% of patients in either arm of CALYPSO underwent post-study therapy, and a majority (68%) of the patients with TC received a crossover of

Table 14.1 Important clinical trials for recurrent ovarian cancer

Study (y)	Drug	*n*	Primary endpoint	RR(%)	PFS(M)	OS(M)	Comments
Platinum-sensitive disease							
Parmar MK et al. (2003)[7]	Platinum (71%: Carboplatin, 17%: CAP)	410	OS	54	13	29	OS was significant (HR 0.82; 95% CI 0.69-0.97; $p = 0.02$). PFS was significant (HR 0.76; 95% CI 0.66-0.89; $p = 0.0004$)
ICON4/OVAR2.2	Platinum+Taxane (80%: TC, 10%: TP)	392		66	10	24	
Pfisterer J et al. (2005) [8]	Carboplatin	178	PFS	47	8.6		PFS was significant (HR 0.72; 95% CI 0.58-0.90; $p = 0.0032$). HR for OS was 0.96 (95% CI 0.75-1.23; $p = 0.7349$).
OVAR2.5	Carboplatin+Gemcitabine	178		31	5.8		
Pujade-Lauraine E et al. (2010)[16]	Carboplatin + Pegylated liposomal doxorubicin	466	PFS	21	11.3	30.7	Test for noninferiority of CD yielding $p < 0.001$.
CALYPSO trial	Pegylated liposomal doxorubicin+Paclitaxel	501		20	9.4	33	
Monk BJ et al. (2010)(2012)[20]	Pegylated liposomal doxorubicin	335	PFS	18.8	5.8	18.9	The trial included 35% platinum-resistant disease. Platinum-sensitive PFS; 9.2M vs7.5M (HR 0.73; 95% CI 0.56-0.95; p = .0170)
	Pegylated liposomal doxorubicin+Trabectedin	337		27.6	7.3	22.2	
Aghajanian C et al. (2012)(2015)[24, 25]	Carboplatin+Gemcitabine	233	PFS	57.4	8.4	32.9	PFS was significant (HR, 0.484; 95% CI 0.388-0.605; $p < 0.0001$). OS was insignificant (HR 0.95; $p = 0.65$)
OCEANS trial	Carboplatin+Gemcitabine+Bevacizumab	247		78.5	12.4	33.6	

Ledermann et al. (2012)[34]	Platinum based chemotherapy	129	PFS		4.8	27.8	Both PFS and OS were significant. In cohort of BRCA mutation was significant (OS:34.9 vs 30.2 months; HR 0·62; $p = 0.025$). In cohort of BRCA wild-type was insignificant (OS:24.5 months with olaparib vs 26.6 months with placebo; HR 0.83 ; $p = 0.37$).
	Platinum based chemotherapy+ maintenance olaparib	136			8.4	29.8	
Liu et al. (2014)[38]	Olaparib	46	PFS		9		PFS was significant (HR 0.42; 95% CI 0·23-0·76; $p = 0{\cdot}005$).
	Olaparib+Cediranib	44			17.7		
Oza A et al. (2015)[28]	Carboplatin+Paclitaxel	75	PFS		9.6		PFS was significant (HR 0.51; $p = 0.0012$), and also significantly improved PFS in BRCA-mutated patients(HR 0.21; $p = 0.0015$). Final OS did not differ between each arm even by the subset analysis only for BRCA mutated patients.
	Carboplatin+Paclitaxel+maintenance olaparib	81			12.2		
Ledermann J et al. (2016)[81]	Platinum based chemotherapy	118	PFS		8.7		

(continued)

Table 14.1 (continued)

Study (y)	Drug	*n*	Primary endpoint	RR(%)	PFS(M)	OS(M)	Comments
ICON6	Platinum based chemotherapy+ cediranib	174			9.9		PFS of maintenance cediranib was more significant than only plainum based chemotherapy (HR 0.56, 95% CI, 0.44–0.72, $p < 0{\cdot}0001$).
	Platinum based chemotherapy+ cediranib+maintenance cediranib	164			11		
Mirza MR et al. (2016) [40]	Platinum based chemotherapy	gBRCA: 65	PFS		5.5		The niraparib group had a significantly longer PFS than the placebo group, regardless of presence (gBRCA cohort, median PFS, 21.0 vs 5.5 months; HR, 0.27) or absence (non-gBRCA without HRD cohort, median PFS, 9.3 vs 3.9 months; HR, 0.45) of gBRCA mutation or HRD status
ENGOT-ov16/NOVA		non-gBRCA:116			3.9		
	Platinum based chemotherapy+niraparib	gBRCA: 138			21		
		non-gBRCA:234			9.3		

Platinum-resistant disease								
Naumann RW et al. (2013)	Pegylated liposomal doxorubicin	31		PFS	15	12		PFS was significant (HR 0.63; 95% CI, 0.41-0.96 ; $p = 0.031$).
PRECEDENT trial	Pegylated liposomal doxorubicin+vintafolide	60			17	22		
Monk BJ et al. (2013) [85, 86]	Weekly-paclitaxel	458		PFS	30	5.4	17.3	PFS was significant (HR 0.66; 95% CI 0·57–0·77; $p < 0{\cdot}0001$). OS was insignificant
TRINOVA 1 trial	Weekly-paclitaxel+trebananib	461			38	7.2	19	
Pujade-Lauraine et al. (2014)[75, 76]	Pegylated liposomal doxorubicin/topotecan/ Weekly-paclitaxel	182		PFS	12	3.4	13.3	PFS was significant (HR 0.484; $p < 0.001$). Overall RR; $p = 0.001$. OS was Insignificant (HR 0.85).
AURELIA trial	Pegylated liposomal doxorubicin/topotecan/ Weekly-paclitaxel+bevacizumab	179			31	6.7	16.6	

RR Response rates, *PFS* Progression-free survival, *OS* Overall survival, *CAP* Cyclophosphamide + adriamycin + cisplatin, *TC* Carboplatin + paclitaxel, *TP* Cisplatin + paclitaxel, *HR* Hazard ratio, *CD* Carboplatin + pegylated liposomal doxorubicin, *HRD* Homologous recombination deficiency

PLD as post-study therapy. The significant influence factors for OS include TFI ≥ 12 months, ECOG PS 0, CA125 < 100Uml, nonmeasurable disease, and one disease site.

CD was reassessed in Japanese patients during a phase II trial in platinum-sensitive ROC [18]. Although the most frequent grades 3–4 toxicities were neutropenia (82%), thrombocytopenia (51%), and anemia (17%), severe non-hematological toxicities were not found. The efficacy of CD reported that 82% of the patients with evaluable CA-125 achieved ≥50% reduction compared with pretreatment results. The overall RR was 52%, and the survival outcomes were almost even (the median PFS and OS rates were 10.7 and 38.8 months) compared to the previous study [16–18].

Adverse effects in both combination regimens were reported. CD was associated with palmar-plantar erythrodysesthesia (PPE) (12 vs. 2.2%) and grades 3–4 thrombocytopenia (15.9 vs. 6.2%). TC was associated with consistent toxicities including alopecia (83.6 vs. 7%), grade 2 or higher neuropathy (26.9 vs. 4.9%), and neutropenia (45.7 vs. 35.2%). Hypersensitivity reaction (HSR) was a serious complication for taxane- and platinum-accumulative patients. A higher percentage of associated ≥ grade 2 HSR occurred in the TC (18.8%) or only carboplatin (23%) groups, whereas CD-induced HSR was only 0–5.6%. Although the mechanism is still unclear, the additional PLD likely reduced HSR [16, 19].

Regarding the non-platinum agent effective for platinum-sensitive ROC, a marine-derived antineoplastic agent of trabectedin was compellingly proved by an OVA-301 phase III RCT under the comparison between trabectedin plus PLD and PLD alone against ROC. This study revealed that median PFS was superior in the group containing trabectedin (7.3 vs. 5.8 months, HR, 0.79; 95% CI, 0.65 to 0.96; $p = 0.019$), although OS was not significant ($p = 0.151$). This study included platinum-resistant (PFI < 6 months)/platinum-sensitive (PFI ≥ 6 months) recurrences. Notably, subsequent analysis of partially sensitive recurrence (PFI from 6 to 12 months) OS in addition to PFS significantly favored the trabectedin plus PLD combination (HR 0.65; 95% CI, 0.45–0.92; $p = 0.0152$) [20, 21].

14.2.2 Targeted Therapies for Platinum-Sensitive Disease

14.2.2.1 Antiangiogenic Agents for Platinum-Sensitive Disease

An angiogenic inhibitor of bevacizumab is a monoclonal antibody against vascular endothelial growth factor (VEGF) and inhibits activity of human VEGF to reduce neovascularization, inhibit tumor growth, and decrease ascite formation. Bevacizumab is the molecular targeted agent, which was initially well proven to have a therapeutic effect for both primary and recurrent ovarian cancers.

Regarding the administration of bevacizumab in ROC, a phase II trial GOG 170 including 41% of platinum-sensitive disease firstly reported the efficacy and tolerability of single-agent bevacizumab. RR was 21%; an additional 52% was reported as stable disease, and 40% were progression-free for a duration of at least 6 months. Platinum sensitivity and prior chemotherapy regimens were not significant influences for PFS under the intravenous bevacizumab therapy [22, 23].

OCEANS is a phase III RCT comparing gemcitabine plus carboplatin with or without bevacizumab in 484 patients of platinum-sensitive ROC. Eligible criteria included no prior chemotherapy in the recurrent stage, no existing measurable disease, and no prior treatment by VEGF pathway-targeted therapy including bevacizumab. The addition of bevacizumab led to a significant increase in PFS compared with placebo (median PFS, 8.4 vs. 12.4 months; $p < 0.0001$). There was also a higher objective RR (78.5% vs. 57.4%; $p < 0.001$) and prolonged duration of response (10.4 vs. 7.4 months; HR = 0.534). GI perforations did not occur during the treatment, but two patients suffered GI perforation after the study treatment, both on the 69th day after the last administration. The final OS was comparable between both arms (GC plus bevacizumab 33.6 months; GC plus placebo 32.9 months; HR = 0.95; $p = 0.65$). Thirty-eight percent of patients in the GC plus placebo arm received subsequent bevacizumab after the trial, making the data difficult to determine a significant improvement in OS [24, 25].

MITO-16/MaNGO OV-2 is an ongoing study to evaluate the efficacy of bevacizumab administered in both first- and second-line therapies. The protocol includes PLD-C or GC or TC with/without bevacizumab as the second-line therapy to platinum-sensitive ROC treated by the first-line therapy including bevacizumab (beyond progression disease (PD)).

14.2.2.2 PARP Inhibitor for Platinum-Sensitive Disease

Olaparib is an oral poly(ADP-ribose) polymerase inhibitor (PARPi), which has successively proven antitumor activity in BRCA1−/BRCA2-mutated cancers, including ROC patients [26–33]. In evaluation of olaparib on tumor response across a spectrum of malignancies in BRCA1−/BRCA2-mutated ROC, RR were 31.1%, and stable disease >8 weeks was 40% even in platinum-resistant cases [29]. The Food and Drug Administration (FDA) in the USA approved olaparib for the fourth-line treatment of BRCA-deficient ovarian cancer. It was permitted based on the efficacy of olaparib monotherapy on 265 patients with platinum-sensitive HGSOC receiving more than two prior regimens of chemotherapy [26, 27, 34]. Almost all patients were examined BRCA status, of whom about half (olaparib, 56%; placebo, 50%) had BRCA mutation. The BRCA-mutated olaparib maintenance cohort significantly improved PFS over placebo (median 11.2 vs. 4.3 months; HR 0.18; $p < 0.0001$); BRCA wild type also showed advantages in PFS compared to placebo (median 7.4 vs. 5.5 months; HR 0.54; $p = 0.0075$). Updated analysis revealed a significant OS advantage in the olaparib cohort of BRCA mutation (median OS, 34.9 vs. 30.2 months; HR, 0.62; $p = 0.025$), although the BRCA wild type in the olaparib group showed no significant changes (median OS, 24.5 vs. 26.6 months; HR, 0.83; $p = 0.37$). Following this retrospective review, a prospective RCT phase II trial was examined [34]. In all patients, PFS was significantly longer in olaparib arm than placebo group (median, 8.4 vs. 4.8 months; $p < 0.001$). OS advantage also appeared in maintenance of olaparib (median, 29·8 vs. 27·8 months) and in the cohort of BRCA mutation (34.9 vs. 30.2 months; HR 0·62; $p = 0·025$). However, OS in patients with BRCA wild type were insignificant (24.5 months with olaparib vs. 26.6 months with placebo; HR 0·83; $p = 0.37$) [27]. Regarding the efficacy of olaparib combined with cytotoxic agents, a phase II trial was performed for platinum-sensitive HGSOC and evaluated oral olaparib plus TC, followed by olaparib as a maintenance therapy [28]. Patients in olaparib plus TC arm had a lower risk of disease progression than the only chemotherapy arm (median PFS, 12.2 vs. 9.6 months; HR 0.51; $p = 0.0012$) and also significantly improved PFS in BRCA-mutated patients (HR 0.21; $p = 0.0015$). Final OS did not differ between each arm even by the subset analysis only for BRCA-mutated patients. At least 10% higher adverse events in the olaparib arm than in the placebo arm were alopecia, nausea, neutropenia, diarrhea, headache, peripheral neuropathy, and dyspepsia. Although 19% of patients had adverse events leading to treatment discontinuation, no fatal adverse events occurred.

Other PARPi drugs include rucaparib and veliparib and have been examined in phase II trials for ROC [35–37]. Various clinical trials of PARPi for ROC are being investigated. Both SOLO-2 (NCT01874353) and ENGOT-ov16/NOVA (NCT01847274) are phase III RCT comparing olaparib (SOLO-2)/niraparib (NOVA) versus placebo in the patients with BRCA mutation, two prior treatments of platinum-based chemotherapy and platinum-sensitive recurrent HGSOC. SOLO-3 (NCT02282020) is comparing olaparib monotherapy versus single-agent chemotherapy in platinum-sensitive ROC. These results have the possibility to alter the standard care for ROC, including the FDA-approved usage of olaparib. The combination of olaparib and cediranib showed survival advantage (PFS, 17.7 vs. 9 months; HR, 0.42; $p = 0.005$) compared to monotherapy, even in either BRCA-unknown status or BRCA wild-type patients (ORR, 76 vs. 32%, $p = 0.006$; PFS, 16.5 vs. 5.7 months; $p = 0.008$) [38]. This combination is now being assessed in two phase III trials for platinum-sensitive ROC with germline BRCA mutation (NCT02446600) and platinum-resistant ROC with no prior antiangiogenic agents (NCT02502266).

Rucaparib is another promising oral PARP1&2i that was proved by a phase II ARIEL trial (NCT01891344) in patients with platinum-sensitive recurrent HGSOC. The trial investigated not only RR but also molecular homologous recombination deficiency (HRD) signature to detect patients with clinical benefit to PARPi. Based on the defined molecular signature by ARIEL2, phase III ARIEL3 trial (NCT1968213) in platinum-sensitive disease stratified three groups before randomization and assessed the rucaparib maintenance compared to placebo.

Niraparib is also PARP1&2i and underwent a phase I study [39], which decided that 300 mg/day is the tolerable dose and achieved 40% RR in HGSOC. Although there is no completed phase II study at present, some phase I–II studies are ongoing (NCT02354586, NCT02354131, NCT02657889). The aforementioned phase III RCT of ENGOT-ov16/NOVA (NCT01847274) evaluated niraparib versus placebo by 553 patients with platinum-sensitive ROC. The niraparib group had a significantly longer PFS than the placebo group, regardless of presence (gBRCA cohort, median PFS, 21.0 vs. 5.5 months; HR, 0.27) or absence (non-gBRCA without HRD cohort, median PFS, 9.3 vs. 3.9 months; HR, 0.45) of gBRCA mutation or HRD status. Interestingly, PFS was also longer in the non-gBRCA cohort with HRD than the placebo group (non-gBRCA with HRD cohort, median PFS, 12.9 vs. 3.8 months; HR, 0.38; 95% CI, 0.24 to 0.5). The reported toxicities of grade 3 or 4 were thrombocytopenia (33.8%), anemia (25.3%), and neutropenia (19.6%) [40].

14.3 Role of Secondary Debulking Surgery in Platinum-Sensitive Disease

In the recurrent cases, the aim of surgery is to prolong survival instead of curing the disease like in the initial therapy. The significance of secondary debulking surgery (SDS) remains poorly defined [41], because of a lack of RCT (Levels 1–2 evidence) assigning patients to suboptimal versus complete cytoreductive surgery. Using additionally analyzed data from the CALYPSO trial [11], OS of patients who had SDS was compared to those treated with chemotherapy alone. Nineteen percent of patients underwent SDS and 80% were treated with only chemotherapy. SDS was associated with improved OS in platinum-sensitive ROC (median OS, 49.9 vs. 29.7 months; HR, 0.68; $p = 0.004$). For patients with SDS, the 3-year OS was 72% for those with no measurable disease and 28% if residual tumors were larger than 5 cm. Patients with favorable prognostic factors benefited the most from SDS (HR, 0.43; $p < 0.001$). In a recent systematic review [12], it was recognized that complete cytoreduction is associated with significant improvement in OS. In cases where cytoreduction was impossible to perform, there was potential to improve the outcome of debulk nodules less than 1 cm. Another report [42] also demonstrated that complete resection was significantly related to overall survival ($p = 0.0019$). As for variables determined before SDS, DFI >12 months, no liver metastasis, solitary tumor, and tumor size <6 cm were independently associated with favorable OS. Patients with three or all four variables ($n = 31$) had significantly better survival compared with the other patients ($n = 13$) (47 vs. 20 months in median survival, $p < 0.0001$). Therefore, the limited patients with longer PFS over 6 months, isolated macroscopic lesions that can be completely resected, and the good performance status were considered for debulking surgery [15]. When SDS is performed, the objective should be complete resection of the tumor when possible [15].

Regarding the QOL assessment, SDS followed by chemotherapy is more tolerable than chemotherapy alone, with the exception of constipation and pain, which only worsen in surgery patients at 3 months [43]. Ongoing phase III RCT with GOG 213 trial (NCT00565851) and DESKTOP III trial (NCT01166737) will clearly define the significance of cytoreductive surgery in ROC. GOG 213 is gathering attention and ongoing to determine the superiority of additional bevacizumab plus TC followed by bevacizumab maintenance to TC alone and the necessity of SDS followed by bevacizumab maintenance in platinum-sensitive ROC for ROC treatment.

14.4 Platinum-Resistant Recurrent Ovarian Cancer

14.4.1 Chemotherapy for Platinum-Resistant Disease

The selection of chemotherapeutic agents should lack cross-resistance to previously used regimens and have a favorable toxicity profile. Single-agent chemotherapy with/without bevacizumab is the standard care for platinum-resistant disease [15]. Combination chemotherapy is not recommended because the survival benefit is not necessarily absolute and adverse effects cumulatively increased. The phase II Japan Gynecologic Oncology Group (JGOG)/West Japan Gynecologic Oncology Group (WJGOG) intergroup study suggested that although docetaxel/irinotecan combination therapy in platinum-refractory/platinum-resistant patients was well tolerated, there was low RR (6.3%) and low survival benefits (median PFS, 12.1 weeks; median OS, 45.3 weeks) especially in platinum–/paclitaxel-refractory tumors (disease control rate, 10%) [44]. Another combination of agents reported by the GOG group, cisplatin (30 mg/m^2) plus gemcitabine (750 mg/m^2), on days 1 and 8, was administered in platinum-resistant patients. It was reported that gemcitabine was reduced (600 mg/m^2) in the second stage because of dense hematologic toxicity. Modest activity was achieved in the median time to progression at 5.4 months and OS at 14.9 months [45].

Although only a limited number of RCTs have been performed, some active agents including irinotecan, gemcitabine, topotecan, docetaxel, paclitaxel, PLD, ifosfamide, oral etoposide, and bevacizumab have been identified. Regarding the effect of irinotecan in platinum-resistant ROC, RR of 29% was achieved even after several prior regimens (median: three regimens). The median time to progression was 17 weeks. Grades 3–4 diarrhea were observed in 10.7% patients, while it was not grade 4 gastrointestinal toxicities [46]. Two phase III studies analyzed single gemcitabine compared with PLD [47, 48]. A research reported [47] that the overall RR of patients with platinum-resistant ROC revealed gemcitabine 6.1% (versus PLD 8.3%; $p = 0.589$), but disease control rate was 60.6% (vs 46.9%; $p = 0.063$). Median PFS (gemcitabine, 3.6 months, vs. PLD, 3.1 months; $p = 0.87$) and median OS with crossover treatment (gemcitabine to PLD, 12.7 months, vs. PLD to gemcitabine, 13.5 months; $p = 0.997$) were comparable in two single regimens. Toxicity profiles with grades 3–4 neutropenia and constipation, nausea, and fatigue were significant but manageable in spite of heavily pretreated ROC patients [47, 49].

PPE was the predominant toxicity in PLD, and 20% of patients experienced grade 2 or 3 PPE in doses of 50 mg/m^2 every 21 or 28 days [47]. In using 40 mg/m^2 every 28 days, a lower incidence of 12% PPE occurred (6/49 patients: grade 2 only) in a nonrandomized phase II study. Notably, PPE developed delayed toxicity secondary to PLD during the administration of the latter regimen even if PPE was not evident during PLD treatment [47]. A phase III non-inferiority trial (JGOG 3018) of PLD 40 mg/m^2 against 50 mg/m^2 for platinum-refractory/platinum-resistant ROC to determine the standard dosage of single PLD administration is now being conducted.

Topotecan is also an active agent for platinum-resistant ROC. A phase III RCT was conducted comparing PLD 50 mg/m^2 every 4 weeks and topotecan 1.5 mg/m^2/day for a succession of 5 days every 3 weeks in ROC including refractory relapse. Although overall PFS was similar in the two groups, only a subgroup of platinum-refractory disease and survival trend in favor of topotecan is compared to PLD ($p = 0.455$) [50]. RR was 12–18%, and the median OS was 7–10 months in resistance ROC [50, 51, 52]. Myelosuppression was the major toxicity, 14–25% of patients with administered 1.5 mg/m^2 for 5 serial days experienced febrile neutropenia [50, 51], and grade 4 neutropenia was observed in 80%. Non-hematological toxicity including gastrointestinal disturbances (nausea, diarrhea, constipation) is relatively mild and noncumulative. Other reports about the single use of topotecan demonstrated that a dose of 1.25 mg/m^2 was safe for Japanese patients without fatal complications like febrile neutropenia or bleeding due to severe myelosuppression, and 7 out of 12 patients could achieve disease control in recurrent ROC. Clinically, a decreased dose level (1 mg/m^2) is recommended for higher-aged patients or complicated renal dysfunction patients [53].

RR for the single use of paclitaxel or docetaxel is 10–45% in platinum-resistant ROC [52, 54–56]. OS was 10–13 months in paclitaxel of tri-weekly 175 mg/m^2 administration [57]. The single 175 mg/m^2 dose of paclitaxel showed no survival benefits and more toxicities in ROC [57]. In a setting where paclitaxel was administered weekly, a recent report showed 4.7 months PFS, and a 21–29% RR, and concluded that weekly paclitaxel was superior in survival and less in toxicity than tri-weekly administrations. Regarding the taxane-free interval in platinum-resistant ROC, patients with the interval of <6 months had 1.8 months lower PFS than ≥6 months group (3.7 vs. 5.5 months) in a phase II trial [58]. Serious toxicities were relatively uncommon in single-agent taxane, such as neuropathy grades 2–3 (25%) and fatigue grade 3 (8%) by paclitaxel [55]. In a Japanese Cooperative Study, a toxicity evaluation of single docetaxel 70 mg/m^2 revealed febrile neutropenia (24%), grades 3–4 anemia (16%), alopecia (68%), mild hypersensitivity reaction (37%), and mild edema (16%) [54].

Oral etoposide (VP-16) is a common and active agent for platinum-resistant ROC. Evidence proved that efficacy of intravenous etoposide had a lower RR (8%) than oral etoposide in ovarian cancer [59] despite previous reports of oral etoposide in platinum-resistant patients of RR 18%–26% [60–62]. The patients dosed at 50–60 mg/m^2/d p.o. for 21 days in a 28-day cycle suffered by 50% grades 3–4 neutropenia and 9% grades 3–4 thrombocytopenia. It has been reported that administration for 14 serial days in a 28-day cycle was active (RR, 18%), in spite of tolerable myelosuppression (grades 3–4 neutropenia, 27%; thrombocytopenia, 18%) and less non-hematologic toxicity [61]. Oral etoposide with intravenous irinotecan was examined based on the results of a positive feasibility study (which showed 44% RR) [63]. However, the phase II trial of JCOG 0503 study showed the regimen was not recommended because of severe myelosuppression [64].

Cyclophosphamide has proven to be another effective choice of oral cytotoxic agents for ROC at a dose of 100 mg/day. Out of 14 patients evaluated, one patient showed partial response (PR) and eight developed stable disease, although moderate gastrointestinal toxicity was observed [65].

14.4.2 Targeted Therapies for Platinum-Resistant Disease

14.4.2.1 Antiangiogenic Agent for Platinum-Resistant Disease

The antiangiogenic agent bevacizumab, which assists the prevention of the development of neovascularization, plays an important role in platinum-resistant ROC. In tumors, elevated VEGF levels cause disorganized and leaky tumor vessels accompanying elevated intrastromal tissue pressure; thus cytotoxic agents cannot reach to the tumor. Bevacizumab has been known to improve drug delivery to the tumor as well as to inhibit neovascularization [66–69]. Thus, a combination with chemotherapy has the potential of synergy for survival in patients with advanced cancer [68, 70].

Single-agent bevacizumab in platinum-resistant ROC was assessed in 44 patients heavily pretreated by cytotoxic agents, 47.7% of patients received 3 prior chemotherapy regimens, and 90% of patients had suspicious of tumor involvement of the GI tract at the time of enrollment. RR was relatively low with 15.9% consisting no complete response (CR) and 7 partial response (PR), and the median PFS was 4.4 months. Due to toxicity, 18.2% of patients discontinued treatment, and serious events occurred in 40.9%. This study was stopped after recruiting 44 patients because of serious toxicities associated with bevacizumab, including GI perforation (11.4%), obstruction (11.3%), and arterial thromboembolic events. All of the patients with GI perforation received three prior chemotherapy regimens and had stable disease at the time of perforation. GI perforation was frequently administered for bowel wall thickening and bowel wall obstruction [71]. Another retrospective report with bevacizumab in combination with cytotoxic chemotherapy in platinum-refractory ROC revealed 9% higher GI perforation, whereas 0–3% of GI perforation were reported in a previous study [22, 72, 73]. Therefore, platinum-resistant ROC, especially heavily pretreated (three prior regimens) patients, tended to have higher incidences of GI perforation. This serious complication could be prevented through examination and exclusion of patients diagnosed with clinical bowel complications, even in patients who underwent multiple prior chemotherapy regimens. Important CT findings that suggest bowel involvement are abnormalities of mesentery blood vessels, decrease or a lack of bowel contrast, and bowel stenosis. While the use of concomitant NSAIDs is also a significant risk factor for GI perforation in colorectal cancer, it is not clearly proved that bevacizumab induced GI perforation because the site was not always around the primary tumor [74]. Other toxicities concerning bevacizumab include fatigue, hypertension, proteinuria, fistula, bleeding, dyspnea, myocardial infarction, venous thromboembolism, and cerebral ischemia.

The open-label randomized phase III AURELIA trial of 360 patients evaluated the combination of bevacizumab and single-agent chemotherapy in platinum-resistant ROC [75]. Patients who had received more than two prior anticancer regimens had refractory disease which was progression during previous platinum-containing therapy or had a history of bowel obstruction and were ineligible. After the physician's choice of chemotherapy was decided (i.e., single-agent paclitaxel, topotecan, PLD), patients were then randomized to receive the selected chemotherapy either alone or in combination with bevacizumab until the disease progression. Upon the progression, patients in the chemotherapy alone arm were eligible to cross over to receive single-agent bevacizumab. PFS was significantly prolonged for patients treated with chemotherapy plus bevacizumab compared with chemotherapy alone (median, 6.7 vs. 3.4 months; HR, 0.484; $p < 0.001$). Overall RR was 27.3% versus 11.8%, respectively ($p = 0.001$). There was no significant difference in OS in any of the chemotherapy cohorts (HR,0.85; median OS; 16.6 vs. 13.3 months). In final OS analysis, 40% of the patients in the chemotherapy only arm had received single-agent bevacizumab after disease progression. GI perforation occurred in 2.2% of bevacizumab-treated patients, and a comparison of QOL revealed the chemotherapy plus bevacizumab arm was over 15% better than chemotherapy alone arm [75, 76].

In colorectal cancer or non-small cell lung cancer (NSCLC), positive survival benefits were evident in readministered bevacizumab at the time of second-line chemotherapy even in disease-progressed patients after the first-line chemotherapy (beyond PD) including bevacizumab [77, 78]. At the time of the AURELIA trial, the usage of bevacizumab for pretreatment was rare, and the study reported that only 7% of patients had previously received bevacizumab. Accordingly, results of the now ongoing JGOG 3023 trial studying the effectiveness of bevacizumab on survival benefit beyond PD in platinum-resistant ROC are being awaited.

There is evidence of other antiangiogenic agents including cediranib, pazopanib, nintedanib, trebananib, sunitinib, and cabozantinib which have shown modest activity in ovarian cancer [23, 79, 80] based on phase II/phase III trials. Cediranib is an orally administered, potent small-molecule inhibitor of several tyrosine kinases and active in patients with both platinum-resistant and platinum-sensitive ROC. Clinical benefits (CR + PR + SD > 16 weeks or CA-125 nonprogression >16 weeks) were 30%, median PFS was 5.2 months, and mean OS was 16.3 months [79]. The phase II trial of ICON6 proved significant survival benefits in PFS (OS was too immature to assess) with platinum-sensitive ROC. The arm with the addition of cediranib 20 mg once daily plus chemotherapy and then continued treatment to progressive disease or excessive toxic effects shows significantly prolonged PFS compared to the arm with placebo plus chemotherapy group or the arm with cediranib plus chemotherapy followed by placebo maintenance (median PFS, 11.0 vs. 8.7 vs. 9.9 months, respectively). However, 32% of patients in the cediranib arm during the chemotherapy phase discontinued treatment due to the common toxicities with diarrhea, neutropenia, hypertension, and voice change [81]. In another phase II trial of platinum-sensitive ROC, it was revealed that cediranib plus olaparib significantly improved median PFS (8.7-month improvement) and overall RR (32% increase in overall RR) over olaparib monotherapy. Some phase II/phase III trials regarding the combination of cediranib and olaparib in recurrent ROC is now ongoing (NCT02340611, NCT02446600, NCT01116648, NCT02345265, NCT02502266).

Sorafenib is a modest activity in ovarian cancer, although patients with chemoresistant clear-cell carcinoma achieved 5–6 months of stable disease in ROC [82, 83]. The angiopoietin inhibitor trebananib is a Tie1/angiopoietin 1 and 2 inhibitor which is expressed on vascular endothelial cells.

A phase II trial with weekly trebananib 10 mg/kg plus paclitaxel may result in prolonged median PFS, and its toxicity profile is distinct from that of VEGF pathway inhibitors such as hypokalemia and peripheral edema [84]. The phase III trial of TRINOVA-1 was investigated with intravenous paclitaxel 80 mg/m^2 plus intravenous trebananib 15 mg/kg or placebo [85]. Results show that trebananib significantly improved median PFS (12.5 vs. 10.9 months; HR, 0.85; $p = 0.024$); although median OS did not differ in each group (19.3 vs. 18.3 months) in intention to treat analysis, the trebananib group was superior in patients with complicated ascites in subset analysis (14.5 vs. 12.3 months; $p = 0.011$) [85, 86]. In addition, the phase III TRINOVA-3 trial of the single-agent trebananib compared to placebo in the first-line chemotherapy of TC in advanced ovarian cancer is now ongoing (NCT01493505).

14.4.2.2 Checkpoint Inhibitors for Platinum-Resistant Disease

Recently, the research as an advanced anticancer strategy testing immune checkpoint inhibitors against ovarian cancer is being examined. The ovarian cancer cells acquire the potential to escape from host immunity mainly via the programmed death 1 (PD-1)/programmed death ligand 1 (PD-L1) pathway and the secondary CTLA-4/B7 pathway in the tumor microenvironment [87–91]. The immune checkpoint inhibitors successively proved anticancer effects on various types of tumors such as melanoma (RR, 28%), renal cancer (RR, 27%), and NSCLC (RR, 18%) through improved local immune activity [92–94].

Several types of checkpoint inhibitors were examined in ROC, and the reported RR in ROC ranged from 6 to 20%. A phase II trial of nivolumab (anti-PD-1 antibody) for platinum-resistant ROC demonstrated 20% RR, including two possible CR cases. The median PFS was 3.5 months, and median OS was 20.0 months. Forty percent of patients experienced grades 3–4 toxicities, and the most frequent toxicity was thyroid dysfunction [95]. The RR by other checkpoint inhibitors includes PD-1 inhibitor pembrolizumab at 11.5% in phase I, CTLA-4 inhibitor ipilimumab at 11% in phases I–II [96], PD-L1 inhibitor avelumab at 10.7% in phase I, and BMS-936559 at 6% in phase I.

Regarding the combination of chemotherapy and a checkpoint inhibitor, it is an interesting phenomenon that chemotherapeutic agents (paclitaxel/gemcitabine) induced overexpression of PD-L1 and paclitaxel combined with PD-1/PD-L1 inhibitor enhanced antitumor effects relative to monotherapy in ovarian cancer [97]. In colorectal cancer, mismatch repair status seems an effective marker for survival. A phase II trial of pembrolizumab revealed that mismatch repair-deficient tumors are more responsive to PD-1 blockade than are mismatch repair tumors [98]. Phase II (NCT02520154) analyzing pembrolizumab plus TC is the only ongoing trial which is investigating first line in ovarian cancer. Several clinical trial combinations of checkpoint inhibitors are now being investigated for ROC (Table 14.2) [99].

Table 14.2 Clinical trials combination of checkpoint inhibitors in ROC (Ref. [94])

	Phase	Platinum response	Trial idetifier
Combination chemotherapies			
Dose-dense paclitaxel + pembrolizumab	2	Resistant	NCT02440425
PLD versus PLD + avelumab versus avelumab	3	Resistant	NCT02580058
PARPi molecules			
Olaparib + tremelimumab	1/2	Sensitive and resistant	NCT02571725
Olaparib + tremelimumab	1/2	Partially sensitive and resistant	NCT02485990
Cediranib + durvalumab versus durvalumab	1/2	Resistant	NCT02484404
Multi-TKI			
ACP-196(TKI) versus ACP-196 + pembrolizumab	2	Sensitive	NCT02537444
Anti-angiogenic agent			
Bevacizumb + atezolizumab	2	Resistant	NCT02659384

ROC recurrent ovarian cancer, *PLD* pegylated liposomal doxorubicin, *PARPi* poly(ADP-ribose) polymerase inhibitor, *TKI* tyrosine kinase inhibitor

14.5 Radiotherapy for Recurrent Ovarian Cancer

Radiotherapy has the potential to be a treatment option for limited patients with ROC. Recent multidimensional radiotherapy techniques allow the decrease of toxicities by minimizing the irradiated critical structure in locally limited recurrent gynecological cancer. There are few prospective studies evaluating the efficacy of ROC. A combination of docetaxel with a low dose (twice weekly, 60 cGy) of whole abdominal radiotherapy in a phase I trial of ROC reported the median PFS in all patients was 3.3 months, 3 out of 10 patients with measurable disease were free of tumor progression after 6 months, and a weekly dose of docetaxel 20 mg/m^2 was well tolerated [100]. A trial of pelvic radiotherapy and concurrent bevacizumab for recurrent gynecological cancer achieved three ROC patients out of 4 relapsed with 1- and 3-year PFS of 80% and 40% in a small prospective feasibility trial [101]. Relatively positive efficacy was reported in palliative radiotherapy in ROC, which achieved response rate ranges at 50–80% and more than 6 months of median PFS [102–106]. Both whole-brain radiation therapy and gamma knife radiosurgery are not only to relieve symptoms but also to prolong survival against brain metastasis [15, 107, 108]. Currently, patients with symptomatic lesion, solitary lesion, brain metastasis, and chemoresistant ROC are worth considering for radiotherapy [15].

Conclusion

The advent of molecular targeting drugs is expected to improve survival outcomes in ROC and have therapeutic effects. It is important to determine the best treatment for each case by having sufficient knowledge about the characteristics of each drug, the effect of using a combination of existing anticancer drugs, and the possible side effects that may occur.

Disclosure Statement We have no disclosures and received no financial supports.

References

1. Heintz AP, Odicino F, Maisonneuve P, Quinn MA, Benedet JL, Creasman WT, et al. Carcinoma of the ovary. FIGO 26th Annual Report on the results of treatment in gynecological cancer. Int J Gynaecol Obstet. 2006;95(Suppl 1):S161–92.
2. Saito T, Katabuchi H. Annual Report of the Committee on Gynecologic Oncology, Japan Society of Obstetrics and Gynecology: Patient Annual Report for 2013 and Treatment Annual Report for 2008. J Obstet Gynaecol Res. 2016;42:1069–79.
3. Ozols RF. Systemic therapy for ovarian cancer: current status and new treatments. Semin Oncol. 2006;33(2 Suppl 6):S3–11.
4. Colombo N, Gore M. Treatment of recurrent ovarian cancer relapsing 6-12 months post platinum-based chemotherapy. Crit Rev Oncol Hematol. 2007;64:129–38.
5. Markman M, Rothman R, Hakes T, Reichman B, Hoskins W, Rubin S, et al. Second-line platinum therapy in patients with ovarian cancer previously treated with cisplatin. J Clin Oncol. 1991;9:389–93.
6. Markman M, Markman J, Webster K, Zanotti K, Kulp B, Peterson G, et al. Duration of response to second-line, platinum-based chemotherapy for ovarian cancer: implications for patient management and clinical trial design. J Clin Oncol. 2004;22:3120–5.
7. Parmar MK, Ledermann JA, Colombo N, du Bois A, Delaloye JF, Kristensen GB, et al. Paclitaxel plus platinum-based chemotherapy versus conventional platinum-based

chemotherapy in women with relapsed ovarian cancer: the ICON4/AGO-OVAR-2.2 trial. Lancet. 2003;361:2099–106.
8. Pfisterer J, Vergote I, Du Bois A, Eisenhauer E, Ago O, Ncic CTG, et al. Combination therapy with gemcitabine and carboplatin in recurrent ovarian cancer. Int J Gynecol Cancer. 2005;15(Suppl 1):36–41.
9. Siegel RL, Miller KD, Jemal A. Cancer statistics, 2015. CA Cancer J Clin. 2015;65:5–29.
10. Matulonis UA, Oza AM, Ho TW, Ledermann JA. Intermediate clinical endpoints: a bridge between progression-free survival and overall survival in ovarian cancer trials. Cancer. 2015;121:1737–46.
11. Lee CK, Lord S, Grunewald T, Gebski V, Hardy-Bessard AC, Sehouli J, et al. Impact of secondary cytoreductive surgery on survival in patients with platinum sensitive recurrent ovarian cancer: analysis of the CALYPSO trial. Gynecol Oncol. 2015;136:18–24.
12. Bristow RE, Puri I, Chi DS. Cytoreductive surgery for recurrent ovarian cancer: a meta-analysis. Gynecol Oncol. 2009;112:265–74.
13. (Guidelines) National Comprehensive Cancer Network (NCCN). Ovarian cancer including fallopian tube cancer and primary peritoneal cancer. 2016.
14. Gonzalez-Martin AJ, Calvo E, Bover I, Rubio MJ, Arcusa A, Casado A, et al. Randomized phase II trial of carboplatin versus paclitaxel and carboplatin in platinum-sensitive recurrent advanced ovarian carcinoma: a GEICO (Grupo Espanol de Investigacion en Cancer de Ovario) study. Ann Oncol. 2005;16:749–55.
15. Komiyama S, Katabuchi H, Mikami M, Nagase S, Okamoto A, Ito K, et al. Japan Society of Gynecologic Oncology guidelines 2015 for the treatment of ovarian cancer including primary peritoneal cancer and fallopian tube cancer. Int J Clin Oncol. 2016;21:435–46.
16. Pujade-Lauraine E, Wagner U, Aavall-Lundqvist E, Gebski V, Heywood M, Vasey PA, et al. Pegylated liposomal Doxorubicin and Carboplatin compared with Paclitaxel and Carboplatin for patients with platinum-sensitive ovarian cancer in late relapse. J Clin Oncol. 2010;28:3323–9.
17. Wagner U, Marth C, Largillier R, Kaern J, Brown C, Heywood M, et al. Final overall survival results of phase III GCIG CALYPSO trial of pegylated liposomal doxorubicin and carboplatin vs paclitaxel and carboplatin in platinum-sensitive ovarian cancer patients. Br J Cancer. 2012;107:588–91.
18. Nakanishi T, Aoki D, Watanabe Y, Ando Y, Tomotsugu N, Sato Y, et al. A Phase II clinical trial of pegylated liposomal doxorubicin and carboplatin in Japanese patients with platinum-sensitive recurrent ovarian, fallopian tube or primary peritoneal cancer. Jpn J Clin Oncol. 2015;45:422–6.
19. Alberts DS, Liu PY, Wilczynski SP, Clouser MC, Lopez AM, Michelin DP, et al. Randomized trial of pegylated liposomal doxorubicin (PLD) plus carboplatin versus carboplatin in platinum-sensitive (PS) patients with recurrent epithelial ovarian or peritoneal carcinoma after failure of initial platinum-based chemotherapy (Southwest Oncology Group Protocol S0200). Gynecol Oncol. 2008;108:90–4.
20. Poveda A, Vergote I, Tjulandin S, Kong B, Roy M, Chan S, et al. Trabectedin plus pegylated liposomal doxorubicin in relapsed ovarian cancer: outcomes in the partially platinum-sensitive (platinum-free interval 6-12 months) subpopulation of OVA-301 phase III randomized trial. Ann Oncol. 2011;22:39–48.
21. Monk BJ, Herzog TJ, Kaye SB, Krasner CN, Vermorken JB, Muggia FM, et al. Trabectedin plus pegylated liposomal Doxorubicin in recurrent ovarian cancer. J Clin Oncol. 2010;28:3107–14.
22. Burger RA, Sill MW, Monk BJ, Greer BE, Sorosky JI. Phase II trial of bevacizumab in persistent or recurrent epithelial ovarian cancer or primary peritoneal cancer: a Gynecologic Oncology Group Study. J Clin Oncol. 2007;25:5165–71.
23. Gadducci A, Lanfredini N, Sergiampietri C. Antiangiogenic agents in gynecological cancer: State of art and perspectives of clinical research. Crit Rev Oncol Hematol. 2015;96:113–28.
24. Aghajanian C, Blank SV, Goff BA, Judson PL, Teneriello MG, Husain A, et al. OCEANS: a randomized, double-blind, placebo-controlled phase III trial of chemotherapy with or without

bevacizumab in patients with platinum-sensitive recurrent epithelial ovarian, primary peritoneal, or fallopian tube cancer. J Clin Oncol. 2012;30:2039–45.
25. Aghajanian C, Goff B, Nycum LR, Wang YV, Husain A, Blank SV. Final overall survival and safety analysis of OCEANS, a phase 3 trial of chemotherapy with or without bevacizumab in patients with platinum-sensitive recurrent ovarian cancer. Gynecol Oncol. 2015;139:10–6.
26. Ledermann J, Harter P, Gourley C, Friedlander M, Vergote I, Rustin G, et al. Olaparib maintenance therapy in patients with platinum-sensitive relapsed serous ovarian cancer: a preplanned retrospective analysis of outcomes by BRCA status in a randomised phase 2 trial. Lancet Oncol. 2014;15:852–61.
27. Ledermann JA, Harter P, Gourley C, Friedlander M, Vergote I, Rustin G, et al. Overall survival in patients with platinum-sensitive recurrent serous ovarian cancer receiving olaparib maintenance monotherapy: an updated analysis from a randomised, placebo-controlled, double-blind, phase 2 trial. Lancet Oncol. 2016;17:1579–89.
28. Oza AM, Cibula D, Benzaquen AO, Poole C, Mathijssen RH, Sonke GS, et al. Olaparib combined with chemotherapy for recurrent platinum-sensitive ovarian cancer: a randomised phase 2 trial. Lancet Oncol. 2015;16:87–97.
29. Kaufman B, Shapira-Frommer R, Schmutzler RK, Audeh MW, Friedlander M, Balmana J, et al. Olaparib monotherapy in patients with advanced cancer and a germline BRCA1/2 mutation. J Clin Oncol. 2015;33:244–50.
30. Fong PC, Yap TA, Boss DS, Carden CP, Mergui-Roelvink M, Gourley C, et al. Poly(ADP)-ribose polymerase inhibition: frequent durable responses in BRCA carrier ovarian cancer correlating with platinum-free interval. J Clin Oncol. 2010;28:2512–9.
31. Audeh MW, Carmichael J, Penson RT, Friedlander M, Powell B, Bell-McGuinn KM, et al. Oral poly(ADP-ribose) polymerase inhibitor olaparib in patients with BRCA1 or BRCA2 mutations and recurrent ovarian cancer: a proof-of-concept trial. Lancet. 2010;376:245–51.
32. Gelmon KA, Tischkowitz M, Mackay H, Swenerton K, Robidoux A, Tonkin K, et al. Olaparib in patients with recurrent high-grade serous or poorly differentiated ovarian carcinoma or triple-negative breast cancer: a phase 2, multicentre, open-label, non-randomised study. Lancet Oncol. 2011;12:852–61.
33. Kaye SB, Lubinski J, Matulonis U, Ang JE, Gourley C, Karlan BY, et al. Phase II, open-label, randomized, multicenter study comparing the efficacy and safety of olaparib, a poly (ADP-ribose) polymerase inhibitor, and pegylated liposomal doxorubicin in patients with BRCA1 or BRCA2 mutations and recurrent ovarian cancer. J Clin Oncol. 2012;30:372–9.
34. Ledermann J, Harter P, Gourley C, Friedlander M, Vergote I, Rustin G, et al. Olaparib maintenance therapy in platinum-sensitive relapsed ovarian cancer. N Engl J Med. 2012;366:1382–92.
35. Coleman RL, Sill MW, Bell-McGuinn K, Aghajanian C, Gray HJ, Tewari KS, et al. A phase II evaluation of the potent, highly selective PARP inhibitor veliparib in the treatment of persistent or recurrent epithelial ovarian, fallopian tube, or primary peritoneal cancer in patients who carry a germline BRCA1 or BRCA2 mutation - An NRG Oncology/Gynecologic Oncology Group study. Gynecol Oncol. 2015;137:386–91.
36. Drew Y, Ledermann J, Hall G, Rea D, Glasspool R, Highley M, et al. Phase 2 multicentre trial investigating intermittent and continuous dosing schedules of the poly(ADP-ribose) polymerase inhibitor rucaparib in germline BRCA mutation carriers with advanced ovarian and breast cancer. Br J Cancer. 2016;114:723–30.
37. Kummar S, Oza AM, Fleming GF, Sullivan DM, Gandara DR, Naughton MJ, et al. Randomized trial of oral cyclophosphamide and Veliparib in high-grade serous ovarian, primary peritoneal, or fallopian tube cancers, or BRCA-mutant ovarian cancer. Clin Cancer Res. 2015;21:1574–82.
38. Liu JF, Barry WT, Birrer M, Lee JM, Buckanovich RJ, Fleming GF, et al. Combination cediranib and olaparib versus olaparib alone for women with recurrent platinum-sensitive ovarian cancer: a randomised phase 2 study. Lancet Oncol. 2014;15:1207–14.
39. Sandhu SK, Schelman WR, Wilding G, Moreno V, Baird RD, Miranda S, et al. The poly(ADP-ribose) polymerase inhibitor niraparib (MK4827) in BRCA mutation carriers and patients with sporadic cancer: a phase 1 dose-escalation trial. Lancet Oncol. 2013;14:882–92.

40. Mirza MR, Monk BJ, Herrstedt J, Oza AM, Mahner S, Redondo A et al. Niraparib maintenance therapy in platinum-sensitive, recurrent ovarian cancer. N Engl J Med 2016375: 2154–164
41. Horowitz NS, Miller A, Rungruang B, Richard SD, Rodriguez N, Bookman MA, et al. Does aggressive surgery improve outcomes? Interaction between preoperative disease burden and complex surgery in patients with advanced-stage ovarian cancer: an analysis of GOG 182. J Clin Oncol. 2015;33:937–43.
42. Onda T, Yoshikawa H, Yasugi T, Yamada M, Matsumoto K, Taketani Y. Secondary cytoreductive surgery for recurrent epithelial ovarian carcinoma: proposal for patients selection. Br J Cancer. 2005;92:1026–32.
43. Plotti F, Scaletta G, Aloisi A, Luvero D, Capriglione S, Miranda A, et al. Quality of life in platinum-sensitive recurrent ovarian cancer: chemotherapy versus surgery plus chemotherapy. Ann Surg Oncol. 2015;22:2387–94.
44. Ushijima K, Kamura T, Tamura K, Kuzuya K, Sugiyama T, Noda K, et al. Docetaxel/irinotecan combination chemotherapy in platinum/taxane-refractory and -resistant ovarian cancer: JGOG/WJGOG Intergroup Study. Int J Clin Oncol. 2013;18:126–31.
45. Brewer CA, Blessing JA, Nagourney RA, Morgan M, Hanjani P. Cisplatin plus gemcitabine in platinum-refractory ovarian or primary peritoneal cancer: a phase II study of the Gynecologic Oncology Group. Gynecol Oncol. 2006;103:446–50.
46. Matsumoto K, Katsumata N, Yamanaka Y, Yonemori K, Kohno T, Shimizu C, et al. The safety and efficacy of the weekly dosing of irinotecan for platinum- and taxanes-resistant epithelial ovarian cancer. Gynecol Oncol. 2006;100:412–6.
47. Mutch DG, Orlando M, Goss T, Teneriello MG, Gordon AN, McMeekin SD, et al. Randomized phase III trial of gemcitabine compared with pegylated liposomal doxorubicin in patients with platinum-resistant ovarian cancer. J Clin Oncol. 2007;25:2811–8.
48. Ferrandina G, Ludovisi M, Lorusso D, Pignata S, Breda E, Savarese A, et al. Phase III trial of gemcitabine compared with pegylated liposomal doxorubicin in progressive or recurrent ovarian cancer. J Clin Oncol. 2008;26:890–6.
49. Watanabe Y, Koike E, Nakai H, Etoh T, Hoshiai H. Phase II study of single-agent gemcitabine in heavily pretreated Japanese patients with recurrent ovarian cancer. Int J Clin Oncol. 2008;13:345–8.
50. Gordon AN, Fleagle JT, Guthrie D, Parkin DE, Gore ME, Lacave AJ. Recurrent epithelial ovarian carcinoma: a randomized phase III study of pegylated liposomal doxorubicin versus topotecan. J Clin Oncol. 2001;19:3312–22.
51. Kudelka AP, Tresukosol D, Edwards CL, Freedman RS, Levenback C, Chantarawiroj P, et al. Phase II study of intravenous topotecan as a 5-day infusion for refractory epithelial ovarian carcinoma. J Clin Oncol. 1996;14:1552–7.
52. ten Bokkel Huinink W, Lane SR, Ross GA. International Topotecan Study G. Long-term survival in a phase III, randomised study of topotecan versus paclitaxel in advanced epithelial ovarian carcinoma. Ann Oncol. 2004;15:100–3.
53. Shimamoto K, Saito T, Nagayama R, Yamaguchi S, Shimada T, Ariyoshi K, et al. Nogitecan hydrochloride treatment for patients with recurrent ovarian cancer. Gan To Kagaku Ryoho. 2015;42:821–5.
54. Katsumata N, Tsunematsu R, Tanaka K, Terashima Y, Ogita S, Hoshiai H, et al. A phase II trial of docetaxel in platinum pre-treated patients with advanced epithelial ovarian cancer: a Japanese cooperative study. Ann Oncol. 2000;11:1531–6.
55. Gynecologic Oncology G, Markman M, Blessing J, Rubin SC, Connor J, Hanjani P, et al. Phase II trial of weekly paclitaxel (80 mg/m2) in platinum and paclitaxel-resistant ovarian and primary peritoneal cancers: a Gynecologic Oncology Group study. Gynecol Oncol. 2006;101:436–40.
56. Kita T, Kikuchi Y, Takano M, Suzuki M, Oowada M, Konno R, et al. The effect of single weekly paclitaxel in heavily pretreated patients with recurrent or persistent advanced ovarian cancer. Gynecol Oncol. 2004;92:813–8.

57. Omura GA, Brady MF, Look KY, Averette HE, Delmore JE, Long HJ, et al. Phase III trial of paclitaxel at two dose levels, the higher dose accompanied by filgrastim at two dose levels in platinum-pretreated epithelial ovarian cancer: an intergroup study. J Clin Oncol. 2003;21:2843–8.
58. McNeish IA, Ledermann JA, Webber L, James L, Kaye SB, Hall M, et al. A randomised, placebo-controlled trial of weekly paclitaxel and saracatinib (AZD0530) in platinum-resistant ovarian, fallopian tube or primary peritoneal cancerdagger. Ann Oncol. 2014;25:1988–95.
59. Eckhardt S, Hernadi Z, Thurzo L, Telekes A, Sopkova B, Mechl Z, et al. Phase II clinical evaluation of etoposide (VP-16-213, Vepesid) as a second-line treatment in ovarian cancer. Results of the South-East European Oncology Group (SEEOG) Study. Oncology. 1990;47:289–95.
60. Hoskins PJ, Swenerton KD. Oral etoposide is active against platinum-resistant epithelial ovarian cancer. J Clin Oncol. 1994;12:60–3.
61. Alici S, Saip P, Eralp Y, Aydiner A, Topuz E. Oral etoposide (VP16) in platinum-resistant epithelial ovarian cancer (EOC). Am J Clin Oncol. 2003;26:358–62.
62. Rose PG, Blessing JA, Mayer AR, Homesley HD. Prolonged oral etoposide as second-line therapy for platinum-resistant and platinum-sensitive ovarian carcinoma: a Gynecologic Oncology Group study. J Clin Oncol. 1998;16:405–10.
63. Nishio S, Sugiyama T, Shouji T, Yoshizaki A, Kitagawa R, Ushijima K, et al. Pilot study evaluating the efficacy and toxicity of irinotecan plus oral etoposide for platinum- and taxane-resistant epithelial ovarian cancer. Gynecol Oncol. 2007;106:342–7.
64. Matsumoto K, Katsumata N, Shibata T, Satoh T, Saitou M, Yunokawa M, et al. Phase II trial of oral etoposide plus intravenous irinotecan in patients with platinum-resistant and taxane-pretreated ovarian cancer (JCOG0503). Gynecol Oncol. 2015;136:218–23.
65. Watanabe Y, Etoh T, Koike E, Mizuno Y, Wang WM, Hoshiai H. Feasibility study of oral cyclophosphamide salvage therapy for the treatment of heavily pretreated patients with recurrent epithelial ovarian cancer. Int J Clin Oncol. 2010;15:468–71.
66. Jain RK. Normalizing tumor vasculature with anti-angiogenic therapy: a new paradigm for combination therapy. Nat Med. 2001;7:987–9.
67. Willett CG, Boucher Y, di Tomaso E, Duda DG, Munn LL, Tong RT, et al. Direct evidence that the VEGF-specific antibody bevacizumab has antivascular effects in human rectal cancer. Nat Med. 2004;10:145–7.
68. Hurwitz H, Fehrenbacher L, Novotny W, Cartwright T, Hainsworth J, Heim W, et al. Bevacizumab plus irinotecan, fluorouracil, and leucovorin for metastatic colorectal cancer. N Engl J Med. 2004;350:2335–42.
69. Giantonio BJ, Catalano PJ, Meropol NJ, O'Dwyer PJ, Mitchell EP, Alberts SR, et al. Bevacizumab in combination with oxaliplatin, fluorouracil, and leucovorin (FOLFOX4) for previously treated metastatic colorectal cancer: results from the Eastern Cooperative Oncology Group Study E3200. J Clin Oncol. 2007;25:1539–44.
70. Sandler A, Gray R, Perry MC, Brahmer J, Schiller JH, Dowlati A, et al. Paclitaxel-carboplatin alone or with bevacizumab for non-small-cell lung cancer. N Engl J Med. 2006;355:2542–50.
71. Cannistra SA, Matulonis UA, Penson RT, Hambleton J, Dupont J, Mackey H, et al. Phase II study of bevacizumab in patients with platinum-resistant ovarian cancer or peritoneal serous cancer. J Clin Oncol. 2007;25:5180–6.
72. Wright JD, Hagemann A, Rader JS, Viviano D, Gibb RK, Norris L, et al. Bevacizumab combination therapy in recurrent, platinum-refractory, epithelial ovarian carcinoma: A retrospective analysis. Cancer. 2006;107:83–9.
73. Garcia AA, Hirte H, Fleming G, Yang D, Tsao-Wei DD, Roman L, et al. Phase II clinical trial of bevacizumab and low-dose metronomic oral cyclophosphamide in recurrent ovarian cancer: a trial of the California, Chicago, and Princess Margaret Hospital phase II consortia. J Clin Oncol. 2008;26:76–82.
74. Hatake K, Doi T, Uetake H, Takahashi Y, Ishihara Y, Shirao K. Bevacizumab safety in Japanese patients with colorectal cancer. Jpn J Clin Oncol. 2016;46:234–40.

75. Pujade-Lauraine E, Hilpert F, Weber B, Reuss A, Poveda A, Kristensen G, et al. Bevacizumab combined with chemotherapy for platinum-resistant recurrent ovarian cancer: The AURELIA open-label randomized phase III trial. J Clin Oncol. 2014;32:1302–8.
76. Husain A, Wang Y, Hanker LC, Ojeda B, Anttila M, Breda E, et al. Independent radiologic review of AURELIA, a phase 3 trial of bevacizumab plus chemotherapy for platinum-resistant recurrent ovarian cancer. Gynecol Oncol. 2016;142:465–70.
77. Bennouna J, Sastre J, Arnold D, Osterlund P, Greil R, Van Cutsem E, et al. Continuation of bevacizumab after first progression in metastatic colorectal cancer (ML18147): a randomised phase 3 trial. Lancet Oncol. 2013;14:29–37.
78. Takeda M, Yamanaka T, Seto T, Hayashi H, Azuma K, Okada M, et al. Bevacizumab beyond disease progression after first-line treatment with bevacizumab plus chemotherapy in advanced nonsquamous non-small cell lung cancer (West Japan Oncology Group 5910L): An open-label, randomized, phase 2 trial. Cancer. 2016;122:1050–9.
79. Matulonis UA, Berlin S, Ivy P, Tyburski K, Krasner C, Zarwan C, et al. Cediranib, an oral inhibitor of vascular endothelial growth factor receptor kinases, is an active drug in recurrent epithelial ovarian, fallopian tube, and peritoneal cancer. J Clin Oncol. 2009;27:5601–6.
80. Friedlander M, Hancock KC, Rischin D, Messing MJ, Stringer CA, Matthys GM, et al. A Phase II, open-label study evaluating pazopanib in patients with recurrent ovarian cancer. Gynecol Oncol. 2010;119:32–7.
81. Ledermann JA, Embleton AC, Raja F, Perren TJ, Jayson GC, Rustin GJ, et al. Cediranib in patients with relapsed platinum-sensitive ovarian cancer (ICON6): a randomised, double-blind, placebo-controlled phase 3 trial. Lancet. 2016;387:1066–74.
82. Matsumura N, Mandai M, Okamoto T, Yamaguchi K, Yamamura S, Oura T, et al. Sorafenib efficacy in ovarian clear cell carcinoma revealed by transcriptome profiling. Cancer Sci. 2010;101:2658–63.
83. Koshiyama M, Matsumura N, Baba T, Yamaguchi K, Yoshioka Y, Konishi I. Two cases of recurrent ovarian clear cell carcinoma treated with sorafenib. Cancer Biol Ther. 2014;15:22–5.
84. Karlan BY, Oza AM, Richardson GE, Provencher DM, Hansen VL, Buck M, et al. Randomized, double-blind, placebo-controlled phase II study of AMG 386 combined with weekly paclitaxel in patients with recurrent ovarian cancer. J Clin Oncol. 2012;30:362–71.
85. Monk BJ, Poveda A, Vergote I, Raspagliesi F, Fujiwara K, Bae DS, et al. Anti-angiopoietin therapy with trebananib for recurrent ovarian cancer (TRINOVA-1): a randomised, multicentre, double-blind, placebo-controlled phase 3 trial. Lancet Oncol. 2014;15:799–808.
86. Monk BJ, Poveda A, Vergote I, Raspagliesi F, Fujiwara K, Bae DS, et al. Final results of a phase 3 study of trebananib plus weekly paclitaxel in recurrent ovarian cancer (TRINOVA-1): long-term survival, impact of ascites, and progression-free survival-2. Gynecol Oncol. 2016;143:27–34.
87. Okazaki T, Chikuma S, Iwai Y, Fagarasan S, Honjo T. A rheostat for immune responses: the unique properties of PD-1 and their advantages for clinical application. Nat Immunol. 2013;14:1212–8.
88. Kooi S, Zhang HZ, Patenia R, Edwards CL, Platsoucas CD, Freedman RS. HLA class I expression on human ovarian carcinoma cells correlates with T-cell infiltration in vivo and T-cell expansion in vitro in low concentrations of recombinant interleukin-2. Cell Immunol. 1996;174:116–28.
89. Hamanishi J, Mandai M, Iwasaki M, Okazaki T, Tanaka Y, Yamaguchi K, et al. Programmed cell death 1 ligand 1 and tumor-infiltrating CD8+ T lymphocytes are prognostic factors of human ovarian cancer. Proc Natl Acad Sci U S A. 2007;104:3360–5.
90. Zou W, Chen L. Inhibitory B7-family molecules in the tumour microenvironment. Nat Rev Immunol. 2008;8:467–77.
91. Keir ME, Butte MJ, Freeman GJ, Sharpe AH. PD-1 and its ligands in tolerance and immunity. Annu Rev Immunol. 2008;26:677–704.
92. Topalian SL, Hodi FS, Brahmer JR, Gettinger SN, Smith DC, McDermott DF, et al. Safety, activity, and immune correlates of anti-PD-1 antibody in cancer. N Engl J Med. 2012;366:2443–54.

93. Robert C, Long GV, Brady B, Dutriaux C, Maio M, Mortier L, et al. Nivolumab in previously untreated melanoma without BRAF mutation. N Engl J Med. 2015;372:320–30.
94. Borghaei H, Paz-Ares L, Horn L, Spigel DR, Steins M, Ready NE, et al. Nivolumab versus Docetaxel in advanced nonsquamous non-small-cell lung cancer. N Engl J Med. 2015;373:1627–39.
95. Hamanishi J, Mandai M, Ikeda T, Minami M, Kawaguchi A, Murayama T, et al. Safety and antitumor activity of Anti-PD-1 antibody, Nivolumab, in patients with platinum-resistant ovarian cancer. J Clin Oncol. 2015;33:4015–22.
96. Hodi FS, Butler M, Oble DA, Seiden MV, Haluska FG, Kruse A, et al. Immunologic and clinical effects of antibody blockade of cytotoxic T lymphocyte-associated antigen 4 in previously vaccinated cancer patients. Proc Natl Acad Sci U S A. 2008;105:3005–10.
97. Peng J, Hamanishi J, Matsumura N, Abiko K, Murat K, Baba T, et al. Chemotherapy induces programmed cell death-ligand 1 overexpression via the nuclear factor-kappab to foster an immunosuppressive tumor microenvironment in ovarian cancer. Cancer Res. 2015;75:5034–45.
98. Le DT, Uram JN, Wang H, Bartlett BR, Kemberling H, Eyring AD, et al. PD-1 blockade in tumors with mismatch-repair deficiency. N Engl J Med. 2015;372:2509–20.
99. Hamanishi J, Mandai M, Konishi I. Immune checkpoint inhibition in ovarian cancer. Int Immunol. 2016;28:339–48.
100. Kunos CA, Sill MW, Buekers TE, Walker JL, Schilder JM, Yamada SD, et al. Low-dose abdominal radiation as a docetaxel chemosensitizer for recurrent epithelial ovarian cancer: a phase I study of the Gynecologic Oncology Group. Gynecol Oncol. 2011;120:224–8.
101. Viswanathan AN, Lee H, Berkowitz R, Berlin S, Campos S, Feltmate C, et al. A prospective feasibility study of radiation and concurrent bevacizumab for recurrent endometrial cancer. Gynecol Oncol. 2014;132:55–60.
102. Yahara K, Ohguri T, Imada H, Yamaguchi S, Kawagoe T, Matsuura Y, et al. Epithelial ovarian cancer: definitive radiotherapy for limited recurrence after complete remission had been achieved with aggressive front-line therapy. J Radiat Res. 2013;54:322–9.
103. Lee SW, Park SM, Kim YM, Kim YS, Choi EK, Kim DY, et al. Radiation therapy is a treatment to be considered for recurrent epithelial ovarian cancer after chemotherapy. Tumori. 2011;97:590–5.
104. Chundury A, Apicelli A, DeWees T, Powell M, Mutch D, Thaker P, et al. Intensity modulated radiation therapy for recurrent ovarian cancer refractory to chemotherapy. Gynecol Oncol. 2016;141:134–9.
105. Machida S, Takei Y, Yoshida C, Takahashi Y, Koyanagi T, Sato N, et al. Radiation therapy for chemotherapy-resistant recurrent epithelial ovarian cancer. Oncology. 2014;86:232–8.
106. Fujiwara K, Suzuki S, Yoden E, Ishikawa H, Imajo Y, Kohno I. Local radiation therapy for localized relapsed or refractory ovarian cancer patients with or without symptoms after chemotherapy. Int J Gynecol Cancer. 2002;12:250–6.
107. Lee YK, Park NH, Kim JW, Song YS, Kang SB, Lee HP. Gamma-knife radiosurgery as an optimal treatment modality for brain metastases from epithelial ovarian cancer. Gynecol Oncol. 2008;108:505–9.
108. Ratner ES, Toy E, O'Malley DM, McAlpine J, Rutherford TJ, Azodi M, et al. Brain metastases in epithelial ovarian and primary peritoneal carcinoma. Int J Gynecol Cancer. 2009;19:856–9.

Management of Ovarian Cancer in Adolescents and Young Adults

15

Norihito Yoshioka and Nao Suzuki

Abstract

About 70,000 young people (ages 15–39) called adolescents and young adults (AYAs) are diagnosed with cancer each year in the United States. The numbers of cancers in AYAs are about six times compared with in children ages 0–14. The past 20 years have seen great improvements in cancer treatment for both children and adults. However, the AYAs with cancer typically do not receive as much attention as children and older adults, and marked improvements in the outcomes of cancer treatment in AYAs have not yet been seen. Therefore, cancer treatments for AYAs must be considered by the specialist.

The clinical study of cancer in AYAs has only just begun. As cancer patients of AYAs often suffer from particular types of cancers and exhibit different therapeutic outcomes from those seen in children and adults today.

In this chapter, we will focus on AYAs and review the management of ovarian cancer in this age group.

Keywords

Adolescent • Ovarian cancer • Treatment

15.1 Introduction

The past 20 years have seen great improvements in cancer treatment for both children and adults. However, marked improvements in the outcomes of cancer treatment in adolescents and young adults (AYAs), who comprise the age group

N. Yoshioka, M.D., Ph.D. (✉) • N. Suzuki, M.D., Ph.D.
Department of Obstetrics and Gynecology, St. Marianna University School of Medicine, Kawasaki, Kanagawa, Japan
e-mail: yoshi531@marianna-u.ac.jp

H. Katabuchi (ed.), *Frontiers in Ovarian Cancer Science*, Comprehensive Gynecology and Obstetrics, DOI 10.1007/978-981-10-4160-0_15

between children and adults, have not yet been seen [1]. Cancer strategies for this age group have been recently prioritized with the aim of improving the survivorship of AYAs. Adolescent girls and young women in particular span the age gap between the fields of pediatrics and gynecology, combining the characteristics of both. Therefore, cancer treatments for both of these age groups must be considered.

It was believed that those people diagnosed with cancer in adolescence or young adulthood between 1975 and 1980 had a better prognosis than the younger or older generations. However, establishment of a range of new treatments and clinical trials improved the survival rate for both children and regular adults, without any corresponding improvements in the survival rate for AYAs. This means that survival rates for the latter generations have become comparatively worse [1]. One possible reason for this is the lack of clinical trials of cancer treatments in AYAs [1]. As a result, the National Cancer Institute (NCI) and the Livestrong Foundation's Adolescent and Young Adults Oncology Progress Review Group collaborated between 2004 and 2005 in carrying out a 10-year study on AYA cancer patients in the United States. Therefore, the clinical study of cancer in AYAs has only just begun. As cancer patients of this age group often suffer from particular types of cancers and exhibit different therapeutic outcomes from those seen in younger children and older adults today, cancer in AYAs is an important topic for research. In this chapter, we will focus on AYAs, who comprise the age group between children and adult women and review the management of ovarian cancer in this age group.

15.2 Definition of Adolescent and Young Adult

AYAs are often defined as individuals aged between 15 and 39 years, but this may vary in different studies [2, 3]. Recent definitions of AYAs are summarized in Table 15.1. The Surveillance, Epidemiology, and End Results (SEER) Report published by the NCI in 2006 defined adolescent and young adult oncology patients as those aged 15–29 years [2]. However, in the report of the NCI's Adolescent and Young Adult Oncology Progress Review Group and the 2016 National Comprehensive Cancer Network (NCCN) Guidelines, they were defined as those aged 15–39 years [2]. Thus, the current mainstream view is to regard those aged 15–39 years as AYAs and to deal with them separately from both younger children and older adults. In our description in this chapter, we will regard AYAs as those aged between 15 and 39 years.

Table. 15.1 Definition of adolescent and young adult

SEER (NCI)	15–29-year-old
Adolescent and young Adult Oncology Progress Review Group	15–39-year-old
NCCN	15–39-year-old

15.3 Cancer in AYAs Worldwide Including Ovarian Cancer

In the United States, 70,000 AYAs are diagnosed with cancer every year, which is seven times more than the number of cancer patients aged under 15 years [4]. In 2014, there were 5330 cancer diagnoses and 610 cancer deaths among adolescents [5]. Keegan et al. used the SEER 13 registry data from 2002 to 2006 to report the 5-year survival rates for various cancers in 45,232 children, AYAs, and older adults [2]. According to that study, the most common cancers among AYAs were breast carcinoma (14.4%), thyroid carcinoma (12.1%), and melanoma (11.2%). The cancers with the best 5-year survival rates were thyroid carcinoma (99.7%), testicular cancer (96.1%), and melanoma (95.5%). Those with the worst 5-year survival rates were hepatic carcinoma (22.8%), gastric carcinoma (26.3%), and pancreatic carcinoma (33.0%), while the other forms of cancer for which the 5-year survival rates were under 50% included high-grade astrocytoma, lung carcinoma, rhabdomyosarcoma, and acute myeloid leukemia. Ovarian cancer occurred in 919 AYAs of the 45,232 included in the study (2.0%), with a 5-year survival rate of 79.5%, which is a much better outcome than the 41.4% 5-year survival rate for older adults aged over 40 years. Thus, survival rate for ovarian cancer in AYAs is not lower than that for other cancers and is higher than that in older adult women. This high survival rate in AYAs suggests that the choice of treatment method should prioritize improving the quality of life (QOL) of the patients.

15.4 Incidence of Ovarian Cancer in AYAs in Japan

As shown in Table 15.2 the Gynecological Cancer Committee carried out a study on 2832 ovarian cancer patients who had started treatment in 2009 at 182 institutions according to clinical statistics. Patients who underwent preoperative chemotherapy and those whose stage was unknown were excluded. Included patients were classified into one of three age groups (under 19, 20–39, and over 40 years), and their ovarian cancer stage was compared. Of the total 2832 patients with ovarian cancer, 25 (0.88%) were aged under 19 years, 283 (10.0%) were aged 20–39 years, and 2524 (89.1%) were aged over 40 years, with the latter accounting for over 90% of the cases. Proportion of patients aged under 39 years with ovarian cancer was 10.88%, and those aged under 19 years was only 0.88%, indicating that this disease is extremely rare in the latter age group. An investigation of the characteristics of ovarian cancer by age group found that of the 2524 patients aged over 40 years, 1152 (45.6%) had Stage I, 275 (10.9%) had Stage II, 884 (35.0%) had Stage III, and 213 (8.5%) had Stage IV cancers. Stages I and III were the most common cancer stages, which is also similar to the general statistics for ovarian cancer, with little difference between the proportions of Stage I and Stage III patients. Of the 308 patients aged under 39 years, 204 (66.2%) had Stage I, 27 (8.8%) had Stage II, 66 (21.4%) had Stage III, and 11 (3.6%) had Stage IV cancers. For the patients aged over 40 years, most cancers were discovered at either Stage I or III, but among those aged under 39 years, a higher proportion was discovered at Stage I. In terms of the

Table 15.2 Characteristics of ovarian cancer stage by age group (Data of JSOG)

	Age	~19		20 ~ 39		40~		Total
FIGO stage		case	%	case	%	case	%	
I	A	8	32	76	26.8	446	17.6	530
	B	1	4	1	0.4	24	1.0	26
	C(b)	4	16	68	24.0	381	15.1	453
	C (1)	0	0	5	1.8	27	1.1	32
	C (2)	1	4	13	4.6	116	4.6	130
	C(a)	4	16	23	8.1	158	6.3	185
II	A	0	0	3	1.1	28	1.1	31
	B	0	0	4	1.4	29	1.1	33
	C(b)	0	0	11	3.9	62	2.5	73
	C (1)	0	0	0	0	7	0.3	7
	C (2)	0	0	3	1.1	59	2.3	62
	C(a)	0	0	6	2.1	90	3.6	96
III	A	1	4	5	1.8	50	2.0	56
	B	0	0	10	3.5	97	3.8	107
	C	4	16	46	16.2	737	29.2	787
IV		2	8	9	3.2	213	8.4	224
total		25		283		2524		2832

substaging of Stage I ovarian cancers among those aged under 39 years, 84 patients (27.2%) had Stage IA, 2 (0.6%) had Stage IB, and 118 (38.3%) had Stage IC cancers, with Stage IC tending to be more common. Further, an investigation of those aged under 19 years (25 patients) found that 18 (72%) had Stage I, 0 (0%) had Stage II, 5 (20%) had Stage III, and 2 (8%) had Stage IV cancers, with a higher proportion of Stage I cancers compared with the other two age groups.

Figure 15.1 shows a summary of the yearly numbers of ovarian cancer patients reported by the Gynecological Cancer Committee of the JSOG (2003–2014) [6, 7]. An investigation on the 49,513 ovarian cancer patients registered in these annual patient reports found that 4895 (9.9%) were AYAs (this statistic included those aged under 15 years as AYAs). These 4895 AYA patients were then classified according to whether their tumor was epithelial, sex cord-stromal, germ cell, or others, and the results were plotted on a graph by age group (Fig. 15.1). As shown in Fig. 15.1, there were 363 ovarian cancer patients aged under 19 years, accounting for 7.4% of AYA ovarian cancer patients. Germ cell tumors were present in 285 cases (78.5%), followed by epithelial tumors in 64 cases (17.6%). There were 1128 ovarian cancer patients aged 20–29 years, accounting for 23.0% of AYA ovarian cancer patients. Epithelial tumors were present in 639 cases (56.6%), followed by germ cell tumors in 471 cases (41.6%). There were 3404 ovarian cancer patients aged 30–39 years, accounting for 69.5% of AYA ovarian cancer patients. Epithelial tumors were present in 2995 cases (88.0%), followed by germ cell tumors in 354 cases (10.4%).

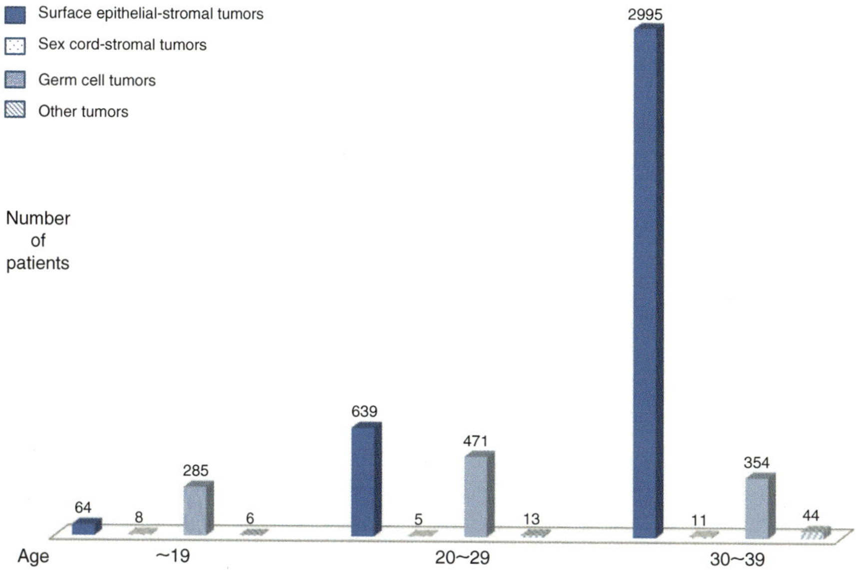

Fig. 15.1 Pathological characteristics of ovarian cancer in AYAs (Data of JSOG)

Bringing together all the AYA ovarian cancer patient data available to date, AYAs account for approximately 9.9% of all ovarian cancer patients, with the highest proportion aged 30–39 years (69.5%), followed by those aged 20–29 years (23.0%) and under 19 years (7.4%). Almost all cancer tumors in AYA ovarian cancer patients were either epithelial tumors or germ cell tumors. Epithelial tumors accounted for the great majority of cancers among those aged 30–39 years, which is similar to ovarian cancer patients aged over 40 years. For those aged 20–29 years, epithelial tumors and germ cell tumors accounted for around half of the cases each. Those aged under 19 years, however, exhibited different characteristics from those aged 20–29 years, with germ cell tumors accounting for 78.5% of the cases.

15.5 Treatment of AYA Ovarian Cancer Patients

From the perspective of improving survivorship, the most important point in the treatment of AYA ovarian cancer patients is to spare their fertility. AYAs are generally defined as those aged between 15 and 39 years, and as members of this age group who may either be considering pregnancy in the future or already want to have children, treatment methods must always be chosen with the conservation of fertility in mind.

The recommended basic fertility-sparing surgical technique for ovarian cancer patients is the ipsilateral salpingo-oophorectomy with omentectomy and laparoscopic cytology. Ipsilateral ovarian biopsy with para-aortic lymph node or pelvic lymph node dissection or biopsy and intraperitoneal biopsy may also be performed as staging laparotomy [8, 9]. Because most AYA ovarian cancer cases are known to comprise either epithelial tumors or germ cell tumors, we will provide an overview of the fertility-sparing surgery for patients with these two types of cancer tumors.

15.5.1 Treatment of Epithelial Tumors

The Japan Clinical Oncology Group (JCOG) reported data from a joint study carried out in 30 institutions in 2010 [10]. Their analysis covered 211 Stage IA or Stage IC ovarian cancer patients who underwent fertility-sparing treatments. They found that fertility-sparing surgeries are recommended for ovarian cancer patients with highly differentiated (G1) or moderately differentiated (G2) Stage IA non-clear cell carcinoma [10]. They also reported that fertility can be spared in cases of Stage IA ovarian clear cell carcinoma or G1/G2 Stage IC non-clear cell carcinoma with ipsilateral lesions as long as an adjuvant chemotherapy is performed [10]. However, the fertility-sparing surgeries are not recommended for G3 Stage I non-clear cell carcinoma and Stage IC clear cell carcinoma patients [10, 11]. Although it may be possible to preserve fertility by carrying out an adjuvant chemotherapy, this may be assumed to deplete the ovarian reserve, depending on the patient's age. Ovarian toxicity of anticancer agents will be discussed below.

15.5.2 Treatment of Germ Cell Tumors

Germ cell tumors are rare tumors that account for less than 5% of all malignant ovarian cancers [11, 12]. However, as these tend to occur in the younger age group (10–29 years) [11, 13], are highly sensitive to chemotherapy, and are ipsilateral in over 95% of the cases [11, 14], they do not frequently provide opportunities to consider the issue of conserving the fertility of AYA ovarian cancer patients. When sparing fertility, detailed peritoneal investigation in addition to ipsilateral salpingo-oophorectomy with omentectomy and laparoscopic cytology is recommended. Some experts consider that tumor debulking is useful for patients with Stage III or IV advanced cancers, but organ damage and combined resection must be avoided and chemotherapy must be started as soon as possible. Fertility-sparing surgeries are not believed to affect the prognosis of patients with advanced cancers [15], and for younger individuals such as AYAs, a procedure that preserves ovarian function and fertility should be chosen. If the patient does not wish to conserve her fertility, the procedure for the initial surgery for ovarian carcinoma should be followed. Germ cell tumors grow rapidly; therefore, it is important that they be diagnosed early and their treatment be started rapidly.

BEP (bleomycin, etoposide and cisplatin) therapy with bleomycin, etoposide, and cisplatin is strongly recommended as a postoperative adjuvant chemotherapy [11, 16–19]. A study of malignant ovarian germ cell tumors in the early 1970s, before the development of the current chemotherapy, found that the cure rate for patients with advanced cancers who underwent surgery alone was almost 0% and that for those with Stage I cancer, it was only 5–20% [20]. Subsequent clinical trials of BEP therapy for testicular germ cell tumors, which are ten times more common than ovarian germ cell tumors, resulted in its establishment as the standard treatment for ovarian germ cell tumors as well. The reported cure rate of BEP therapy for ovarian germ cell tumors is almost 100% for early-stage tumors and over 75% even in advanced cases [18], making it highly effective as postoperative adjuvant chemotherapy. Although there are some concerns about the ovarian toxicity of chemotherapy, BEP therapy does not include any drugs that are severely toxic to the ovaries [21]. Chemotherapy can be omitted for Stage IA undifferentiated germ cell tumors and G1 Stage I immature teratomas [15, 22]. In such cases, prognosis is reportedly good if a treatment strategy of rigorous monitoring and the use of BEP therapy in the event of recurrence is followed [20]. Thus, fertility-sparing surgeries are the treatment of choice for such germ cell tumors in AYAs, and the use of BEP therapy as a postoperative adjuvant chemotherapy or recurrence therapy is recommended.

15.6 Fertility Preservation Treatment in AYAs

Young cancer patients and those with autoimmune diseases may suffer from irreversible reproductive dysfunctions from the anticancer agents or radiotherapy used to treat them. The concept of oncofertility, bringing together the fields of oncology and reproductive medicine to resolve gonadal failure, loss of fertility, and other reproductive issues following cancer treatment, was proposed by Woodruff et al. in 2006. Conservation of fertility must always be a matter of concern for cancer patients in the AYA age group, and oncofertility treatment is very often indicated. Here, we will describe the current status and future prospects of the oncofertility treatment required for ovarian cancer in AYAs.

15.6.1 Chemotherapy-Induced Ovarian Toxicity

Although surgery is an important treatment for ovarian cancer, anticancer drug therapy is also extremely important. In AYA cancer patients, it is both important to perform fertility-sparing surgeries and to consider gonadal toxicity if chemotherapy is required. However, the gonadal tissue is extremely vulnerable to chemotherapy, and the resulting damage is permanent. Oligomenorrhea, amenorrhea, anovulation, and other forms of ovarian dysfunction resulting from the use of chemotherapy are termed "chemotherapy-induced amenorrhea" and occur with a reported incidence of 20–100% [23]. Frequency of chemotherapy-induced amenorrhea has been found to depend on the choice of drug used, duration of treatment, and its total dose [24]. Incidence of premature menopause is reportedly lower in younger patients, who still have a large number of primordial follicles remaining, than in older adults [25]. Table 15.3 [26] shows the risk categories for the ovarian toxicity of anticancer agents. Alkylating agents are the best-known cytotoxic anticancer agents, and

Table 15.3 Classification of chemotherapy-induced ovarian toxicity

Risk	Chemotherapy
High risk	Cyclophosphamide
	Ifosfamide
	Dacarbazine
Intermediate risk	Cisplatin
	Carboplatin
	Doxorubicin
	Etoposide
Low risk	Actinomycin D
	Vincristine
	Methotrexate
	Fluorouracil
	Bleomycin
No data	Paclitaxel
	Docetaxel
	Gemcitabine
	Irinotecan

cyclophosphamide and ifosfamide are among the most commonly used drugs of this type. As shown in Table 15.3, cyclophosphamide is classified as a particularly high-risk agent, as it causes severe ovarian toxicity and is believed to entail a high risk of refractory infertility [27]. Risk of cyclophosphamide-induced amenorrhea increases after the age of 35 years and reportedly exceeds 80% over the age of 40 years [28]. These drugs are seldom included in the regimens currently used for ovarian cancer treatment. Doxorubicin, the best-known anthracycline anticancer agent, exerts its antitumor effect by suppressing RNA and DNA biosynthesis. As shown in Table 15.3, it is categorized as an intermediate risk agent and may be included in second-line and subsequent regimens. Doxorubicin-induced ovarian toxicity results in amenorrhea in 96% of women aged 40–49 years [23], but its incidence in younger age groups was reportedly less than 10% [29]. Platinum-based anticancer agents, which act by inhibiting DNA replication and inducing apoptosis, include cisplatin, carboplatin, and nedaplatin. The only reports of ovarian toxicity involve cisplatin, for which the incidence of amenorrhea is reportedly related to the total dose administered [30]. Basic experiments have also shown that cisplatin reduces the ovulation rate in rats and diminishes the concentrations of anti-Mullerian hormone (AMH) and inhibin-α in the blood [31]. BEP therapy, as described above as the first treatment of choice for germ cell tumors, includes cisplatin and is used to treat AYAs [16–19]. A study on 41 Stage I germ cell tumor patients treated with BEP therapy after fertility-sparing surgeries found that normal menstrual cycles were preserved in 71.4% of the cases, and no patient developed primary ovarian insufficiencies (POI) [32]. Thus, fertility may be comparatively well preserved following BEP therapy.

Taxane anticancer agents, such as paclitaxel and docetaxel, are used in the standard regimens for the treatment of surface epithelial-stromal tumors. Animal experiments in rats have also shown that paclitaxel reduces the number of primordial ovarian follicles [33] but does not exert severe ovarian toxicities in this animal model [34]. Further, a prospective study that compared anthracycline and taxane anticancer agents found that the incidence of amenorrhea was higher when taxanes were used [35]. However, as shown in Table 15.3, they are classified in the risk category of "no data." Thus, more data must be gathered on their effect on fertility after chemotherapy for ovarian cancer.

15.6.2 Radiotherapy-Induced Ovarian Toxicity

As described above, surface epithelial-stromal and germ cell tumors account for the vast majority of ovarian cancers in AYAs. These forms of ovarian cancer are mainly treated by surgery and chemotherapy, with radiotherapy used in only a few cases. If complete remission is not achieved after initial treatments for surface epithelial-stromal tumors, then maintaining the patient's QOL is prioritized, with complaints of pain particularly requiring proactive treatments. Further, radiotherapy for palliative purposes is reportedly effective [36, 37]. Among germ cell tumors, one tumor for which radiotherapy is effective is dysgerminoma. Like the seminoma in the testes, dysgerminoma is highly sensitive to radiation, and until the late 1980s, radiotherapy was frequently used to treat patients with this type of tumor. From then on, good therapeutic outcomes were obtained from chemotherapy, and as radiotherapy makes fertility preservation difficult and causes acute toxicity to organs such as those in the gastrointestinal tract, it is now very seldom used to treat dysgerminoma. Thus, it is now rare for AYAs to undergo radiotherapies for ovarian cancer. In this chapter, we will also describe radiation-induced ovarian toxicities in general.

The testes and ovaries, which are the gonads responsible for reproductive function, are exceptionally sensitive to radiation. Toxicity is induced by far lower doses of radiation than those tolerated by many other healthy tissues. When these tissues fall within the radiation field, it has an extremely strong effect, and even outside the radiation field, the threshold is often exceeded by trace amounts of scattered radiation. Radiation exposure of 4–6 Gy in adults and 10–20 Gy in children is generally regarded as sufficient doses to reduce ovarian function, and studies have found that irreversible ovarian failure is caused by radiation exposure exceeding 18.5 Gy at age 10 years, 16.5 Gy at age 20 years, and 14.3 Gy at age 30 years [38]. Generally, the best-known disease for which ovarian function is affected by radiotherapy is leukemia, in which patients undergo 12 Gy total body irradiation (TBI) before bone marrow transplantation. Other situations for which ovary management is a matter of great concern during treatment planning include total pelvic irradiation for cervical cancer, Wilms tumor in children, neuroblastoma, and postoperative irradiation for abdominal rhabdomyosarcoma. The ovaries can be preserved in some cases of cervical cancer in young women. If the ovaries have been spared, ovarian displacement should be considered to move the ovaries out of the radiation field to avoid their exposure during postoperative radiotherapies. Ovarian function after ovarian displacement is generally good [39], with reported rates of ovarian function maintenance of 41 [40], 50 [41], 60 [42], and 71% [43]. If the radiation dose to the displaced ovaries is less than 3 Gy, ovarian function is reportedly maintained in 90% of the patients [41], although measures must be taken to anchor the ovaries after their displacement.

15.7 Fertility Preservation Treatment

Although the prevalence of cancer has been recently increasing, development of multimodal therapies has enabled many patients to overcome their disease. In particular, the 5-year survival rate for pediatric cancer patients aged under 15 years and for those in the AYA age group now exceeds 80%, and consideration of fertility preservation in younger cancer patients is progressing on a daily basis. From the viewpoint of improving the survivorship and QOL of younger cancer patients, the use of fertility preservation treatments before multimodal therapies are implemented is one method of avoiding fertility loss. There are three possible choices of fertility preservation methods in women: cryopreserved embryos, cryopreserved eggs, and cryopreserved ovarian tissue. Which of these is chosen will depend on considerations including (1) the type of cancer, (2) how advanced it is, (3) the types of anticancer agents used, (4) when chemotherapy is started, (5) age at the start of treatment, and (6) whether or not the patient is married. Each method has its own advantages and disadvantages and must be implemented with a full understanding of its indications and precautions, including the medical and social contexts. It is important to inform patients that fertility preservation treatment does not guarantee that pregnancy can be achieved and that its use in cancer patients entails some risk. Additionally, we should obtain their full understanding. It is also imperative to prioritize cancer treatments above all else and to offer fertility preservation treatments in such a way that the treatment of underlying diseases is not delayed, with the doctors only providing it if they judge it to be feasible. As ovarian cancer means that cancer cells are present in the ovarian tissue itself, ovarian tissue cryopreservation is contraindicated because of its risk of minimal residual disease (MRD) development. However, the first live birth resulting from an embryo generated by the harvesting of immature oocytes from surgically extracted ovarian tissue, in vitro maturation and fertilization, and subsequent embryo implantation has been recently reported in a case that indicates the potential for oncofertility treatment use in advanced medical institutions [44].

Conclusion

Ovarian cancer in AYAs has specific characteristics compared with the same disease in other age groups. Preservation of fertility must always be taken into account when considering treatments, but this must be handled carefully as this is an area in which sufficient evidence has yet to be established. Close collaboration between pediatricians and obstetricians/gynecologists, including during the post-treatment period, is required in the future to gather evidence on the treatment of ovarian cancer in this age group and provide better treatment.

References

1. Bleyer A. O'Leary M BR, Ries L. Cancer epidemiology in older adolescents and young adults 15 to 29 years of age, including SEER incidence and survivals: 1975–2000. National Cancer Institute, NIH Pub 2006.
2. Keegan TH, Ries LA, Barr RD, et al. Comparison of cancer survival trends in the United States of adolescents and young adults with those in children and older adults. Cancer. 2016;122:1009–16.
3. Sender L, Zabokrtsky KB. Adolescent and young adult patients with cancer: a milieu of unique features. Nat Rev Clin Oncol. 2015;12:465–80.
4. U.S. Department of Health and Human Services, National Institutes of Health, National Cancer Institute, Livestrong Young Adult Alliance. Closing the gap: research and care imperatives for adolescents and young adults with cancer: report of the adolescent and young adults oncology progress review group. U.S. Department of Health and Human Services, National Institutes of Health, National Cancer Institute, Livestrong Young Adult Alliance, 2006.
5. Ward E, DeSantis C, Robbins A, Kohler B, Jemal A. Childhood and adolescent cancer statistics, 2014. CA Cancer J Clin. 2014;64:83–103.
6. Yamagami W, Aoki D. Annual report of the Committee on Gynecologic Oncology, the Japan Society of Obstetrics and Gynecology. J Obstet Gynaecol Res. 2015;41:1861–9.
7. Saito T, Katabuchi H. Annual Report of the Committee on Gynecologic Oncology, Japan Society of Obstetrics and Gynecology: Patient Annual Report for 2013 and Treatment Annual Report for 2008. J Obstet Gynaecol Res. 2016;42:1069–79.
8. Lee IH, Choi CH, Hong DG, et al. Clinicopathologic characteristics of granulosa cell tumors of the ovary: a multicenter retrospective study. J Gynecol Oncol. 2011;22:188–95.
9. Zhang M, Cheung MK, Shin JY, et al. Prognostic factors responsible for survival in sex cord stromal tumors of the ovary--an analysis of 376 women. Gynecol Oncol. 2007;104:396–400.
10. Satoh T, Hatae M, Watanabe Y, et al. Outcomes of fertility-sparing surgery for stage I epithelial ovarian cancer: a proposal for patient selection. J Clin Oncol. 2010;28:1727–32.
11. Komiyama S, Katabuchi H, Mikami M, et al. Japan Society of Gynecologic Oncology guidelines 2015 for the treatment of ovarian cancer including primary peritoneal cancer and fallopian tube cancer. Int J Clin Oncol. 2016;21:435–46.
12. Parker SL, Tong T, Bolden S, Wingo PA. Cancer statistics, 1997. CA Cancer J Clin. 1997;47:5–27.
13. Chan JK, Tewari KS, Waller S, et al. The influence of conservative surgical practices for malignant ovarian germ cell tumors. J Surg Oncol. 2008;98:111–6.
14. Mahdi H, Swensen RE, Hanna R, et al. Prognostic impact of lymphadenectomy in clinically early stage malignant germ cell tumour of the ovary. Br J Cancer. 2011;105:493–7.
15. Patterson DM, Murugaesu N, Holden L, Seckl MJ, Rustin GJ. A review of the close surveillance policy for stage I female germ cell tumors of the ovary and other sites. Int J Gynecol Cancer. 2008;18:43–50.
16. Gershenson DM, Morris M, Cangir A, et al. Treatment of malignant germ cell tumors of the ovary with bleomycin, etoposide, and cisplatin. J Clin Oncol. 1990;8:715–20.
17. Brown J, Shvartsman HS, Deavers MT, et al. The activity of taxanes compared with bleomycin, etoposide, and cisplatin in the treatment of sex cord-stromal ovarian tumors. Gynecol Oncol. 2005;97:489–96.
18. Williams S, Blessing JA, Liao SY, Ball H, Hanjani P. Adjuvant therapy of ovarian germ cell tumors with cisplatin, etoposide, and bleomycin: a trial of the Gynecologic Oncology Group. J Clin Oncol. 1994;12:701–6.
19. Kang H, Kim TJ, Kim WY, et al. Outcome and reproductive function after cumulative high-dose combination chemotherapy with bleomycin, etoposide and cisplatin (BEP) for patients with ovarian endodermal sinus tumor. Gynecol Oncol. 2008;111:106–10.
20. Gershenson DM. Management of ovarian germ cell tumors. J Clin Oncol. 2007;25:2938–43.

21. Loren AW, Mangu PB, Beck LN, et al. Fertility preservation for patients with cancer: American Society of Clinical Oncology clinical practice guideline update. J Clin Oncol. 2013;31:2500–10.
22. Billmire DF, Cullen JW, Rescorla FJ, et al. Surveillance after initial surgery for pediatric and adolescent girls with stage I ovarian germ cell tumors: report from the Children's Oncology Group. J Clin Oncol. 2014;32:465–70.
23. Bines J, Oleske DM, Cobleigh MA. Ovarian function in premenopausal women treated with adjuvant chemotherapy for breast cancer. J Clin Oncol. 1996;14:1718–29.
24. Wallace WH, Anderson RA, Irvine DS. Fertility preservation for young patients with cancer: who is at risk and what can be offered? Lancet Oncol. 2005;6:209–18.
25. Anderson RA, Rosendahl M, Kelsey TW, Cameron DA. Pretreatment anti-Mullerian hormone predicts for loss of ovarian function after chemotherapy for early breast cancer. Eur J Cancer. 2013;49:3404–11.
26. Donnez J, Martinez-Madrid B, Jadoul P, Van Langendonckt A, Demylle D, Dolmans MM. Ovarian tissue cryopreservation and transplantation: a review. Hum Reprod Update. 2006;12:519–35.
27. Rodriguez-Wallberg KA, Oktay K. Options on fertility preservation in female cancer patients. Cancer Treat Rev. 2012;38:354–61.
28. Parulekar WR, Day AG, Ottaway JA, et al. Incidence and prognostic impact of amenorrhea during adjuvant therapy in high-risk premenopausal breast cancer: analysis of a National Cancer Institute of Canada Clinical Trials Group Study – NCIC CTG MA.5. J Clin Oncol. 2005;23:6002–8.
29. Brusamolino E, Lunghi F, Orlandi E, et al. Treatment of early-stage Hodgkin's disease with four cycles of ABVD followed by adjuvant radio-therapy: analysis of efficacy and long-term toxicity. Haematologica. 2000;85:1032–9.
30. Wallace WH, Shalet SM, Crowne EC, Morris-Jones PH, Gattamaneni HR, Price DA. Gonadal dysfunction due to cis-platinum. Med Pediatr Oncol. 1989;17:409–13.
31. Yeh J, Kim B, Liang YJ, Peresie J. Mullerian inhibiting substance as a novel biomarker of cisplatin-induced ovarian damage. Biochem Biophys Res Commun. 2006;348:337–44.
32. Park JY, Kim DY, Suh DS, et al. Outcomes of pediatric and adolescent girls with malignant ovarian germ cell tumors. Gynecol Oncol. 2015;137:418–22.
33. Yucebilgin MS, Terek MC, Ozsaran A, et al. Effect of chemotherapy on primordial follicular reserve of rat: an animal model of premature ovarian failure and infertility. Aust N Z J Obstet Gynaecol. 2004;44:6–9.
34. Tarumi W, Suzuki N, Takahashi N, et al. Ovarian toxicity of paclitaxel and effect on fertility in the rat. J Obstet Gynaecol Res. 2009;35:414–20.
35. Fornier MN, Modi S, Panageas KS, Norton L, Hudis C. Incidence of chemotherapy-induced, long-term amenorrhea in patients with breast carcinoma age 40 years and younger after adjuvant anthracycline and taxane. Cancer. 2005;104:1575–9.
36. Tinger A, Waldron T, Peluso N, et al. Effective palliative radiation therapy in advanced and recurrent ovarian carcinoma. Int J Radiat Oncol Biol Phys. 2001;51:1256–63.
37. E C, Quon M, Gallant V, Samant R. Effective palliative radiotherapy for symptomatic recurrent or residual ovarian cancer. Gynecol Oncol. 2006;102:204–9.
38. Ginsberg JP. New advances in fertility preservation for pediatric cancer patients. Curr Opin Pediatr. 2011;23:9–13.
39. Fujiwara K, Mohri H, Yoshida T, Yamauchi H, Kohno I. Subcutaneous transposition of the ovary following hysterectomy. Int J Gynaecol Obstet. 1997;58:223–8.
40. Buekers TE, Anderson B, Sorosky JI, Buller RE. Ovarian function after surgical treatment for cervical cancer. Gynecol Oncol. 2001;80:85–8.
41. Feeney DD, Moore DH, Look KY, Stehman FB, Sutton GP. The fate of the ovaries after radical hysterectomy and ovarian transposition. Gynecol Oncol. 1995;56:3–7.

42. Morice P, Juncker L, Rey A, El-Hassan J, Haie-Meder C, Castaigne D. Ovarian transposition for patients with cervical carcinoma treated by radiosurgical combination. Fertil Steril. 2000;74:743–8.
43. Chambers SK, Chambers JT, Kier R, Peschel RE. Sequelae of lateral ovarian transposition in irradiated cervical cancer patients. Int J Radiat Oncol Biol Phys. 1991;20:1305–8.
44. Prasath EB, Chan ML, Wong WH, et al. First pregnancy and live birth resulting from cryopreserved embryos obtained from in vitro matured oocytes after oophorectomy in an ovarian cancer patient. Hum Reprod. 2014;29:276–8.

Management of Ovarian Cancer in the Elderly Population

16

Masanori Kaneuchi and Hideaki Masuzaki

Abstract

Ovarian cancer is the second leading cause of female-specific cancer death in women over the age of 65 years, and almost half of newly diagnosed cases are in this age group. Many elderly people live with disability and various comorbidities and are vulnerable to stressors. Primary cytoreductive surgery followed by adjuvant chemotherapy is the conventional treatment strategy for advanced ovarian cancer. The increased likelihood of physical comorbidities in elderly patients is thought to be associated with a higher risk of postoperative morbidities and severe side effects from cytotoxic agents. Therefore, elderly patients might be undertreated and miss the opportunity to receive the conventional treatment because of concern about its risks on the part of clinicians. However, guidelines specific for the treatment of elderly patients with ovarian cancer have not been adequately developed. Although treatment strategies for these patients need to be based on relatively limited evidence, appropriate criteria for decision-making regarding treatment have been studied. Appropriate assessments of geriatric patients with cancer to predict the risks of treatment have also been proposed. In this chapter, we outline the current evidence for surgery, chemotherapy, the newer anticancer agents, and comprehensive geriatric assessment to assist gynecologists treating elderly patients with ovarian cancer.

Keywords

Ovarian cancer • Elderly • Cytoreduction • Chemotherapy • Geriatric assessment

M. Kaneuchi, M.D., Ph.D. (✉) • H. Masuzaki, M.D., Ph.D.
Department of Obstetrics and Gynecology, Nagasaki University Hospital, 1-7-1 Sakamoto, Nagasaki City 852-8501, Japan
e-mail: mkaneuc@nagasaki-u.ac.jp

H. Katabuchi (ed.), *Frontiers in Ovarian Cancer Science*, Comprehensive Gynecology and Obstetrics, DOI 10.1007/978-981-10-4160-0_16

16.1 Introduction

Ovarian cancer is the second leading cause of female-specific cancer death in women over the age of 65 years in both the USA and Japan. The most recent Surveillance, Epidemiology, and End Results (SEER) data indicate that the age-adjusted incidence rate of ovarian cancer was 11.9 per 100,000 women per year in 2009–2013 and that the number of deaths in this period was 7.5 per 100,000 women per year [1]. The median age at diagnosis of ovarian cancer was 63 years, and 45.2% of newly diagnosed cases were in women aged ≥65 years. The Japan Society of Obstetrics and Gynecology (JSOG) reported similar trends in their annual report of the committee on gynecologic oncology. Patients aged 60–69 and ≥70 years accounted for 26.9% and 17.4%, respectively, of all patients [2]. Although the World Health Organization does not define a clear cutoff point for chronological old age because of regional variations in factors affecting aging, 65 years is commonly accepted as elderly in most developed countries [3]. Therefore, it is considered that almost half of cases of ovarian cancer occur in older women.

Nearly half of ovarian cancer are diagnosed in the advanced stages and have peritoneal carcinomatosis at this time. The mainstay of treatment for advanced ovarian cancer continues to be maximal PCS (primary cytoreductive surgery) followed by adjuvant chemotherapy. These aggressive treatments have the possibility to increase the risk of peri-treatment morbidities for elderly patients, because elderly people are often in the state of frailty, living with disability and various comorbidities, and are vulnerable to stressors. Although evidences to define the treatment strategies for these patients are still limited, appropriate guidelines or criteria for decision-making regarding treatment have been studied. We would like to describe the current evidences and researches in treatment and geriatric assessment for elderly women with ovarian cancer.

16.2 Treatment-Related Risks in the Elderly

The risk of treatment-related complications increases in the elderly. Conditions such as hypertension, hypercholesterolemia, and hyperglycemia become more common as people age and increase the risk of postoperative morbidity, including delirium, infection, cardiac disease, and venous thromboembolism. There have been reports of significantly higher postoperative morbidity and mortality rates in men and women aged ≥80 years undergoing various types of surgery when compared with their younger counterparts [4, 5]. The increased likelihood of physical comorbidities in elderly patients is also associated with a greater risk of side effects from cytotoxic agents because of the altered pharmacokinetics in this age group. Therefore, conventional chemotherapy might be inadvisable in older patients with comorbidities. Further, even in the absence of definite comorbidity, elderly patients are potentially more vulnerable to physical and psychological stressors. A recent retrospective study of patients with stage III ovarian cancer in six of the Gynecologic Oncology Group (GOG) trials showed that 267 (14.1%) of 1895 enrolled patients who underwent primary cytoreductive surgery (PCS) followed by chemotherapy including paclitaxel plus cisplatin were aged ≥70 years [6]. This study showed that increasing age was associated with increased risks of disease progression (hazard ratio [HR] 1.06, 95% confidence interval [CI] 1.02–1.11 for every 10-year increment in age) and death (HR 1.12, 95% CI 1.06–1.18). This study also showed that chronological age was an independent risk factor for a poorer outcome over and above the factors already known to be associated with a poorer prognosis, namely, the histology of the cancer and size of the residual tumor after primary surgery. However, the evidence is mixed in this regard, and it is still unclear whether chronological age itself should be considered a risk factor in the context of treatment of ovarian cancer. Either way, there is concern that elderly patients with cancer might be undertreated and miss the opportunity for outcomes similar to those that can be achieved in younger patients because of concern about the risks of treatment on the part of clinicians.

16.3 Primary Therapy for Elderly Women with Ovarian Cancer

16.3.1 Primary Cytoreductive Surgery

Over half of patients diagnosed with epithelial ovarian cancer have peritoneal carcinomatosis. Therefore, complete PCS is considered key in treatment of the disease. A systematic review of studies about postoperative mortality after PCS for advanced ovarian cancer reported a mean postoperative mortality rate of 3.7% (range 2.5–4.8%) in population-based studies and an overall mean postoperative mortality rate of 2.8% [7]. Another cohort study reported that patients aged ≥65 years with stage III or IV ovarian cancer who underwent PCS had an overall 30-day mortality rate of 8.2% [8]. Although the 30-day mortality rate was 5.6% in patients in the above studies who underwent elective surgery, it was 12.7% in those aged ≥75 years. Compared with the overall average mortality rate shown in the systematic review [7], the mortality rate of the elderly patients in this cohort study was high, especially in the patients aged ≥75 years.

There is a significant relationship between the volume of residual cancer and survival after cytoreductive surgery in patients with advanced ovarian cancer. Therefore, the question arises regarding how radical cytoreductive surgery should be in this age group, given that elderly patients are considered to be at a generally increased risk of perioperative morbidity and mortality. There is some evidence that surgical treatment may be less radical in older women with ovarian cancer. A review of the SEER database found that the rate of optimal cytoreduction for advanced ovarian cancer decreased from 43.7% in women aged <60 years to 29.5 and 21.7% in those aged 60–79 years and ≥80 years, respectively [9]. However, there are reports showing that similar levels of cytoreductive surgery can be achieved in both younger and older patients [10, 11]. An analysis of 2870 patients who underwent surgery for ovarian cancer in the National Surgical Quality Improvement Program database for 2005–2012, 701 (24.4%) of whom were aged ≥70 years, showed perioperative complication rates of 9.5, 9.7, 13.4, and 14.6% in patients aged <50, 50–59, 60–69, and ≥70 years, respectively [12]. Compared with patients aged ≤50 years, those aged ≥70 years had a significantly higher rate of prolonged hospitalization (16.5% vs. 32.5%, $P < 0.0001$), nonroutine discharge (2.2% vs. 16.8%, $P < 0.0001$), transfusion (26.1% vs. 39.2%, $P < 0.0001$), and death (0.9% vs. 2.7%, $P < 0.001$). Although advanced age alone was not associated with an increased rate of perioperative complications, age ≥ 70 years and a higher American Society of Anesthesiologists score were significantly associated with prolonged hospitalization and nonroutine discharge ($P < 0.05$).

Given the abovementioned increased risks of perioperative morbidity and mortality and the evidence suggesting an increased probability of incomplete cytoreductive surgery in the elderly, it would seem preferable that these high-risk patients be treated in specialized high-volume hospitals. There is some evidence in support of this concept. In one study, 58, 51, and 40% of cytoreductive surgical procedures undertaken in patients aged ≥65 years with advanced ovarian cancer were performed by gynecologic oncologists, general gynecologists, and general surgeons, respectively [13]. Although surgeons specialized in gynecologic oncology were significantly more likely to perform radical surgery in these patients, there was no significant difference in survival between patients treated by gynecologic oncology surgeons and those treated by general gynecologists. Further, in the patients with stage III ovarian cancer, the rate of complete cytoreductive surgery achieved by gynecologic oncology surgeons was significantly higher than that achieved by general gynecologists (24% vs. 12%; $P = 0.02$). There has also been a report of a significantly improved 5-year survival rate in patients treated by gynecologic oncology surgeons, but only when patients aged >75 years were excluded from this analysis [14]. A meta-analysis of 19 studies demonstrated a better outcome in patients with ovarian cancer treated by a gynecologic oncology surgeon or in a specialized hospital, but with the caveats of potential publication bias, insufficient information provided about the effect of specialized care and hospital characteristics, and heterogeneity in each study [15]. However, given the potential disadvantages of this type of surgery, which are unpredictable in nature, it would be difficult to perform a randomized controlled study. However, there is a report showing that elderly patients (≥75 years) were just as likely as younger patients to want curative surgery [16]. Considering recent developments in anesthesiology and in surgical techniques and devices, we should seek to perform cytoreductive surgery for advanced ovarian cancer in all patients, regardless of age.

16.3.2 Chemotherapy

16.3.2.1 Concerns About Chemotherapy in Elderly Patients

Chemotherapy has a key role in the treatment of ovarian cancer, particularly in advanced disease. However, because aging is associated with decreased renal, hepatic, and/or bone marrow function, there are inevitable concerns about potentially severe side effects of cytotoxic agents in the elderly. Several analyses of the SEER-Medicare database have highlighted the disadvantages of chemotherapy in elderly patients with ovarian cancer. One analysis, which included 9361 patients aged ≥65 years with stage I–IV ovarian cancer identified between 1991 and 2002, showed that patients aged ≥80 years accounted for 47.2% of all patients who did not receive chemotherapy and only 16.0–19.2% of those who did receive chemotherapy [17]. A more recent analysis of the SEER database identified 4617 patients with stage II–IV ovarian cancer diagnosed between 2001 and 2005, and showed that 28.8% of those aged ≥65 years received no chemotherapy, 24.7% received a partial course of chemotherapy, and only 46.5% received a full course of chemotherapy [18]. This report also showed that chemotherapy was more likely to be incomplete in patients aged ≥75 years than in those aged 65–74 years (odds ratio [OR] 1.64; 95% CI 1.33–2.04). Analysis of a Phase III clinical trial of triplet chemotherapy (GOG 182) reported that being aged ≥70 years was associated with less likelihood of receiving all eight cycles of chemotherapy [19]. As mentioned earlier, it is generally believed that older women with a diagnosis of ovarian cancer are likely to have more comorbidities present. A significant association between the presence of two or more comorbidities and incomplete chemotherapy (OR 1.83, 95% CI 1.34–2.50) was also reported [18]. Another study, albeit in a small number of patients (90 aged 70–79 years and 41 aged ≥80 years) covering the period 1996–2004 showed that 87% of patients aged 70–79 years received combination chemotherapy (a taxane and platinum) and only 46% of those aged ≥80 years received combination chemotherapy even though the comorbidities in the two age groups were similar [20]. The abovementioned reports consistently indicate that elderly patients are less likely to receive standard chemotherapy.

16.3.2.2 Primary Intravenous Chemotherapy

The current standard chemotherapeutic regimen for ovarian cancer is a combination of intravenous carboplatin and paclitaxel [21, 22]. Until the late 1990s, a combination of cisplatin (or carboplatin) and cyclophosphamide was the preferred regimen. In Europe, Groupe d'Investigateurs Nationaux pour l'Etude des Cancers Ovariens (GINECO) performed a prospective study in elderly women treated for advanced ovarian cancer between 1998 and 2000 to determine the feasibility of chemotherapy in this age group [22]. Eighty-three patients aged >70 (median 76) years received six cycles of intravenous carboplatin (area under the curve [AUC] 5) and cyclophosphamide (600 mg/m^2) every 4 weeks. Sixty (72%) of the 83 patients received their six cycles of chemotherapy without severe toxicity or tumor progression. Multivariate analysis showed that symptoms of depression at baseline ($P = 0.006$), dependence ($P = 0.048$), and a performance status ≤2 ($P = 0.026$) were independent predictors of severe toxicity. Symptoms of depression ($P = 0.003$), FIGO (International Federation of Gynecology and Obstetrics) stage IV ($P = 0.007$), and more than six different comedications per day ($P = 0.043$) were identified as independent prognostic factors for overall survival (OS). This study concluded that the comprehensive geriatric assessment tool, which includes evaluation of comorbidities, comedications per day, and patient autonomy, could predict severe toxicity and

OS in elderly patients with advanced ovarian cancer. GINECO went on to perform a retrospective extension of this study using the same eligibility criteria to add a further 75 patients from 2001–2004 who were treated with combination chemotherapy consisting of carboplatin (AUC 5) and paclitaxel (175 mg/m^2) every 3 weeks [24]. Among the observed grade 3–4 toxicities, rates of leucopenia and neutropenia were significantly higher in the carboplatin-paclitaxel (CP) group than in the carboplatin-cyclophosphamide (CC) group (27.4 and 52.8% vs. 14.0 and 8.1%, respectively). Thrombocytopenia was observed more often in the CC group than in the CP group (39.5% vs. 9.7%). Among the non-hematologic toxicities, alopecia and sensory neuropathy were observed more frequently in the CP group. Although several characteristic toxicities were noted in the CP group, there was no significant difference in the rate of completion of six cycles of chemotherapy without severe toxicities or disease progression between the CC group and the CP group (75.6% and 68.1%, respectively). Therefore, the CP regimen was considered to be as feasible for elderly patients as the CC regimen. However, multivariate analysis indicated that not only age ($P = 0.013$), stage IV disease ($P = 0.001$), and symptoms of depression ($P < 0.001$) but also the CP regimen itself ($P = 0.025$) were independent prognostic factors for poorer OS in this study. The authors speculated that this result might be attributable to the higher rate of toxicities with paclitaxel and administration of chemotherapy for a shorter interval (3 weeks rather than 4 weeks).

The above findings raised the question of whether a decreased dose of chemotherapy with a shorter interval between treatments might be able to improve the safety of a taxane-carboplatin regimen. The Phase II Multicentre Italian Trial in Ovarian cancer (MITO-5) study performed in 2003–2005 investigated the tolerability of a weekly schedule of CP in 26 patients aged ≥70 (median 77) years [25]. The patients received intravenous carboplatin (AUC 2) and paclitaxel (60 mg/m^2) on days 1, 8, and 15 every 4 weeks. Seventeen (65%) of the patients completed six cycles of chemotherapy. Fourteen patients had two or more comorbidities. Although no febrile neutropenia was observed, grade 3–4 neutropenia was observed in 6 (23%) of the patients. Sensory neuropathy was observed in two patients (8%); however, the severity of neurotoxicity was grade 1. Median estimated progression-free survival (PFS) was 13.6 months and median OS was 32.0 months. The authors concluded that weekly administration of CP had a favorable toxicity profile. Another multicenter study retrospectively compared the toxicity profiles and outcomes in 100 patients aged ≥70 years with stage II–IV ovarian or primary peritoneal cancer treated with a standard-dose CP regimen (carboplatin AUC 5–6 and paclitaxel 175 mg/m^2 every 3 weeks) or a reduced-dose CP regimen (carboplatin AUC 4–5 and paclitaxel 135 mg/m^2 every 3 weeks) from 1994 to 2005 [26]. Twenty-six patients (median age 77.0 years) received the reduced-dose regimen, and 74 patients (median age 74.7 years) received the standard-dose regimen. Significant higher rates of grade 3–4 neutropenia, cumulative toxicities, and delays in therapy were observed in the patients who received standard-dose chemotherapy ($P = 0.002$, $P = 0.003$, and $P = 0.05$, respectively). However, there was no significant difference in PFS or OS between the two regimens. Although the number of patients included in this study was small, it appeared that the reduced-dose CP regimen had an acceptable safety profile and was as effective as the standard CP regimen for elderly patients. Similar results were obtained in studies of patients aged ≥65 years [27] and ≥70 years [28] who received platinum-taxane chemotherapy for advanced ovarian cancer. A Phase III study (MITO-7) then compared the efficacy of carboplatin (AUC 6) and paclitaxel (175 mg/m^2) every 3 weeks (tri-weekly CP) for six cycles with that of weekly carboplatin (AUC 2) and weekly paclitaxel (60 mg/m^2) for 18 weeks (weekly CP) [29]. Of the 822 patients enrolled, data for 404 patients (median age 59 years, 86% with stage III or IV disease) who received tri-weekly CP and 406 patients (median age 60 years, 85% with stage III or IV disease) who received weekly CP were available for analysis. The study included 151 patients aged ≥70 years. There was no significant difference in PFS between the tri-weekly and weekly regimens (17.3 months vs. 18.3 months, $P = 0.066$). Evaluation of quality of life (QoL) using the Functional Assessment of Cancer Therapy-Ovarian (FACT-O) questionnaire showed that the weekly CP regimen was more feasible than the tri-weekly CP regimen. Moreover, the weekly CP regimen was associated with a significant lower risk of febrile neutropenia (0.5% vs. 3%), grade ≥ 3 thrombocytopenia (1% vs. 7%), and grade ≥ 2 neuropathy (6% vs. 17%). Subgroup analysis revealed no heterogeneity of treatment effect according to patient age (younger or older than 70 years) or size of the treating institution (large, ≥90 patients; intermediate, 20–89 patients; small, <20 patients). The authors commented that a weekly regimen of CP might be a reasonable first-line treatment option for women with advanced ovarian cancer. Although the MITO-7 study did not include a specific analysis of data for elderly patients, it suggested that a weekly chemotherapy regimen may be appropriate for this age group. Of note, weekly administration of the CP regimen has since been mentioned as a promising regimen for elderly patients and those with poorer performance status in the National Comprehensive Cancer Network (NCCN) guidelines [21].

Thus far, there has been limited prospective elderly-specific research on ovarian cancer. The first such trial in the USA is GOG 273, which was initiated in 2011 to assess both tolerance of chemotherapy and the characteristics predictive of the ability to complete chemotherapy in women aged ≥70 years with stage III–IV ovarian cancer. A geriatric assessment scoring tool is included to predict toxicity and assess QoL. In this study, the physician can choose between two treatment regimens (carboplatin AUC 5 and paclitaxel 135 mg/m^2 every 3 weeks or carboplatin AUC 5 every 3 weeks). The preliminary data suggested that women who received CP every 3 weeks had better rates of completion without dose delay or reductions than those who received carboplatin alone. A multivariate analysis showed that treatment with carboplatin alone, administration of neoadjuvant chemotherapy (NAC), and limited participation in social activities were associated with less likelihood of completion of 4 cycles of chemotherapy. However, given that both treatments improved QoL in these elderly patients, there may be a good chance of benefit using either of these treatment regimens in this age group. In 2013, a further choice of chemotherapeutic regimen (paclitaxel 60 mg/m^2 weekly and carboplatin AUC 5 every 3 weeks) was added. The GOG 273 trial has now reached its accrual target and is closed to further recruitment [19, 30, 31]. Further analyses of this trial are awaited.

16.3.2.3 Neoadjuvant Chemotherapy

Maximum cytoreductive surgery to decrease the residual tumor volume is important in the treatment of advanced ovarian cancer. Aggressive surgical resection, including resection of the bowel and/or other organs is often needed, and high-risk patients (including the elderly and those with multiple comorbidities) are less likely to be considered for such extensive surgery because of the increased risk of perioperative morbidity. Therefore, NAC may be performed to reduce the tumor volume before radical surgery to improve the completeness of cytoreductive surgery and might be considered an attractive treatment approach by both patients and their treating clinicians.

Unfortunately, meta-analyses assessing the benefits of NAC in advanced ovarian cancer have not shown a definite conclusion. One meta-analysis reported that NAC was associated with inferior OS when compared with upfront surgery and suggested that the likely reason for this was that definitive operative intervention was not undertaken sooner [32]. However, another meta-analysis reported that NAC contributed to an increased rate of optimal cytoreduction and that survival outcomes were non-inferior to those achieved by upfront PCS [33].

The European Organization for Research and Treatment of Cancer (EORTC) performed a randomized prospective study (EORTC 55971) to compare the effectiveness of NAC followed by interval cytoreductive surgery with that of PCS followed by adjuvant chemotherapy [34]. Although a higher rate of complete cytoreduction and lower postoperative morbidity and mortality rates were achieved in the NAC group, no significant difference in OS or PFS was found between the group that underwent NAC followed by interval cytoreductive surgery and the group that underwent PCS followed by adjuvant chemotherapy (29 months and 30 months, respectively, for OS, and 12 months for PFS in both groups). This finding indicated that NAC followed by interval cytoreductive surgery was non-inferior to PCS followed by chemotherapy as a treatment option for patients with advanced ovarian cancer. This study included patients aged ≥70 years (55 in the PCS group and 70 in the NAC group). Although analysis of the elderly age group in this study was limited, there did not appear to any difference in OS between NAC and PCS in the older women.

Further, there has been a retrospective study that used inclusion criteria similar to those in EORTC 55971 and reported better survival outcomes after PCS than after NAC [35]. In this study, 285 (90%) of 316 enrolled patients received PCS. Although 87% of the patients had stage IIIC ovarian cancer, optimal cytoreduction (residual tumor diameter ≤1 cm) was achieved in 71% of cases, with a median OS of 50 months and a median PFS of 17 months. The authors mentioned that the higher rate of optimal cytoreduction achieved in their study when compared with that in EORTC 55971 (71% vs. 42%) might have accounted for their results. Their conclusion was that PCS should continue to be the preferred initial management for advanced ovarian cancer and that NAC followed by interval cytoreductive surgery should be reserved for patients who are unlikely to tolerate PCS and/or for whom optimal cytoreduction is not feasible. A retrospective study from a single institution also showed achieving better median OS and PFS with PCS followed by platinum-based chemotherapy than with NAC followed by cytoreductive surgery (72 months and 22 months vs. 43 months and 14 months, respectively) [36]. In this institution, the proportion of patients who received NAC increased significantly from 22% before publication of the results of the EORTC trial to 30% afterward when the selection criteria for each treatment strategy became more stringent. Therefore, the better survival outcomes reported for PCS in that study might stem from high-risk patients being selected more effectively for NAC.

Recently, contrary to the reports described above, association of NAC treatment with shorter OS compared to PCS for stage IIIC ovarian cancer (33 months vs. 43 months of median OS; HR 1.40, 95% CI 1.11–1.77) was shown in the multi-institutional study of NCCN ovarian cancer outcomes database project [37]. Because this was retrospective analysis differently from EORTIC trial, further studies to evaluate the effectiveness of NAC treatment will be needed. It was also shown in this study that proportion of NAC treatment for stage IIIC and IV ovarian cancer significantly increased from 16% to 34% similarly to the above report [36]. In total, patients aged >74 years received NAC more frequently compared to patients aged 18–54 years in both stage IIIC (33% vs. 23%; OR 2.25, 95% CI 1.21–4.16) and IV (56% vs. 36%; OR 2.64, 95% CI 1.14–6.10) [37]. Although no precise description about this trend was shown, it might be the result of attending doctor's decision considering chronological age and/or higher risk of perioperative morbidity in elderly patients.

There have been a few retrospective elderly-specific studies of the effectiveness of NAC, albeit from single institutions with small patient numbers. A retrospective analysis comparing the therapeutic outcome of NAC with that of PCS in 175 patients aged ≥65 years treated between 1997 and 2007 was reported [38]. This study included 141 (81%) patients aged 65–79 years and 34 (19%) aged ≥80 years. A comparison of PCS and NAC found no significant difference in surgical complication rates (58.8% vs. 64.0%; OR 0.80, 95% CI 0.37–1.75) or in chemotherapy-related complication rates (55.2% vs. 60.3%; OR 0.79, 95% CI 0.34–1.90). There was also no significant difference in surgical complication rates between patients aged 65–79 years and those aged ≥80 years (63.1% vs. 52.9%; OR 1.01, 95% CI 0.79–1.18) or in chemotherapy-related complication rates (57.1% vs. 32.2%; OR 1.04, 95% CI 0.82–1.27). Further, there was no significant difference in median disease-specific survival between patients aged ≥80 years and those aged 65–79 years (24 months vs. 35 months, $P = 0.15$). The findings of this study suggest that patients aged ≥80 years and those aged 65–79 years have a similar risk of surgical and chemotherapeutic complications and comparable survival. Another retrospective cohort analysis also reported the benefit of NAC in 104 patients aged ≥70 years who were treated with PCS ($n = 62$, 60%, mean age 75.9 years) or NAC (n = 42, 40%, mean age 76.9 years) for stage III or IV ovarian cancer between 1996 and 2009 [39]. The rate of complete cytoreduction with no macroscopic residual tumor was significantly higher in the NAC group (71.4%) than in the PCS group (28.1%, $P < 0.001$). Further, NAC was associated with significantly fewer perioperative complications, including less blood loss ($P = 0.01$), less requirement for small bowel resection ($P = 0.009$), a shorter intensive care unit (ICU) stay ($P = 0.02$), and a shorter hospital stay ($P = 0.04$). Median OS and PFS in the NAC group were not inferior to those in the PCS group (25 months vs. 39 months, $P = 0.947$, and 25 months vs. 19 months, $P = 0.078$, respectively). Interestingly, there has been a cost-utility analysis of NAC in elderly patients based on the randomized controlled study [34] comparing NAC and PCS that showed NAC to be a cost-saving treatment when compared with PCS for patients aged ≥65 years with ovarian cancer [40]. According to this analysis, if the survival effect is assumed to be equal for NAC and PCS, NAC yields a cost savings of US$5616.

As already mentioned, NAC followed by cytoreductive surgery is an attractive therapeutic option, but its efficacy remains controversial. The clinical practice guideline for NAC published by the Society of Gynecologic Oncology and the American Society of Clinical Oncology outlines appropriate criteria for identifying patients who are not suitable for PCS and in whom NAC could be considered and advises that chronological age should also be taken into account in the decision-making [41].

16.3.2.4 Intraperitoneal Chemotherapy

Intraperitoneal (IP) chemotherapy is considered to have pharmacokinetic characteristics that differ from those associated with intravenous chemotherapy, including a more direct effect on cancerous lesions. Therefore, IP administration of cytotoxic agents in patients with ovarian cancer and peritoneal carcinomatosis could be expected to have advantages. Two large Phase III studies investigated the survival outcomes in women who received IP taxane-platinum-based chemotherapy. One was the intergroup (a coalition of the GOG, Southwestern Oncology Group [SWOG], and Eastern Cooperative Oncology Group) Phase III (GOG 114/SWOG 9227) trial published in 2001 [42], and the other was the GOG 172 trial published in 2006 [43]. Both studies showed significantly better median OS and median PFS in the groups that received IP chemotherapy, although the rates of G3–G4 hematologic, gastrointestinal, and general toxicities were significantly higher than in those who received intravenous chemotherapy. However, controversy persists regarding whether the better survival outcomes and higher rates of treatment toxicity seen in these studies reflect the increased total amount of cytotoxic agents administered in the IP arms.

Although approximately 10% of the patients enrolled in the above two studies were aged ≥70 years, no elderly-specific analysis was performed in either study. Given the complicated nature of the procedure and the higher rates of toxicity involved, most oncologists would hesitate to administer chemotherapy via the IP route in their elderly patients, particularly at the doses described above. However, two studies have demonstrated that IP treatment is feasible in both younger and older patients. Both these studies used an IP regimen similar to that in the GOG 172 trial. A multi-institutional retrospective analysis was performed in 109 patients with ovarian, fallopian tube, or primary peritoneal cancer who received IP treatment from 2006 to 2009 [44]. Eighty-six patients were aged <70 years and 23 were aged ≥70 years. No significant increase in grade 3–4 chemotherapy-related complications was observed in the older patients. Further, although the older patients were significantly less likely to complete their planned number of cycles (OR 0.30, 95% CI 0.10–0.87), there was no significant difference in OS or PFS between the patients aged <70 years and those who were older. The median PFS was 14.5 months in patients aged <70 years and 19.0 months in those who were older ($P = 0.68$). Therefore, the authors considered that chronological age alone should not limit access to IP chemotherapy. They also compared the toxicity of intravenous vs. IP treatment in their patients aged ≥70 years and found significantly more comorbidities in the intravenous group than in the IP group. However, the finding of less toxicity with IP chemotherapy might simply reflect the reluctance of physicians to embark on the IP route for fear of increased toxicity in patients with multiple comorbidities. Therefore, given the lack of significant differences in complication rates or survival outcomes, the intravenous route seems preferable to the IP route in elderly patients with multiple comorbidities. There is another report that showed the results similar to those of report shown above [44] for the IP chemotherapy route with regard to treatment completion rate, toxicity, and survival outcome in their analysis of 200 patients (100 aged <65 years and 100 aged ≥65 years) [45].

In a retrospective study of patients with stage III ovarian cancer in the two GOG trials, which enrolled a combined total of 845 patients who received optimal PCS followed by IP chemotherapy (paclitaxel plus cisplatin), chronological age was found to be a significant independent predictor of poorer OS (HR 1.00, 95% CI 1.02–1.03; $P = 0.012$) [46]. The authors found that the risk of death increased 1.01 times for each 1-year increment in age. However, the age range in the GOG trials was 49–64 years, so elderly patients were not actually included in this study. The results of recent trials from the Japan Gynecologic Oncology Group [47] and the National Cancer Institute of Canada Clinical Trials Group (NCIC CTG) [48], in which the same doses of cytotoxic agents administered via the intravenous route were given via the IP route, are eagerly awaited.

The NCCN guideline for ovarian cancer recommends IP treatment in patients with stage III disease who have undergone PCS and have a residual tumor diameter of <10 mm [21]. Therefore, we should not hesitate to provide IP treatment for elderly patients satisfying these criteria.

16.4 Treatment of Relapsed Ovarian Cancer

16.4.1 Secondary Cytoreductive Surgery

Secondary cytoreductive surgery (SCS) aims to achieve maximum resection of residual cancer after primary treatment or of relapsed cancer. The strategy used to treat relapsed disease depends on the time that has elapsed since treatment with a platinum-based agent. In general, a surgical approach is not recommended as the initial treatment for a relapse that is platinum refractory or resistant because the benefits are minimal [49, 50]. However, SCS has been reported to be beneficial for platinum-sensitive relapse in carefully selected patients [51, 52] and is now recommended for these patients in the NCCN guideline [21]. The *D*escriptive *E*valuation of preoperative *S*election *K*ri*T*eria for *OP*erability in recurrent *OVAR*ian cancer (DESKTOP OVAR) trial reported that a combination of good performance status (Eastern Cooperative Oncology Group 0), early FIGO stage (I or II) at initial diagnosis or no residual tumor after primary surgery, and an estimated low volume of ascites (<500 ml) can predict complete resection in 79% of patients [53]. A retrospective analysis performed at the Mayo Clinic showed that these criteria (together known as the AGO score) had a positive predictive value of 84.3% for complete SCS. However, complete SCS was also achieved in 64.4% of patients with a negative AGO score [54]. Phase III trials, including DESKTOP III and GOG 213, are presently further investigating the ability of the AGO score to select patients for SCS and the effectiveness of SCS followed by adjuvant chemotherapy [52].

To date, no trial has specifically investigated the feasibility or survival outcomes of SCS in elderly patients. Chronological age was not identified as a significant factor associated with completion of SCS in either univariate or multivariate analysis in the DESKTOP OVAR trial, so SCS might be an option for elderly patients who have platinum-sensitive relapse and meet the above criteria.

16.4.2 Chemotherapy

Platinum sensitivity is considered to be key in chemotherapy for relapsed ovarian cancer. For the treatment of platinum-sensitive relapsed ovarian cancer, combination chemotherapy that includes a platinum agent has been reported to be superior to chemotherapy using a platinum agent alone. The International Collaborative Ovarian Neoplasm 4 / Arbeitsgemeinschaft Gynaekologische Onkologie Studiengruppe Ovarialkarzinom (ICON4/AGO-OVAR-2.2)-2.2 trial evaluated the effectiveness of combination paclitaxel-platinum therapy in 802 women with platinum-sensitive relapsed ovarian cancer, 239 (29.8%) of whom were aged ≥65 years [55]. Both OS and PFS were significantly better in women who received combination chemotherapy than in those who received a platinum agent alone (HR 0.82, 95% CI 0.69–0.67; $P = 0.023$, and HR 0.76, 95% CI 0.66–0.89; $P = 0.0004$, respectively). Subgroup analysis showed no significant age-related difference in OS or PFS. The results for platinum-based combination chemotherapy containing gemcitabine are similar. An Intergroup (AGO-OVAR, NCIC CTG, EORTC GCG) trial reported significantly improved PFS in women who received gemcitabine-carboplatin chemotherapy when compared with those who received carboplatin alone (HR 0.72, 95% CI 0.58–0.90; $P = 0.0031$), but no significant improvement in OS (HR 0.96, 95% CI 0.75–1.23; $P = 0.735$) [56]. The response rate for gemcitabine-carboplatin chemotherapy was significantly higher than that for carboplatin alone (47.2% vs. 30.9%; $P = 0.0016$). Although hematologic toxicity and need for granulocyte-colony stimulating factor were significantly more frequent in the women who received combination chemotherapy, their QoL was not worsened. One hundred (28.1%) of the 356 patients enrolled in this study were aged ≥65 years, and subgroup analysis showed no significant age-related difference in PFS.

Comparisons of the effectiveness of other types of combination chemotherapy in women with relapsed ovarian cancer have also been reported. The Caelyx in Platinum Sensitive Ovarian patients (CALYPSO) trial compared the efficacy and safety of combination chemotherapy containing pegylated liposomal doxorubicin and carboplatin (C-PLD) with that of a CP regimen in 976 women with platinum-sensitive relapsed ovarian cancer and demonstrated significantly better PFS in the C-PLD group (HR 082, 95% CI 0.72–0.94; $P = 0.005$) [57]. A subsequent analysis of the 157 patients (16.1%) in the CALYPSO trial who were aged ≥70 years showed no significant difference in hematologic toxicity between younger (<70 years) and older (≥70 years) patients in either treatment group [58]. Sensory neuropathy (grade ≥ 2) was significantly more common in the elderly patients (24.4% vs. 15.5%, $P = 0.007$), whereas allergic reactions were observed more frequently in the younger patients (13.9% vs. 5.8%, $P = 0.005$). The toxicity profile (i.e., grade ≥ 2 alopecia, sensory neuropathy, arthralgia, and hand-foot syndrome) in the elderly women was not different from that observed in the CALYPSO study population overall. Further, in the women aged ≥70 years, there was no significant difference in median PFS between the C-PLD and CP regimens (11.6 months vs. 10.3 months, $P = 0.44$). The authors concluded that chemotherapy containing carboplatin and pegylated liposomal doxorubicin achieved a survival outcome similar to that achieved by the CP regimen in elderly patients but with less toxicity.

Relapsed ovarian cancer refractory or resistant to platinum is usually treated with a single non-platinum agent [19, 21], such as pegylated liposomal doxorubicin, topotecan, irinotecan, gemcitabine, docetaxel, or weekly paclitaxel. However, as yet there is no definitive study performed in elderly patients with platinum-resistant relapsed ovarian cancer. In general, the response rate for these agents in platinum-resistant relapse is 20%–30% at most. Considering the poor prognosis in these patients, it might be better at this point to switch from chemotherapy to hospice care for maintenance of QoL, particularly in elderly patients.

16.5 Molecular Targeted Therapy for Ovarian Cancer

Bevacizumab (anti-vascular endothelial growth factor monoclonal antibody) is the only agent that has been demonstrated to improve survival in patients with advanced or recurrent ovarian cancer. The activity of bevacizumab as primary chemotherapy for ovarian cancer has been studied in two major Phase III trials, i.e., GOG 218 [59] and ICON-7 [60], which, respectively, included 430 (23%) and 150 (10%) women aged ≥70 years. In the bevacizumab arms of GOG 218 and ICON-7, the oldest patients were aged 89 years and 82 years, respectively. Two further Phase III trials in platinum-sensitive Ovarian Cancer Study Comparing Efficacy and Safety of Chemotherapy and Anti-Angiogenic Therapy in Platinum-Sensitive Recurrent Disease (OCEANS) [61] and platinum-resistant Avastin Use in Platinum-Resistant Epithelial Ovarian Cancer (AURELIA) [62] relapsed ovarian cancer have also shown better PFS in patients treated with bevacizumab. However, none of these four trials performed a specific subset analysis for elderly patients. To date, no study has specifically investigated the effectiveness and feasibility of chemotherapy including bevacizumab for elderly patients with ovarian cancer. However, hypertension, proteinuria, thromboembolism, and hemorrhage are the well-known major toxicities of bevacizumab, and gastrointestinal perforation is reported to be the most life-threatening toxicity [63]. Clearly, these toxicities should be kept in mind when considering the use of bevacizumab in elderly patients with physical comorbidities.

Olaparib, a poly (ADP-ribose) polymerase inhibitor, has been reported to be a potentially effective agent in patients with ovarian cancer harboring BRCA mutations [64, 65]. Olaparib is now approved by the US Food and Drug Administration for patients who have received three or more lines of chemotherapy and is listed as one of the preferred agents in the NCCN guideline [21]. The results of further investigations showing the effectiveness and feasibility of this agent in elderly patients with ovarian cancer are awaited.

16.6 Comprehensive Geriatric Assessment

16.6.1 Frailty

Frailty in elderly people is defined as a state of vulnerability to various kinds of stressors and is attributable to the age-related decrease in physiological reserve. Frailty in an elderly person manifests as a number of symptoms and signs, including weakness, fatigue, weight loss, poor balance, low levels of physical activity, slowed motor processing and performance, social withdrawal, mild cognitive changes, and increased vulnerability to stressors, culminating in disability, loss of independence, diminished QoL, and mortality (Fig. 16.1) [66]. In the pathway to frailty, various molecular alterations and physiological reactions are considered to be associated (Fig. 16.2) [67]. Frailty may also be associated with psychological and financial problems.

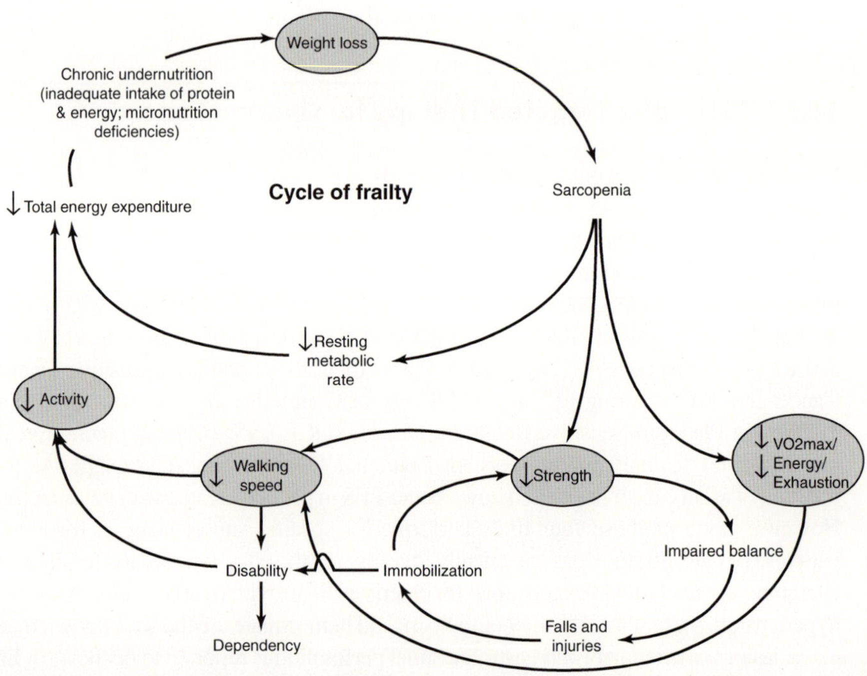

Fig. 16.1 Cycle of frailty [66], reprinted with permission of Oxford University Press

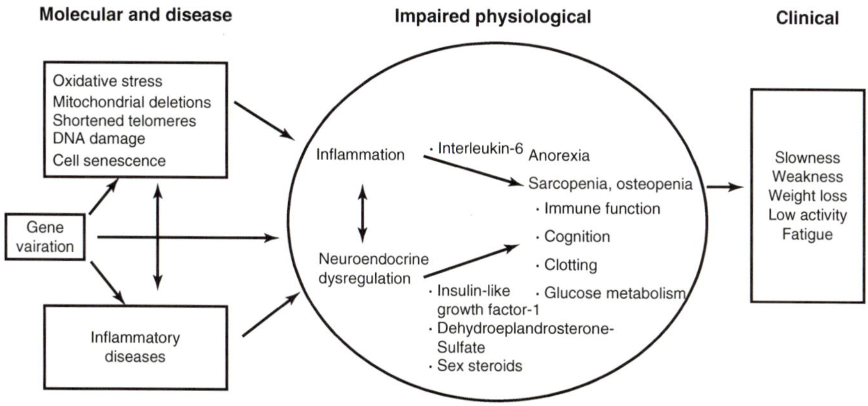

Fig. 16.2 Hypothesized molecular and physiological association with frailty [67], reprinted with permission of John Wiley and Sons

The question rises as to the best way of assessing elderly patients to determine if they are frail or not. Some useful criteria in this regard has been proposed based on the findings of the Cardiovascular Health Study, in which 5317 people aged 65–101 years (57.9% female, 14.8% African American) were evaluated to define the phenotype of frailty [68]. Five components of frailty were investigated, including unintentional weight loss (4.5 kg in the past year), weakness (grip strength, stratified by sex and body mass index), poor endurance (self-reported in response to two questions from the Center for Epidemiological Studies-Depression Scale [69]), slowness (walking speed, stratified by sex and height), and low physical activity (weighted score of kilocalories expended per week). Individuals who satisfied three or more of the above five criteria were defined as frail and those who met one or two criteria were categorized as pre-frail. Using these criteria, 368 people (6.9%) in this population were characterized as frail and 2480 (46.6%) as pre-frail. Mortality rates at 3 and 7 years in frail people were 18% and 43%, respectively, whereas those in non-frail people were 3 and 12%. This frailty phenotype could independently predict the risks of incident falls, worsened mobility or disability in activities of daily living, incident hospitalization, and death over 3 or 7 years, with hazard ratios ranging from 1.82 to 4.46 and from 1.28 to 2.10 for the frail and intermediate groups, respectively. Similar models of frailty have been proposed by the Women's Health and Aging Study [70], the Edmonton Frail Scale [71], and others [72].

16.6.2 Pretreatment Evaluation in Elderly Patients

16.6.2.1 Score to Predict Peri-treatment Morbidities

Although medical frailty is a concept with a relatively short history, a frail state is clearly associated with poorer health outcomes in the elderly. Therefore, appropriate assessment of elderly patients is necessary to predict the risk of severe peri-treatment morbidities or an unexpected worse outcome when considering treatment for any type of cancer. Several systematic reviews have revealed that appropriate assessment has adequate feasibility and high sensitivity for predicting frailty in elderly patients with cancer. However, the types of assessment used have not always been useful for prediction of adverse outcomes or had high specificity or negative predictive value [73–75]. Therefore, it is possible that the assessment methods presently used to guide therapeutic decision-making may be inadequate for elderly patients with cancer.

16.6.2.2 Assessment to Predict Perioperative Morbidities

Efforts to evaluate the effectiveness of the assessment protocols proposed for elderly patients with ovarian cancer are ongoing. The Modified Frailty Index (mFI) consists of 11 variables derived from the Canadian Study of Health and Aging Frailty Index and was reported to predict morbidities requiring ICU admission in patients scheduled for colectomy (Table 16.1) [76]. The usefulness of the mFI as a predictor of the risk of morbidities has also been investigated in a retrospective study of 6551 patients who were identified in the National Surgical Quality Improvement Program data for 2008–2011 as having undergone surgery for gynecologic cancer (although the exact number with ovarian cancer was not reported) [77]. One hundred and eighty-eight (2.9%) of these women developed life-threatening complications requiring management in ICU or resulting in death within 30 days postoperatively. The complication rates were 2, 2.7, 4.4, 7.4, and 24.4% for mFI scores of 0, 1, 2, 3, and ≥4, respectively, and were significantly higher in patients with a score ≥ 3 than those with a score ≤ 2 ($P < 0.001$). In multivariate analysis, significant predictors of severe complications were a preoperative albumin level < 3 g/dl (OR 6.5, 95% CI 4.31–9.96), longer operating time (OR 1.003 per minute increase, 95% CI 1.001–1.004), non-laparoscopic surgery (OR 3.3, 95% CI 1.56–8.83), and an mFI score ≥ 2 (score 2, OR 1.91, 95% CI 1.17–3.11; score 3, OR 2.33, 95% CI 1.05–5.19; score ≥ 4, OR 12.5, 95% CI 4.77–32.76). When the women were categorized as low-risk and high-risk groups on the basis of a preoperative albumin level ≤ 3 g/dl

Table 16.1 Eleven variables to calculate Modified Frailty Index (mFI) based upon patient's medical record [76, 77]

Variables for Modified Frailty Index (mFI)	
1.	Nonindependent functional status
2.	History of diabetes mellitus
3.	History of either chronic obstructive pulmonary disease or pneumonia
4.	History of congestive heart failure
5.	History of myocardial infarction
6.	History of percutaneous coronary intervention, cardiac surgery, or angina
7.	Hypertension requiring the use of medications
8.	Peripheral vascular disease or rest pain
9.	Impaired sensorium
10.	Transient ischemic attack or cerebrovascular accident without deficit
11.	Cerebrovascular accident with deficit

and/or an mFI score ≥ 4, the high-risk group showed a higher (≥10%) rate of severe perioperative complications when compared with the low-risk group (≤10%). The authors concluded that the mFI criteria could identify patients with gynecologic malignancy who were at high risk for perioperative complications that require management in ICU or are fatal.

An ovarian cancer-specific investigation has since been performed for 751 patients aged ≥65 years identified in the National Surgical Quality Improvement Program database as having undergone PCS between 2005 and 2016 [78]. One hundred and twenty-three (16.4%) of these patients encountered complications of the same level of severity as those described in the previous report [77]. A number of variables, including patient demographics (age, body mass index, race), preoperative laboratory values (creatinine, hematocrit, platelet count, white blood cell count, albumin), and comorbidities (hypertension, cigarette smoking, diabetes, chronic obstructive pulmonary disease, history of cerebrovascular accident, myocardial infarction within the previous 6 months, history of transient ischemic attack), were compared between patients with and without severe morbidities. Eight variables identified to be significant were chosen for a model to predict the probability of postoperative complications in patients aged ≥65 years undergoing PCS for ovarian cancer (Table.16.2). The variables chosen for the proposed predictive model were ascites (present or absent), current smoking (yes or no), race (white vs. nonwhite), preoperative creatinine (≥1.5 mg/dL or <1.5 mg/dL), preoperative platelet count (≥450 × 10^9/L or <450 × 10^9/L), preoperative hematocrit (≥30% or <30%), preoperative white blood cell count (≥10 × 10^9/L or <10 × 10^9/L), and preoperative albumin (≥3.5 g/dL or <3.5 g/dL). The area under the receiver-operating characteristic curve for the model was 0.725, indicating fair (not poor but not good) performance. This model could predict a 35% probability of severe postoperative complications with 21.8% sensitivity and 92.6% specificity. When the threshold of prediction was decreased to 50% probability, the sensitivity decreased to 9.8% although specificity increased to 98.0%. These findings indicate that preoperative evaluation to identify patients with the highest risk of severe postoperative complications is not easy. However, the high specificity of this model means that patients who can undergo PCS safely could be identified, including those who are elderly.

Table. 16.2 Eight variables for the model to predict the major postoperative complication [78]

Variables for the predictive model	
Physical status or habit	
Ascites	Yes or No
Current smoker	Yes or No
Race	White or Non-white
Preoperative laboratory data	
Creatinine (mg/dL)	<1.5 or ≥1.5
Platelet (×10^9/L)	<450 or ≥450
Hematocrit (%)	<30 or ≥30
White blood cell (×10^9/L)	<10 or ≥10
Albumin (g/dL)	<3.5 or ≥3.5

16.6.2.3 Assessment to Predict Tolerance of Chemotherapy

A GINECO study has reported a comprehensive geriatric assessment tool that can predict the risk of severe treatment-related toxicities in elderly patients with ovarian cancer [23]. Based on their study findings, the authors devised a geriatric vulnerability score (GVS), calculated from five criteria, namely, a low activities of daily living score (<6), a low instrumental activities of daily living score (<25), hypoalbuminemia (<3.5 g/dL), lymphopenia at inclusion ($<1 \times 10^9$/L), and a high Hospital Anxiety and Depression Scale score (>14). GVS is sum of these variables of each patient. The patients aged ≥70 years with ovarian cancer were separated into two groups using a cutoff point of 3. Patients with a GVS ≥3 were significantly less likely to complete their planned chemotherapy than those with a GVS <3 (OR 0.41, 95% CI 0.17–0.99; $P = 0.044$) and were significantly more likely to have more severe (grade ≥ 3) non-hematologic toxicities (OR 4.40; 95% CI 1.92–10.08; $P = 0.0002$), more serious adverse events (OR 2.79, 95% CI 1.27–6.11; $P = 0.009$), and more unplanned hospital admissions (OR 2.57, 95% CI 1.17–5.63; $P = 0.017$) [79]. Since the chemotherapy administered in this study was carboplatin alone, further investigation is needed to evaluate the predictive accuracy of the GVS in elderly patients with ovarian cancer who receive combination chemotherapy with a taxane and a platinum agent.

Conclusion

Nearly half of all patients with ovarian cancer are diagnosed in the advanced stages of the disease and have peritoneal carcinomatosis at this time. The mainstay of treatment for advanced ovarian cancer continues to be maximal PCS followed by adjuvant chemotherapy. Clearly, the improvements in supportive care for patients and in the surgical devices available, as well as innovative cytotoxic and supportive agents, have contributed to the improved treatment of ovarian cancer. However, it should be acknowledged that the development of clinical guidelines has played a very important part in these improvements. Clinical evidence concerning the treatment of various types of cancer in the elderly has been steadily accumulating in recent years, and general guidelines for geriatric medicine have been proposed [80–82]. However, guidelines specific for the treatment of each type of cancer have not been adequately developed for elderly patients because of the difficulties inherent in performing clinical trials in this age group. Therefore, our treatment strategies for these patients have to be based on relatively limited evidence from analyses of subgroups in the major clinical trials.

The current evidence indicates that every effort should be made to perform PCS followed by chemotherapy in patients with advanced ovarian cancer, regardless of the patient's chronological age. A weekly chemotherapeutic regimen or single-agent chemotherapy is recommended for elderly patients and those with poorer performance status. However, the issues of frailty and the higher risk of peri-treatment morbidities do need to be considered in these patients. There is increasing awareness of the importance of appropriate assessment of geriatric patients with cancer, and a variety of scoring systems to predict the risks of treatment have been proposed.

It is now time to leave behind the concept that elderly patients are only eligible for palliative treatment because of their chronological age. Further studies, based on the accumulation of evidence from clinical trials that have included elderly patients, will be invaluable for increasing the reliability of geriatric assessment protocols and for predicting patients who can tolerate standard treatments.

References

1. Surveillance, Epidemiologyand End Results Program. National Cancer Institute, Rockville, 2016. http://seer.cancer.gov/statfacts/html/ovary.html Accessed 10 Dec 2016.
2. Saito T, Katabuchi H. Annual Report of the Committee on Gynecologic Oncology, Japan Society of Obstetrics and Gynecology: Patient Annual Report for 2013 and Treatment Annual Report for 2008. J Obstet Gynaecol Res. 2016;42:1069–79.
3. World Health Organization. Definition of an older or elderly person. Geneva: World Health Organization; 2002. http://www.who.int/healthinfo/survey/ageingdefnolder/en/ Accessed 10 Dec 2016.
4. Hamel MB, Henderson WG, Khuri SF, Daley J. Surgical outcomes for patients aged 80 and older: morbidity and mortality from major noncardiac surgery. J Am Geriatr Soc. 2005;53:424–9.
5. Turrentine FE, Wang H, Simpson VB, Jones RS. Surgical risk factors, morbidity, and mortality in elderly patients. J Am Coll Surg. 2006;203:865–77.
6. Winter WE 3rd, Maxwell GL, Tian C, Carlson JW, Ozols RF, Rose PG, Gynecologic Oncology Group Study, et al. Prognostic factors for stage III epithelial ovarian cancer: a Gynecologic Oncology Group Study. J Clin Oncol. 2007;25:3621–7.
7. Gerestein CG, Damhuis RA, Burger CW, Kooi GS. Postoperative mortality after primary cytoreductive surgery for advanced stage epithelial ovarian cancer: a systematic review. Gynecol Oncol. 2009;114:523–7.
8. Thrall MM, Goff BA, Symons RG, Flum DR, Gray HJ. Thirty-day mortality after primary cytoreductive surgery for advanced ovarian cancer in the elderly. Obstet Gynecol. 2011;118:537–47.
9. Pignata S, Vermorken JB. Ovarian cancer in the elderly. Crit Rev Oncol Hematol. 2004;49:77–86.
10. Wright JD, Herzog TJ, Powell MA. Morbidity of cytoreductive surgery in the elderly. Am J Obstet Gynecol. 2004;190:1398–400.
11. Sharma S, Driscoll D, Odunsi K, Venkatadri A, Lele S. Safety and efficacy of cytoreductive surgery for epithelial ovarian cancer in elderly and high-risk surgical patients. Am J Obstet Gynecol. 2005;193:2077–82.
12. Patankar S, Burke WM, Hou JY, Tergas AI, Huang Y, Ananth CV, et al. Risk stratification and outcomes of women undergoing surgery for ovarian cancer. Gynecol Oncol. 2015;138:62–9.
13. Earle CC, Schrag D, Neville BA, Yabroff KR, Topor M, Fahey A, et al. Effect of surgeon specialty on processes of care and outcomes for ovarian cancer patients. J Natl Cancer Inst. 2006;98:172–80.
14. Engelen MJ, Kos HE, Willemse PH, Aalders JG, de Vries EG, Schaapveld M, et al. Surgery by consultant gynecologic oncologists improves survival in patients with ovarian carcinoma. Cancer. 2006;106:589–98.
15. Vernooij F, Heintz P, Witteveen E, van der Graaf Y. The outcomes of ovarian cancer treatment are better when provided by gynecologic oncologists and in specialized hospitals: a systematic review. Gynecol Oncol. 2007;105:801–12.
16. Nordin AJ, Chinn DJ, Moloney I, Naik R, de Barros Lopes A, Monaghan JM. Do elderly cancer patients care about cure? Attitudes to radical gynecologic oncology surgery in the elderly. Gynecol Oncol. 2001;81:447–55.

17. Nurgalieva Z, Liu CC, Du XL. Risk of hospitalizations associated with adverse effects of chemotherapy in a large community-based cohort of elderly women with ovarian cancer. Int J Gynecol Cancer. 2009;19:1314–21.
18. Fairfield KM, Murray K, Lucas FL, Wierman HR, Earle CC, Trimble EL, et al. Completion of adjuvant chemotherapy and use of health services for older women with epithelial ovarian cancer. J Clin Oncol. 2011;29:3921–6.
19. Tew WP. Ovarian cancer in the older woman. J Geriatr Oncol. 2016;7:354–61.
20. Uyar D, Frasure HE, Markman M, von Gruenigen VE. Treatment patterns by decade of life in elderly women (> or =70 years of age) with ovarian cancer. Gynecol Oncol. 2005;98:403–8.
21. Ovarian cancer including fallopian tube cancer and primary peritoneal cancer. Version 1, 2016. NCCN Clinical Practice Guidelines in Oncology. Fort Washington, PA, 2016. https://www.nccn.org/professionals/ physician_gls/ pdf/ovarian.pdf.
22. Komiyama S, Katabuchi H, Mikami M, Nagase S, Okamoto A, Ito K, et al. Japan Society of Gynecologic Oncology guidelines 2015 for the treatment of ovarian cancer including primary peritoneal cancer and fallopian tube cancer. Int J Clin Oncol. 2016;21:435–46.
23. Freyer G, Geay JF, Touzet S, Provencal J, Weber B, Jacquin JP, et al. Comprehensive geriatric assessment predicts tolerance to chemotherapy and survival in elderly patients with advanced ovarian carcinoma: a GINECO study. Ann Oncol. 2005;16:1795–800.
24. Trédan O, Geay JF, Touzet S, Delva R, Weber B, Cretin J, Groupe d'Investigateurs Nationaux pour l'Etude des Cancers Ovariens, et al. Carboplatin/cyclophosphamide or carboplatin/paclitaxel in elderly patients with advanced ovarian cancer? Analysis of two consecutive trials from the Groupe d'Investigateurs Nationaux pour l'Etude des Cancers Ovariens. Ann Oncol. 2007;18:256–62.
25. Pignata S, Breda E, Scambia G, Pisano C, Zagonel V, Lorusso D, et al. A phase II study of weekly carboplatin and paclitaxel as first-line treatment of elderly patients with advanced ovarian cancer. A Multicentre Italian Trial in Ovarian cancer (MITO-5) study. Crit Rev Oncol Hematol. 2008;66:229–36.
26. Fader AN, von Gruenigen V, Gibbons H, Abushahin F, Starks D, Markman M, et al. Improved tolerance of primary chemotherapy with reduced-dose carboplatin and paclitaxel in elderly ovarian cancer patients. Gynecol Oncol. 2008;109:33–8.
27. Eisenhauer EL, Tew WP, Levine DA, Lichtman SM, Brown CL, Aghajanian C, et al. Response and outcomes in elderly patients with stages IIIC-IV ovarian cancer receiving platinum-taxane chemotherapy. Gynecol Oncol. 2007;106:381–7.
28. Hilpert F, du Bois A, Greimel ER, Hedderich J, Krause G, Venhoff L, et al. Feasibility, toxicity and quality of life of first-line chemotherapy with platinum/paclitaxel in elderly patients aged >or=70 years with advanced ovarian cancer – a study by the AGO OVAR Germany. Ann Oncol. 2007;18:282–7.
29. Pignata S, Scambia G, Katsaros D, Gallo C, Pujade-Lauraine E, De Placido S, et al. Multicentre Italian Trials in Ovarian cancer (MITO-7).; Groupe d'Investigateurs Nationaux pour l'Etude des Cancers Ovariens et du sein (GINECO), Mario Negri Gynecologic Oncology (MaNGO), European Network of Gynaecological Oncological Trial Groups (ENGOT-OV-10), Gynecologic Cancer InterGroup (GCIG) Investigators. Carboplatin plus paclitaxel once a week versus every 3 weeks in patients with advanced ovarian cancer (MITO-7): a randomised, multicentre, open-label, phase 3 trial. Lancet Oncol. 2014;15:396–405.
30. Troso-Sandoval TA, Lichtman SM. Chemotherapy of ovarian cancer in elderly patients. Cancer Biol Med. 2015;12:292–301.
31. Ahmed A. Gynecologic cancer in the older patient: the activities of the Elderly Working Group of NRG Oncology. Alexandria, VA: American Society of Clinical Oncology; 2016. http://www.ascopost.com/issues/july-25-2015/gynecologic-cancer-in-the-older-patient-the-activities-of-the-elderly-working-group-of-nrg-oncology/ Accessed Dec 11, 2016.
32. Bristow RE, Chi DS. Platinum-based neoadjuvant chemotherapy and interval surgical cytoreduction for advanced ovarian cancer: a meta-analysis. Gynecol Oncol. 2006;103:1070–6.
33. Kang S, Nam BH. Does neoadjuvant chemotherapy increase optimal cytoreduction rate in advanced ovarian cancer? Meta-analysis of 21 studies. Ann Surg Oncol. 2009;16:2315–20.

34. Vergote I, Tropé CG, Amant F, Kristensen GB, Ehlen T, Johnson N, European Organization for Research and Treatment of Cancer-Gynaecological Cancer Group, NCIC Clinical Trials Group, et al. Neoadjuvant chemotherapy or primary surgery in stage IIIC or IV ovarian cancer. N Engl J Med. 2010;363:943–53.
35. Chi DS, Musa F, Dao F, Zivanovic O, Sonoda Y, Leitao MM, et al. An analysis of patients with bulky advanced stage ovarian, tubal, and peritoneal carcinoma treated with primary debulking surgery (PDS) during an identical time period as the randomized EORTC-NCIC trial of PDS vs neoadjuvant chemotherapy (NACT). Gynecol Oncol. 2012;124:10–4.
36. Mueller JJ, Zhou QC, Iasonos A, O'Cearbhaill RE, Alvi FA, El Haraki A, et al. Neoadjuvant chemotherapy and primary debulking surgery utilization for advanced-stage ovarian cancer at a comprehensive cancer center. Gynecol Oncol. 2016;140:436–42.
37. Meyer LA, Cronin AM, Sun CC, Bixel K, Bookman MA, Cristea MC, et al. Use and effectiveness of neoadjuvant chemotherapy for treatment of ovarian cancer. J Clin Oncol. 2016;34:3854–63.
38. McLean KA, Shah CA, Thompson SA, Gray HJ, Swensen RE, Goff BA. Ovarian cancer in the elderly: outcomes with neoadjuvant chemotherapy or primary cytoreduction. Gynecol Oncol. 2010;118:43–6.
39. Glasgow MA, Yu H, Rutherford TJ, Azodi M, Silasi DA, Santin AD, et al. Neoadjuvant chemotherapy (NACT) is an effective way of managing elderly women with advanced stage ovarian cancer (FIGO Stage IIIC and IV). J Surg Oncol. 2013;107:195–200.
40. Rowland MR, Lesnock JL, Farris C, Kelley JL, Krivak TC. Cost-utility comparison of neoadjuvant chemotherapy versus primary debulking surgery for treatment of advanced-stage ovarian cancer in patients 65 years old or older. Am J Obstet Gynecol. 2015;212:763.e1–8.
41. Wright AA, Bohlke K, Armstrong DK, Bookman MA, Cliby WA, Coleman RL, et al. Neoadjuvant chemotherapy for newly diagnosed, advanced ovarian cancer: Society of Gynecologic Oncology and American Society of Clinical Oncology Clinical Practice Guideline. J Clin Oncol. 2016;34:3460–73.
42. Markman M, Bundy BN, Alberts DS, Fowler JM, Clark-Pearson DL, Carson LF, et al. Phase III trial of standard-dose intravenous cisplatin plus paclitaxel versus moderately high-dose carboplatin followed by intravenous paclitaxel and intraperitoneal cisplatin in small-volume stage III ovarian carcinoma: an Intergroup study of the Gynecologic Oncology Group, Southwestern Oncology Group, and Eastern Cooperative Oncology Group. J Clin Oncol. 2001;19:1001–7.
43. Armstrong DK, Bundy B, Wenzel L, Huang HQ, Baergen R, Lele S, Gynecologic Oncology Group, et al. Intraperitoneal cisplatin and paclitaxel in ovarian cancer. N Engl J Med. 2006;354:34–43.
44. Kothari R, Nagel C, Koopmeiners JS, Ivy JJ, Geller M, Salani R, et al. The effect of age on the tolerability of intraperitoneal chemotherapy, complication rate, and survival in patients with ovarian cancer. Gynecol Oncol. 2010;119:491–5.
45. O'Cearbhaill R, Li D, Shi W, Thaler H, Sabbatini PJ, Konner J, et al. Intraperitoneal chemotherapy in older women with epithelial ovarian cancer. J Geriatr Oncol. 2012;3:189–95.
46. Landrum LM, Java J, Mathews CA, Lanneau GS Jr, Copeland LJ, Armstrong DK, et al. Prognostic factors for stage III epithelial ovarian cancer treated with intraperitoneal chemotherapy: a Gynecologic Oncology Group study. Gynecol Oncol 2013;130:12–18.
47. Fujiwara K, Aotani E, Hamano T, Nagao S, Yoshikawa H, Sugiyama T, et al. A randomized Phase II/III trial of 3 weekly intraperitoneal versus intravenous carboplatin in combination with intravenous weekly dose-dense paclitaxel for newly diagnosed ovarian, fallopian tube and primary peritoneal cancer. Jpn J Clin Oncol. 2011;41:278–82.
48. Mackay HJ, Provencheur D, Heywood M, Tu D, Eisenhauer EA, Oza AM, Meyer R. Phase II/III study of intraperitoneal chemotherapy after neoadjuvant chemotherapy for ovarian cancer: ncic ctg ov.21. Curr Oncol. 2011;18:84–90.
49. Morris M, Gershenson DM, Wharton JT. Secondary cytoreductive surgery in epithelial ovarian cancer: nonresponders to first-line therapy. Gynecol Oncol. 1989;33:1–5.
50. Tebes SJ, Sayer RA, Palmer JM, Tebes CC, Martino MA, Hoffman MS. Cytoreductive surgery for patients with recurrent epithelial ovarian carcinoma. Gynecol Oncol. 2007;106:482–7.

51. Bristow RE, Puri I, Chi DS. Cytoreductive surgery for recurrent ovarian cancer: a meta-analysis. Gynecol Oncol. 2009;112:265–74.
52. Suh DH, Kim HS, Chang SJ, Bristow RE. Surgical management of recurrent ovarian cancer. Gynecol Oncol. 2016;142:357–67.
53. Harter P, du Bois A, Hahmann M, Hasenburg A, Burges A, Loibl S, Arbeitsgemeinschaft Gynaekologische Onkologie Ovarian Committee, AGO, Ovarian Cancer Study Group, et al. Surgery in recurrent ovarian cancer: the Arbeitsgemeinschaft Gynaekologische Onkologie (AGO) DESKTOP OVAR trial. Ann Surg Oncol. 2006;13:1702–10.
54. Janco JM, Kumar A, Weaver AL, McGree ME, Cliby WA. Performance of AGO score for secondary cytoreduction in a high-volume U.S. center. Gynecol Oncol. 2016;141:140–7.
55. Parmar MK, Ledermann JA, Colombo N, du Bois A, Delaloye JF, Kristensen GB, ICON and AGO Collaborators, et al. Paclitaxel plus platinum-based chemotherapy versus conventional platinum-based chemotherapy in women with relapsed ovarian cancer: the ICON4/AGO-OVAR-2.2 trial. Lancet. 2003;361:2099–106.
56. Pfisterer J, Plante M, Vergote I, du Bois A, Hirte H, Lacave AJ, et al. AGO-OVAR, NCIC CTG, EORTC GCG. Gemcitabine plus carboplatin compared with carboplatin in patients with platinum-sensitive recurrent ovarian cancer: an intergroup trial of the AGO-OVAR, the NCIC CTG, and the EORTC GCG. J Clin Oncol. 2006;24:4699–707.
57. Pujade-Lauraine E, Wagner U, Aavall-Lundqvist E, Gebski V, Heywood M, Vasey PA, et al. Pegylated liposomal doxorubicin and carboplatin compared with paclitaxel and carboplatin for patients with platinum-sensitive ovarian cancer in late relapse. J Clin Oncol. 2010;28:3323–9.
58. Kurtz JE, Kaminsky MC, Floquet A, Veillard AS, Kimmig R, Dorum A, Gynecologic Cancer Intergroup, et al. Ovarian cancer in elderly patients: carboplatin and pegylated liposomal doxorubicin versus carboplatin and paclitaxel in late relapse: a Gynecologic Cancer Intergroup (GCIG) CALYPSO sub-study. Ann Oncol. 2011;22:2417–23.
59. Burger RA, Brady MF, Bookman MA, Fleming GF, Monk BJ, Huang H, Gynecologic Oncology Group, et al. Incorporation of bevacizumab in the primary treatment of ovarian cancer. N Engl J Med. 2011;365:2473–83.
60. Perren TJ, Swart AM, Pfisterer J, Ledermann JA, Pujade-Lauraine E, Kristensen G, ICON7 Investigators, et al. A phase 3 trial of bevacizumab in ovarian cancer. N Engl J Med. 2011;365:2484–96.
61. Aghajanian C, Blank SV, Goff BA, Judson PL, Teneriello MG, Husain A, et al. OCEANS: a randomized, double-blind, placebo-controlled phase III trial of chemotherapy with or without bevacizumab in patients with platinum-sensitive recurrent epithelial ovarian, primary peritoneal, or fallopian tube cancer. J Clin Oncol. 2012;30:2039–45.
62. Pujade-Lauraine E, Hilpert F, Weber B, Reuss A, Poveda A, Kristensen G, et al. Bevacizumab combined with chemotherapy for platinum-resistant recurrent ovarian cancer: the AURELIA open-label randomized phase III trial. J Clin Oncol. 2014;32:1302–8.
63. Cannistra SA, Matulonis UA, Penson RT, Hambleton J, Dupont J, Mackey H, et al. Phase II study of bevacizumab in patients with platinum-resistant ovarian cancer or peritoneal serous cancer. J Clin Oncol. 2007;25:5180–6.
64. Ledermann J, Harter P, Gourley C, Friedlander M, Vergote I, Rustin G, et al. Olaparib maintenance therapy in patients with platinum-sensitive relapsed serous ovarian cancer: a preplanned retrospective analysis of outcomes by BRCA status in a randomized phase 2 trial. Lancet Oncol. 2014;15:852–61.
65. Kaufman B, Shapira-Frommer R, Schmutzler RK, Audeh MW, Friedlander M, Balmaña J, et al. Olaparib monotherapy in patients with advanced cancer and a germline BRCA1/2 mutation. J Clin Oncol. 2015;33:244–50.
66. Xue QL, Bandeen-Roche K, Varadhan R, Zhou J, Fried LP. Initial manifestations of frailty criteria and the development of frailty phenotype in the Women's Health and Aging Study II. J Gerontol A Biol Sci Med Sci. 2008;63:984–90.
67. Walston J, Hadley EC, Ferrucci L, Guralnik JM, Newman AB, Studenski SA, et al. Research agenda for frailty in older adults: toward a better understanding of physiology and etiology:

summary from the American Geriatrics Society/National Institute on Aging Research conference on Frailty in Older Adults. J Am Geriatr Soc. 2006;54:991–1001.
68. Fried LP, Tangen CM, Walston J, Newman AB, Hirsch C, Gottdiener J, Cardiovascular Health Study Collaborative Research Group, et al. Frailty in older adults: evidence for a phenotype. J Gerontol A Biol Sci Med Sci. 2001;56:M146–56.
69. Orme JG, Reis J, Herz EJ. Factorial and discriminant validity of the Center or Epidemiological Studies Depression (CES-D) scale. J Clin Psychol. 1986;42:28–33.
70. Bandeen-Roche K, Xue QL, Ferrucci L, Walston J, Guralnik JM, Chaves P, et al. Phenotype of frailty: characterization in the women's health and aging studies. J Gerontol A Biol Sci Med Sci. 2006;61:262–6.
71. Rolfson DB, Majumdar SR, Tsuyuki RT, Tahir A, Rockwood K. Validity and reliability of the Edmonton Frail Scale. Age Ageing. 2006;35:526–9.
72. Xue QL. The frailty syndrome: definition and natural history. Clin Geriatr Med. 2011;27:1–15.
73. Puts MT, Hardt J, Monette J, Girre V, Springall E, Alibhai SM. Use of geriatric assessment for older adults in the oncology setting: a systematic review. J Natl Cancer Inst. 2012;104:1133–63.
74. Hamaker ME, Jonker JM, de Rooij SE, Vos AG, Smorenburg CH, van Munster BC. Frailty screening methods for predicting outcome of a comprehensive geriatric assessment in elderly patients with cancer: a systematic review. Lancet Oncol. 2012;13:e437–44.
75. Puts MT, Santos B, Hardt J, Monette J, Girre V, Atenafu EG, et al. An update on a systematic review of the use of geriatric assessment for older adults in oncology. Ann Oncol. 2014;25:307–15.
76. Obeid NM, Azuh O, Reddy S, Webb S, Reickert C, Velanovich V, et al. Predictors of critical care-related complications in colectomy patients using the National Surgical Quality Improvement Program: exploring frailty and aggressive laparoscopic approaches. J Trauma Acute Care Surg. 2012;72:878–83.
77. Uppal S, Igwe E, Rice LW, Spencer RJ, Rose SL. Frailty index predicts severe complications in gynecologic oncology patients. Gynecol Oncol. 2015;137:98–101.
78. Barber EL, Rutstein S, Miller WC, Gehrig PA. A preoperative personalized risk assessment calculator for elderly ovarian cancer patients undergoing primary cytoreductive surgery. Gynecol Oncol. 2015;139:401–6.
79. Falandry C, Weber B, Savoye AM, Tinquaut F, Tredan O, Sevin E, et al. Development of a geriatric vulnerability score in elderly patients with advanced ovarian cancer related with first-line carboplatin: a GINECO prospective trial. Ann Oncol. 2013;24:2808–13.
80. Extermann M, Aapro M, Bernabei R, Cohen HJ, Droz JP, Lichtman S, et al. Use of comprehensive geriatric assessment in older cancer patients: recommendations from the task force on CGA of the International Society of Geriatric Oncology (SIOG). Crit Rev Oncol Hematol. 2005;55:241–52.
81. Decoster L, Van Puyvelde K, Mohile S, Wedding U, Basso U, Colloca G, et al. Screening tools for multidimensional health problems warranting a geriatric assessment in older cancer patients: an update on SIOG recommendations. Ann Oncol. 2015;26:288–300.
82. NCCN. Older adult oncology. Version 2, 2016. NCCN clinical practice guidelines in oncology. Fort Washington, PA, 2016. https://www.nccn.org/professionals/physician_gls/pdf/senior.pdf

Palliative Medicine in the Management of Ovarian Cancer

17

Masaki Fujimura

Abstract

In patients with ovarian cancer, almost half of them die from the disease. Thus, patients with advanced ovarian cancer should be treated with palliative care. In palliative settings, most patients need care particularly for malignant bowel obstruction and ascites. Importantly, surgical and conservative treatment modalities should be considered for these patients. This chapter presents the current status of palliative care of ovarian cancer patients in Japan and across the world.

Keywords

Ovarian cancer patients • Malignant bowel obstruction • Palliative care • Octreotide

17.1 Introduction

Ovarian cancer patients represent only 1.3% of all cancer patients in the USA. However, their survival rates are relatively low such that their 5-year survival rate (5YSR) in 2008 was less than 50% [1]. The same trend is observed in Japan. According to the Japan Society of Obstetrics and Gynecology oncology statistics, 5792 ovarian cancer cases, which represent approximately 26% of three major gynecologic malignancies, were registered in 2013, and the 5YSR was calculated as approximately 59% in patients initially treated in 2008 [2]. These figures indicate that almost half of ovarian cancer patients eventually die from the disease. With this situation, gynecologic oncologists have the responsibility to manage and provide

M. Fujimura, M.D., Ph.D.
Department of Obstetrics and Gynecology, Tokyo Medical University, Ibaraki Medical Center, 3-20-1 Amimachi-Chuo, Inashiki-Gun, Ibaraki, Japan
e-mail: masakif@tokyo-med.ac.jp

H. Katabuchi (ed.), *Frontiers in Ovarian Cancer Science*, Comprehensive Gynecology and Obstetrics, DOI 10.1007/978-981-10-4160-0_17

care to many terminal ovarian cancer patients. Once ovarian cancer recurs in such patients after the initial treatment, a complete cure is difficult to achieve with any treatment modality. Thus, the treatment goal for these patients should be changed from achieving a complete cure to prolongation of their lifespan. Moreover, considerable attention should be paid to enhancing their quality of life (QOL) as part of their end-of-life care. In fact, it is now mandatory that all physicians taking care of ovarian cancer patients must know palliative medicine and care.

17.2 Palliative Care Necessary for Specific Recurrence Symptom in Ovarian Cancer Patients

Recurrence in the abdominal cavity is most frequently observed in ovarian cancer patients, making them distinct in terms of having a specific recurrence symptom compared with other patients with gynecologic malignancies such as cervical cancer or corpus cancer. In patients with advanced or end-stage ovarian cancer, bowel obstruction is most frequently encountered as a result of the so-called peritonitis carcinomatosa, which represents ascites producing peritonitis caused by peritoneal disseminated cancer cells. Additionally, attention should be given to terminal cases of women with specific psychosocial problems such as anxiety as a mother who has to take care of the children, as a wife who has to attend to the needs of her husband and family, and as a woman with social responsibilities in a particular residential district. In this chapter, specific bowel obstructive symptoms and distinct psychosocial problems of women with ovarian cancer are discussed.

17.2.1 Bowel Obstruction

For bowel obstruction cases in gynecologic malignancy patients, 71% of these cases were reported to be caused by ovarian cancer, 20% by uterine corpus cancer, 5.7% by peritoneal cancer, and 2.9% by uterine cervical cancer [3]. Ovarian cancer is the most common cause of bowel obstruction in gynecologic malignancy. Also, 5–35% of ovarian cancer patients eventually develop bowel obstruction owing to the spread of the disease, which is referred to as malignant bowel obstruction (MBO) [4]. These obstructions occur in the small intestine (44–61%), large intestine (18–46%), and both the small and large intestines (6–22%) [3–5]. In terms of bowel obstruction, the small intestine is the most frequently involved area. MBO particularly causes various symptoms such as nausea and vomiting resulting from fluid retention in the obstructed bowel, as well as abdominal pain resulting from bowel distension. Body weight loss and dehydration subsequently follow after prolonged bowel obstruction. If these symptoms persist, the QOL and nutritional condition of the patients would deteriorate.

17.2.1.1 Management of MBO

Two types of management can be provided for bowel obstruction. The first is surgical treatment consisting of the so-called bypass operation and colostomy in case of large bowel obstruction. The second is nonoperative conservative treatment using medications such as corticosteroids or octreotide. These modalities are discussed in the Japan Society of Gynecologic Oncology (JSGO) guidelines 2015 for the treatment of ovarian cancer including primary peritoneal cancer and fallopian tube cancer [6].

17.2.1.2 Management of MBO: Surgical Treatment

This type of management includes bowel-to-bowel bypass operation and colostomy in the case of large bowel obstruction. About 40–80% of small bowel obstructed patients who received bypass operation were reported to have successfully gained relief from their obstruction symptom; however, obstruction recurred in 10–50% of the patients [7]. On the other hand, patients with multiple sites of intestinal obstruction and those with rapidly progressive disease are not good candidates for surgery, but patients with relatively limited tumor burdens, those with a single site of intestinal obstruction, and those with a reasonable chance of responding to subsequent chemotherapy are better candidates for surgery [8]. Pothuri et al. reported that 84% of 64 MBO cases with recurrent ovarian cancer were successfully operable and that 71% of the MBO cases experienced symptom relief by operation. Although the mobility and motility rates after the operations were 22 and 6%, respectively, the median survival time (MST) was 11.6 months in cases of successful bowel operation; however, the MST was only 3.9 months in cases of non-successful bowel operation. Furthermore, they reported that home care and solid food intake were manageable in patients with successful operation [9]. Also, 54% of 90 cases of MBO patients with ovarian cancer required emergent operation, and their postoperative mobility and motility rates were 27 and 18%, respectively. They documented that 66% of the patients who had operation experienced symptom relief when they were free of ascites [10]. The efficacy of bowel operation for recurrent MBO was also documented. A previous report stated that 50% of ten cases of recurrent MBO after bowel operation apparently had a successful second bowel operation and that 30% of the cases experienced symptom relief [11]. Taking these factors into consideration, the indications for MBO bowel operations would be as follows: (1) the patient's general condition is good, (2) the patient understands the purpose of the operation, (3) the operation will likely be accomplished, (4) the patient understands the operative risks, (5) sufficient lifespan (>3–6 M) is expected, (6) the patient has no ascites, and (7) the patient aspires to recover from the condition (unpublished data: author's personal opinion).

Percutaneous endoscopic gastrostomy (PEG) could be another surgical option for MBO patients [12]. PEG allows enteral nutrition in patients despite bypassing the mouth particularly when their own intestine must be avoided. Thus, its indication is limited to a small number of candidate cases in whom MBO bowel operation could not be indicated and the estimated lifespan is limited. However, it has also been reported that after PEG introduction, about half of the patients could swallow a meal, and the rest could swallow liquid [13]. These findings have been similarly reported by other authors [14]. After tube placement, 92.5% of cases experienced relief of symptoms, and 91% tolerated some form of oral intake [14]. A recent report demonstrated the use of venting gastrostomy (VG) at home for MBO patients with advanced ovarian cancer. Specifically, *a* conclusion was drawn that VG may be beneficial in controlling nausea and vomiting in such patients [15]. They also stated that VG tube placement was associated with minimal complications which is apparently the most important consideration for MBO patients.

17.2.1.3 Management of MBO: Conservative Treatment

The use of anticancer agents is usually not encouraged in ovarian cancer patients with MBO because many of them are already exhausted from several courses of anticancer drug treatment and their MBO condition. In a retrospective comparison of surgical and conservative interventions in MBO patients, the survival periods in both treatment modalities showed no statistically significant difference [16], although the study design was not randomized.

Octreotide is one of the potentially effective octapeptides for MBO patients. Watari et al. previously examined the antiemetic effects of octreotide given at 300–600 μg/day under continuous delivery. Of 22 ovarian cancer patients with MBO, 68% had complete antiemetic activity. This antiemetic effect was eventually observed in 82% of all the patients and lasted for about 3 days [17]. Octreotide is superior to scopolamine butylbromide (SB) in terms of providing relief from gastrointestinal symptoms as described in a previous report [18]. This finding was corroborated by other investigators who described the superior effects of octreotide over SB in their study of 97 MBO patients with ovarian cancer [19]. Specifically, they compared the effects of octreotide (0.3 mg/day) with the effects of SB (60 mg/day) both administered through continuous subcutaneous infusion.

Corticosteroids are another possible alternative for providing MBO symptom relief. Philip et al. previously demonstrated the effects of dexamethasone (8 mg/day) in 13 MBO cases associated with gynecologic malignancy [20]. Symptom relief was obtained in 69% of the 13 cases, and the effect lasted until the patients' death in 78% of these cases. They concluded that corticosteroid administration can be considered for inoperable MBO patients without exception. Meta-analysis of two systemic reviews comparing the placebo and corticosteroid groups for 98 MBO patients concluded that dexamethasone given intravenously at 6–16 mg/day is effective for reducing MBO-induced emesis [21].

17.2.1.4 Surgical Treatment or Conservative Treatment for MBO: Which Is Better?

Bais et al. reported that 79% of operable MBO patients could survive for more than 60 days with a median survival time of 109 days, whereas 39% of conservatively treated cases could survive only for an average of 37 days. Also, 68% of cases with operation could be discharged from hospital. Thus, they concluded that operative intervention should be performed before other treatment modalities in operable MBO cases [22]. A study involving 47 MBO patients with ovarian cancer compared 27 operated patients with 20 patients conservatively treated with octreotide. The physical status (PS) of the patients in the operation group was superior to the PS of the patients in the conservatively treated group, and it was concluded that operative intervention should be considered as the first choice of treatment in operable patients [23]. Considering these results, operation would ideally be carried out for MBO patients with ovarian cancer if they are operable. However, octreotide and corticosteroid treatments with considerable liquid infusion would alternatively be used for MBO patients with ovarian cancer if their conditions are not conducive for surgical intervention.

17.2.2 Ascites Accumulation-Management of Ascites

Ultrasound-guided paracentesis has been routinely adopted for managing massive ascites in patients with ovarian cancer. This procedure can be performed in an outpatient setting or even at home. About 2–4 liters of ascites is withdrawn in one procedure, which is recommended to be performed once or once every 2 weeks. Another treatment option is the introduction of cell-free and concentrated ascites reinfusion therapy (CART). The effect of CART on 37 patients with massive ascites was previously reported by Ito et al. who showed that various symptoms related to malignant ascites, particularly fatigue, improved within a 24-h period following CART [24]. When available in an institution, CART would be a strong treatment modality for the relief of distress due to massive ascites. An important basic component for managing ascites that usually accompanies MBO is the control of fluid infusion. Several reports have demonstrated the survival benefit of home parenteral nutrition for end-stage MBO patients [25–26]. However, in a patient group with a worse general condition, contrary results were obtained. Thirty-two cases of severely ill patients have been monitored for 12 months, and 63% of the patients never experienced any hunger and 62% experienced neither thirst nor slight thirst during their terminal illness [27]. They concluded that food and fluid administration beyond the specific levels requested by the patients may play a minimal role in providing comfort to terminally ill patients. In consideration of these reports, it is therefore important not to infuse a large amount of liquid, as well as to listen attentively to the patients. In the JSGO guidelines previously mentioned, the volume of the infusion solution is limited to <1000 mL/day for patients with abdominal pain due to accumulation of ascites, if their life expectancy is estimated to be 1–2 months or less [6].

17.2.3 Specific Psychosocial Problems of Female Cancer Patients

An important aspect regarding patients who need palliative care for malignant tumor is the recognition of their psychological symptoms. This holds true for patients with gynecologic malignancy. However, female patients may have much more psychosocial problems than male patients because they have more social and personal roles in the society. Women usually take care of the children as a mother more than the fathers do, work as a housewife attending to the needs of the family, or occasionally play a role as a manager in a residential district, among others. When a mother suffers from ovarian cancer, she may feel overburdened of her responsibility for all those things around her, as well as beholden to her husband, children, family members, and the people in her office or residential district. These trends are frequently observed in a

Japanese society in which women are still considered to play a supporting role. This specific aspect of gynecologic cancer patients in the palliative care field is a problem that needs to be further elucidated in the Japanese society. From this background, the Japan Society of Gynecological Palliative Medicine (JSGPM), a nonprofit organization, has recently been founded. Specific psychosocial problems of female patients receiving palliative care should be further investigated.

17.3 Current Status of Palliative Care for Gynecologic Cancer Patients

17.3.1 Status Around the World

In recent years, much attention has been given to the field of gynecologic palliative medicine around the world. Several reports on palliative care education in the field of gynecologic oncology have been recently documented [28–29]. However, studies regarding QOL and palliative care in end-stage gynecologic patients are still sparsely encountered. Lefkowits et al. surveyed the improvement of symptom burden after palliative care consultation in a cohort setting in gynecologic oncology patients and found that the majority of improvements occurred within 1 day of consultation [30]. Regrettably, reports concerning palliative care in the field of gynecologic oncology are still scarce, and the current status of palliative care in this field is not apparently evident around the world.

17.3.2 Status of Palliative Care in Gynecologic Oncology in Asia

A study was performed comparing the quality of life (QOL) of patients who received salvage chemotherapy or were treated with palliative care only for refractory or recurrent epithelial ovarian cancer in Thailand. The patients treated with each treatment modality had comparable QOL scores [31]. Tsubamoto et al. surveyed the roles of palliative chemotherapy and hospice enrollment in late-stage ovarian cancer patients in Japan. They concluded that chemotherapy after the first refraction could be a good option for recurrent ovarian cancer patients, and they encouraged hospice enrollment when patients fall into the terminal stage [32]. Recently, a large-scale survey of palliative care provided in a Japanese gynecologic oncology setting has been performed. Specifically, Futagami et al. performed this large-scale survey in Japan as part of a JSGPM program [33]. They surveyed 393 facilities in which gynecologic cancer treatment was being administered regarding the present situation of providing palliative care. A total of 115 facilities responded to the survey. There were 1134 end-stage patients who were enrolled in the survey, and ovarian cancer patients represented 516 cases (45.5%). In the survey, end-of-life care was managed by the Department of Obstetrics and Gynecology (OB/GYN) in 72% of the facilities, by the palliative care unit in 9%, and by other means which included both the OB/GYN and palliative care unit in 19% (Fig. 17.1a) [33]. End-of-life care is seldom provided in local affiliated hospitals or at home in Japan.

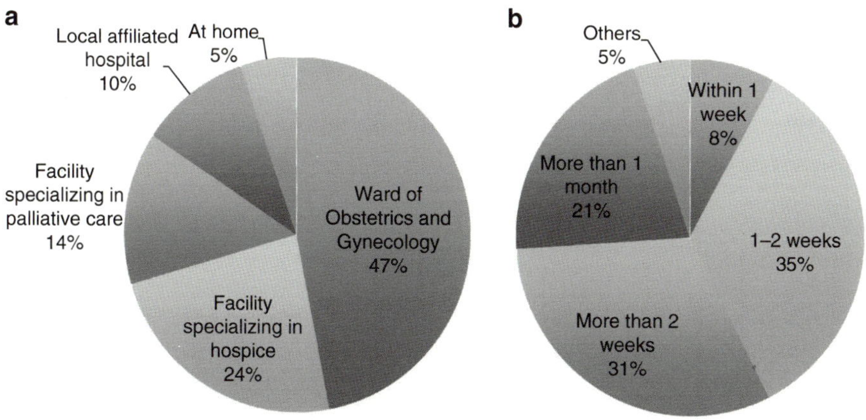

Fig. 17.1 (**a**) Institutions where end-of-life care was provided [33]. (**b**) Waiting periods for transfer to a palliative care unit [33]

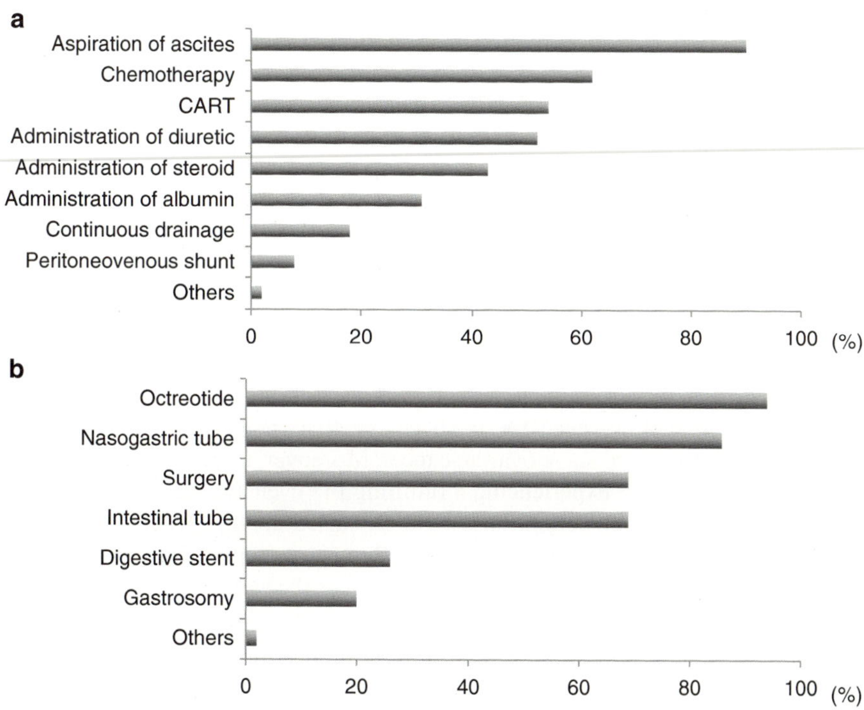

Fig. 17.2 (**a**) Treatment modalities for managing ascites (multiple answers allowed) [33]. (**b**) Treatment modalities for managing MBO (multiple answer allowed) [33]

When patients were referred to a palliative care unit, most of them had to wait for 1–2 weeks before they could be transferred (Fig. 17.1b) [33]. The survey also asked about the treatments for ascites and MBO. In Japan, paracentesis is the most common management followed by chemotherapy and CART (Fig. 17.2a) [33].

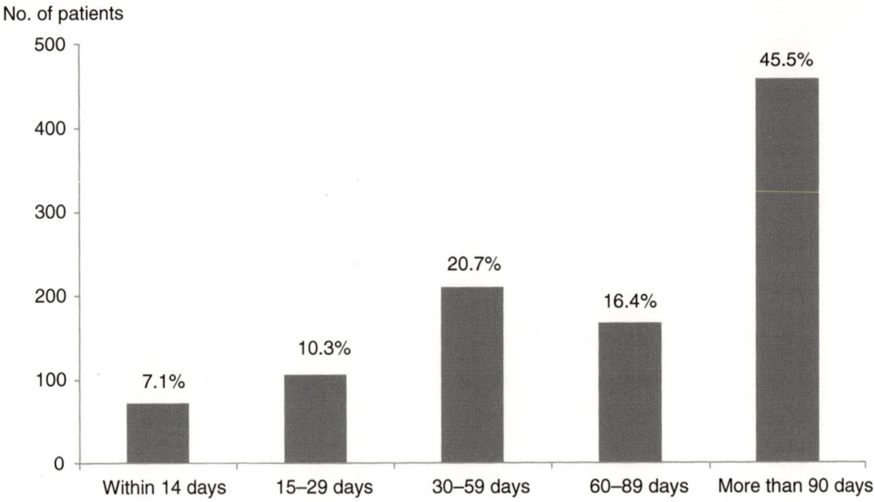

Fig. 17.3 Periods from the date of last chemotherapy to death [33]

Also, octreotide administration is the most commonly applied treatment modality for MBO management, followed by nasogastric tube incursion and surgery (Fig. 17.2b) [33]. In most cases, the last chemotherapy was delivered more than 90 days from the time of death of the patients (45.5%); however, 7.1% of the patients died within 14 days of the last chemotherapy (Fig. 17.3) [33]. They concluded that additional research surveys should be performed in relation to these data drawn using a large-scale survey.

17.4 Future Perspectives in Gynecologic Palliative Care

There is a compelling need for fresh perspectives regarding palliative care in patients with advanced stage ovarian cancer. Moreover, there is a real necessity to develop strategies for experiencing a fulfilling life even among end-stage ovarian cancer patients. Serious attention should be raised among gynecologic oncologists to provide more sophisticated and effective palliative care in the society. Although medical situations differ by areas across the world, gynecologic oncologists have to devote more attention to ways on how to maximally prolong a patient's life instead of resigning to the fact that the patient is terminally ill with cancer. Many patients wish to be at home when their time has come rather than to be in a certain district or hospital. It is the duty of gynecologic oncologists to make every opportunity and create a good environment for discussing end-of-life care provisions such as how to provide care to patients with end-stage ovarian cancer. Some models from other countries around the world are available for giving hope to end-stage patients.

Conclusion

Although the methods may be different for each district in countries across the world, the purpose for providing optimal care to patients is universal, that is, providing patients with a good reason to live their life to the fullest. This should be considered as a universal and primary purpose of gynecologic oncologists.

References

1. http://seer.cancer.gov/statfacts/html/ovary.html.
2. Saito T, Katabuchi H. Annual Report of the Committee on Gynecologic Oncology, Japan Society of Obstetrics and Gynecology: Patient Annual Report for 2013 and Treatment Annual Report for 2008. J Obstet Gynecol Res. 2016;42:1069–79.
3. Caceres A, Zhou Q, Iasonos A, et al. Colorectal stents for palliation of large-bowel obstructions in recurrent gynecologic cancer: an updated series. Gynecol Oncol. 2008;108:482–5.
4. Clarkle-Pearson DL, Chin NO, Delong ER, et al. Surgical management of intestinal obstruction in ovarian cancer. I. Clinical features, postoperative complications, and survival. Gynecol Oncol. 1987;26:11–8.
5. Chi DS, Phaeton R, Miner TJ, et al. A prospective outcomes analysis of palliative procedures performed for malignant intestinal obstruction due to recurrent ovarian cancer. Oncologist. 2009;14:835–9.
6. Komiyama S, Katabuchi H, Mikami M, et al. Japan Society of Gynecologic Oncology (JSGO) guidelines 2015 for the treatment of ovarian cancer including primary peritoneal cancer and fallopian tube cancer. Int J Clin Oncol. 2016;21:435–46.
7. Feuer DJ, Broadley KE, Shepherd JH, et al. Systematic review of surgery in malignant bowel obstruction in advanced gynecological and gastrointestinal cancer. Gynecol Oncol. 1999;75:313–22.
8. Rubin SC. Intestinal obstruction in advanced ovarian cancer: what does the patient want? Gynecol Oncol. 1999;75:311–2.
9. Pothuri B, Vaidya A, Aghajanian C, et al. Palliative surgery for bowel obstruction in recurrent ovarian cancer: an updated series. Gynecol Oncol. 2003;89:306–13.
10. Kolomainen DF, Daponte A, Barton DPJ, et al. Outcomes of surgical management of bowel obstruction in relapsed epithelial ovarian cancer (EOC). Gynecol Oncol. 2012;125:31–6.
11. Pothuri B, Meyer L, Gerardi M, et al. Reoperation for palliation of recurrent malignant bowel obstruction in ovarian carcinoma. Gynecol Oncol. 2004;95:193–5.
12. Meyer L, Pothuri B. Decompressive percutaneous gastrostomy tube use in gynecologic malignancies. Curr Treat Options in Oncol. 2006;7:111–20.
13. Pothuri B, Montemarano M, Gerardi M, et al. Percutaneous endoscopic gastrostomy tube placement in patients with malignant bowel obstruction due to ovarian carcinoma. Gynecol Oncol. 2005;96:330–4.
14. Rath KS, Loseth D, Muscarella P, et al. Outcomes following percutaneous upper gastrointestinal decompressive tube placement for malignant bowel obstruction in ovarian cancer. Gynecol Oncol. 2013;129:103–6.
15. DeEulis TG, Yennurajalingam S. Venting gastrostomy at home for symptomatic management of bowel obstruction in advanced/recurrent ovarian malignancy: a case series. J Palliat Med. 2015;18:722–8.
16. Bryan DN, Radbod R, Berek JS. An analysis of surgical versus chemotherapeutic intervention for the management of intestinal obstruction in advanced ovarian cancer. Int J Gynecol Cancer. 2006;16:125–34.

17. Watari H, Hosaka M, Wakui Y, et al. A prospective study on the efficacy of octreotide in the management of malignant bowel obstruction in gynecologic cancer. Int J Gynecol Cancer. 2012;22:692–6.
18. Mercadante S, Casuccio A, Mangione S. Medical treatment for inoperable malignant bowel obstruction: a qualitative systematic review. J Pain Symptom Manag. 2007;33:217–23.
19. Daniele A, Ferrero A, Fuso L, et al. Palliative care in patients with ovarian cancer and bowel obstruction. Support Care Cancer. 2015;23:3157–63.
20. Philip J, Lickiss N, Grant PT, et al. Corticosteroids in the management of bowel obstruction on a gynecological oncology unit. Gynecol Oncol. 1999;74:68–73.
21. Feuer DJ, Broadley KE. Corticosteroids for the resolution of malignant bowel obstruction in advanced gynaecological and gastrointestinal cancer. Cochrane Database Syst Rev. 2000;(1). Art. No.: CD001219.
22. Bais JMJ, Schilthuis MS, Slors JFM, et al. Intestinal obstruction in patients with advanced ovarian cancer. Int J Gynecol Cancer. 1995;5:346–50.
23. Mangili G, Aletti G, Frigerio L, et al. Palliative care for intestinal obstruction in recurrent ovarian cancer: a multivariate analysis. Int J Gynecol Cancer. 2005;15:830–5.
24. Ito T, Hanafusa N, Iwase S, et al. Effects of cell-free and concentrated ascites reinfusion therapy (CART) on symptom relief of malignancy–related ascites. Int J Clin Oncol. 2015;20:623–8.
25. King LA, Carson LF, Konstantinides N, et al. Outcome assessment of home parenteral nutrition in patients with gynecologic malignancies: what have we learned in a decade of experience? Gynecol Oncol. 1993;51:377–82.
26. Bozzetti F, Cozzaglio L, Biganzoli E, et al. Quality of life and length of survival in advanced cancer patients on home parenteral nutrition. Clin Nutr. 2002;21:281–8.
27. MaCann RM, Hall WJ, Groth-Juncker A. Confort cares for terminally ill patients. The appropriate use of nutrition and hydration. JAMA. 1994;272:1263–6.
28. Ratanakaaew A, Khemapech N, Laurujisawat P. Palliative care education in gynecologic oncology: a survey of gynecologic oncologists and gynecologic oncology fellows in Thailand. Asian Pac J Cancer Prev. 2015;16:6331–4.
29. Eskander RN, Osann K, Dickson E, et al. Assessment of palliative care training in gynecologic oncology: a gynecologic oncology fellow research network study. Gynecol Oncol. 2014;134:3779–384.
30. Lefkowits C, Teuteberg W, Courtney-Brooks M, et al. Improvement in symptom burden within one day after palliative care consultation in a cohort of gynecologic oncology inpatients. Gynecol Oncol. 2015;136:424–8.
31. Srisuttayasathien M, Khemapech N. Quality of life in ovarian cancer patients choosing to receive salvage chemotherapy or palliative treatment. Asian Pac J Cancer Prev. 2013;14:7669–74.
32. Tsubamoto H, Ito Y, Kanazawa R, et al. Benefit of palliative chemotherapy and hospice enrollment in late-stage ovarian cancer patients. J Obstet Gynecol Res. 2014;40:1399–406.
33. Futagami M, Yokoyama Y, Sato T, et al. A survey of palliative care for patients with gynecologic cancer in Japan: a Japan Society of Gynecologic Palliative Medicine (JSGPM) survey. Asian Pac Cancer Prev. 2016;17:4637–42.

Printed by Printforce, the Netherlands